Smartphone and Internet Addiction: Health Concerns and Solutions

Smartphone and Internet Addiction: Health Concerns and Solutions

Editor: Ezra Potter

FOSTER ACADEMICS

www.fosteracademics.com

www.fosteracademics.com

FOSTER ACADEMICS

Cataloging-in-Publication Data

Smartphone and internet addiction : health concerns and solutions / edited by Ezra Potter.
p. cm.
Includes bibliographical references and index.
ISBN 978-1-64646-624-5
1. Nomophobia--Health aspects. 2. Smartphones--Psychological aspects. 3. Internet addiction.
4. Internet addiction--Health aspects. 5. Digital media--Psychological aspects. 6. Compulsive behavior.
7. Psychiatry. I. Potter, Ezra.
RC552.N66 S63 2023
616.858 4--dc23

Foster Academics,
118-35 Queens Blvd., Suite 400,
Forest Hills, NY 11375, USA

ISBN 978-1-64646-624-5 (Hardback)

Contents

Preface

The world is advancing at a fast pace like never before. Therefore, the need is to keep up with the latest developments. This book was an idea that came to fruition when the specialists in the area realized the need to coordinate together and document essential themes in the subject. That's when I was requested to be the editor. Editing this book has been an honour as it brings together diverse authors researching on different streams of the field. The book collates essential materials contributed by veterans in the area which can be utilized by students and researchers alike.

An addiction is a chronic dysfunction of the brain system concerned with reward, motivation and memory. It involves the way a body craves a substance or behavior, especially if it causes a compulsive or obsessive pursuit of reward and lack of concern over consequences. In contemporary times, smartphone and internet addiction has become a major issue of concern. Smart phone addiction is composed of various basic components. These include obsessive phone use, behaviors such as repetitive checking for messages or updates, or feelings of agitation or suffering without the phone. Internet addiction is a type of addiction that involves the inability to control one's internet use. This condition results in serious impairment of various life functions and can result in a variety of health conditions. This book provides a comprehensive understanding of smartphone and internet addiction. It will serve as a reference to a broad spectrum of readers.

Each chapter is a sole-standing publication that reflects each author´s interpretation. Thus, the book displays a multi-facetted picture of our current understanding of application, resources and aspects of the field. I would like to thank the contributors of this book and my family for their endless support.

Editor

1

Mobile Phone Addiction and Risk-Taking Behavior among Chinese Adolescents: A Moderated Mediation Model

Kai Dou [1], Lin-Xin Wang [1], Jian-Bin Li [2,*], Guo-Dong Wang [1], Yan-Yu Li [1] and Yi-Ting Huang [1]

1 Department of Psychology and Research Center of Adolescent Psychology and Behavior, School of Education, Guangzhou University, Guangzhou 510006, China; psydk@gzhu.edu.cn (K.D.); wlx_psy@e.gzhu.edu.cn (L.-X.W.); 1708400055@e.gzhu.edu.cn (G.-D.W.); 2111808175@e.gzhu.edu.cn (Y.-Y.L.); 1666100038@e.gzhu.edu.cn (Y.-T.H.)

2 Department of Early Childhood Education, The Education University of Hong Kong, Hong Kong, China

* Correspondence: lijianbin@eduhk.hk

Abstract: *Objectives*: The mobile phone (MP) is an indispensable digital device in adolescents' daily lives in the contemporary era, but being addicted to MP can lead to more risk-taking behavior. However, little is known about the mediating and moderating mechanisms underlying this relation. To address the gaps in the literature, the present study examined the idea that MP addiction is associated with reduced self-control, which further associates with increased risk-taking behavior. In addition, this study also investigated the moderation effect of adolescent sex in the association between MP addiction and self-control. *Methods*: A three-wave longitudinal study, each wave spanning six months apart, was conducted in a sample of Chinese adolescents (final N = 333, 57.4% girls). *Results*: Results of the moderated mediation model suggest that after controlling for demographic variables and baseline levels of self-control and risk-taking behavior, MP addiction at T1 positively predicted increased risk-taking behavior at T3 through reduced self-control at T2 for girls but not for boys. *Conclusions*: Theoretically, these findings contribute to the understanding about the working processes in the association between MP addiction and risk-taking behavior in adolescents. Practically, the results implied that boosting self-control appeared as a promising way to reduce girls' risk-taking behavior, particularly for those who are addicted to MPs.

Keywords: mobile phone addiction; risk-taking behavior; self-control; sex; adolescents

1. Introduction

Mobile phones (MPs) are ubiquitous in the contemporary era. With the advancement of high-speed internet, MPs become more versatile and play a significant role in people's daily lives. According to a recent report, China's MP users reached 897 million, an increase of 4.2 million compared to 2018 [1]. Adolescents constitute a major proportion of MP users in China. Although the appropriate use of MPs (e.g., looking up useful information and maintaining positive social ties) can be beneficial to adolescents (e.g., feeling higher subjective well-being) [2,3], being addicted to a MP is associated with a wide array of undesirable outcomes in adolescents [4–6]. Among others, a salient undesirable consequence associated with MP addiction is risk-taking behavior [7–10]. MP addiction is a type of addiction to technology and it can be defined as the uncontrolled or excessive use of mobile phones, with an inability to control craving, feeling anxious, withdrawal, and productivity loss as symptoms [11]. Although the association between MP addiction and risk-taking behavior in adolescents has been well documented, scant research has examined how and for whom MP addiction is associated with risk-taking behavior. Examining these issues may shed light on the intervention and prevention of adolescents' risk-taking behavior. In this study, we propose that MP addiction would be related to reduced self-control which further drives them to engage in more risk-taking behavior. In addition, we also explore whether sex would play a role as well, given the sex differences in self-control [12–14] and MP addiction [15,16]. We examined these issues in a sample of Chinese adolescents.

1.1. Mobile Phone Addiction and Risk-Taking Behavior

Risk-taking behavior refers to the actions that may potentially result in adverse consequences [17,18]. Adolescents are more prone to engage in risk-taking behavior compared to their younger peers and adults [19]. According to the dual system model, the socioemotional system of adolescents develops rapidly but the cognitive control system develops relatively more slowly [19]. The rapid development of the socioemotional system enhances adolescents' pursuit of rewarding stimuli, while the slow development of the cognitive control system limits the adolescents' inhibition of risk-taking behavior [20,21]. The imbalance between the development of the socioemotional system and the development of the cognitive control system results in the increase in adolescents' risk-taking behavior.

Compared to computers, the MP is more flexible, mobile and timely. Being addicted to a MP can be associated with risk-taking behavior in adolescents for two reasons [21,22]. First, individuals tend to seek rewarding incentives, novel stimuli and excitement through engaging in risk-taking behavior, common in adolescents [19]. The use of a MP is often accompanied with rewarding incentives, novel stimuli and excitement, and thus MP addiction may exacerbate the adolescents' tendencies of engaging in risk-taking behavior [23,24]. Previous research has indicated that adolescents who frequently use MPs engage in more reckless driving [25], smoking and alcohol abuse [26] than those who are not addicted to MPs. Second, MP addiction may restrain adolescents' cognitive control, which further contributes to their risk-taking behavior. In accordance with this perspective, a previous study has found that those who are addicted to MPs are reluctant to spend cognitive resources and are prone to adopt intuitive thinking in daily lives [27,28]. In the absence of cognitive control and analytical thinking, individuals may have more difficulties in restraining the tendencies of seeking novelty, rewarding incentives, and excitement through risk-taking behavior [29–31]. Taken together, we assume that MP addiction would be related to an increase in risk-taking behavior in adolescents.

1.2. The Mediation Effect of Self-Control

Self-control is defined as the ability that individuals make effort to overcome impulsion and automatic reaction, and to support the pursuit of long-term goals [32,33]. As a vital psychological function, self-control is associated with a number of positive outcomes, including less risk-taking behavior [32–34]. The general theory of crime postulates that individuals with low self-control are inclined to be short-sighted and impulsive, which is a core cause of young people's delinquency [35]. Research has found that adolescents with low self-control are more likely to have excessive drinking [36,37], substance abuse [38], gambling [39,40] and other risk-taking behavior. In addition, the strength model of self-control posits that self-control resource depletion in the previous stage limits the availability of self-control for the next stage, which may increase the likelihood of the occurrence of risk-taking behavior [41,42].

Self-control may play a "bridge" role between MP addiction and adolescents' risk-taking behavior. There could be different pathways from mobile phone addiction to low self-control. On the one hand, MP addiction may reduce cognitive control, distract attention, and make the cognitive control system "lazied" in adolescents, and thus they prefer intuitive cognitive processing [27,28,43]. For instance, in a sample of 1721 adolescents, Hong et al. (2020) found that MP addiction leads to cognitive failures. On the other hand, MPs may provide immediate stimulation and feedback that may activate the socioemotional system, rendering adolescents vulnerable to instant gratification and short-term rewards. Individual differences in low self-control and the temporary depletion of self-control resources due to MP addiction can render adolescents' cognitive resources insufficient to override the tendencies of seeking novelty and excitement, which may be further associated with more risk-taking behavior. On these bases, we assume that MP addiction can indirectly affect adolescents' risk-taking via reduced self-control.

1.3. *The Moderation Effect of Sex*

Previous research has revealed sex differences in the pattern of mobile phone use [15,16]. For instance, girls are more prone to use MPs for social networking, entertainment and shopping [44,45], while boys are more likely to use MPs for work and games [15]. In this sense, compared to boys, girls are considered to be more emotionally involved when using MPs, experience more emotional swifts, and have higher social motivation [15]. In addition, boys are prone to engage in more risk-taking behavior than girls during adolescence [46], because boys have higher sensation-seeking tendencies and lower impulsive control [47,48]. As a relatively malleable personal characteristic, self-control can be affected by environment. Compared to boys, girls are more likely to be susceptible to external factors (e.g., MP addiction) [13]. In line with this, MP addiction could suppress girls' self-control rather than boys. Therefore, we assume that sex would moderate the effect of MP addiction on adolescents' self-control.

1.4. *The Present Study*

Taken together, this three-wave longitudinal study, with each wave spanning six months apart, investigates the association between MP addiction and risk-taking behavior as well as the underlying mechanisms in a sample of Chinese adolescents. Specifically, we would examine the idea that MP addiction would be associated with increased risk-taking behavior through reduced self-control. Moreover, we would examine the moderating role of sex (see in Figure 1). In sum, we hypothesized that: (1) MP addiction would be positively related with adolescent risk-taking behavior; (2) self-control would mediate the relation between MP addiction and risk-taking behavior; (3) sex would moderate the effect of MP addiction on adolescents' self-control, with the negative effect of MP addiction on self-control being stronger for girls than boys; and (4) sex would moderate the mediation effect of self-control, with the mediation effect of self-control being more pronounced for girls than boys. Combining all these hypotheses results in a moderated mediation model (Figure 1).

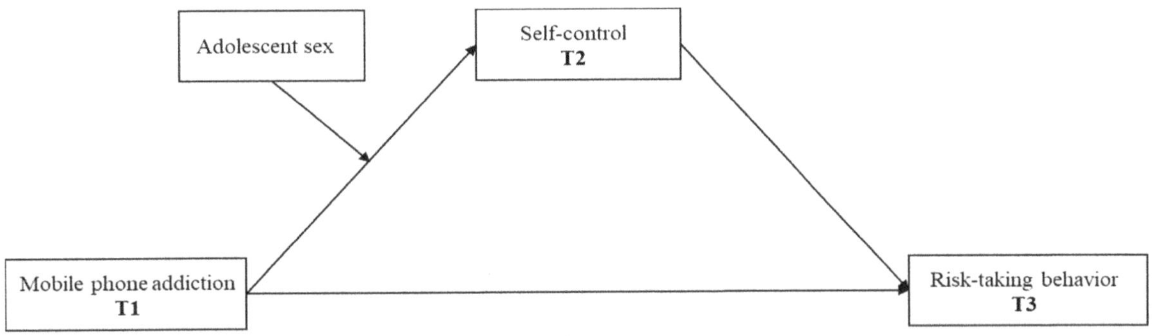

Figure 1. Conceptual moderated mediation model of the association between mobile phone addiction and risk-taking behavior; T1 = Time 1; T2 = Time 2; T3 = Time 3.

2. Method

2.1. *Participants and Procedures*

The data were collected from a public middle school in a large city in southern China. All the procedures involving human participants were reviewed and approved by the research ethics committee in the School of Education at Guangzhou University (Protocol Number: GZHU2019018). Written consent forms from the parents and oral assent from the adolescents were obtained before data collection across the waves. At each wave, two trained research assistants hosted the survey and the participants completed the questionnaires during regular class hours in the classroom. All the participants received a small gift worthy of 15 RMB (approximately 2.5 US Dollars) after completing the questionnaires each time.

A total of 412 parents provided consent for their children's participation. Finally, 399 10th graders (M = 15.37, SD = 0.52, 52.1% girls) participated in the first wave of data collection (Time 1, T1). Of the 399 adolescents, 353 (attrition rate = 11.53%) and 386 (attrition rate = 3.26%) participated in the assessments at Time 2 (T2) and Time 3 (T3), respectively. The time interval of the data collection between each wave was six months. Detailed demographic characteristics of the T1 sample are presented in Table 1.

Table 1. Summary of the demographic variables at T1.

Variables	N	%
Adolescent sex		
Boys	191	47.9%
Girls	208	52.1%
Only child at home		
Yes	198	49.6%
No	201	50.4%
Father's work status		
Unemployment	32	8.0%
Part-time job	45	11.3%
Full-time job	322	80.7%
Mother's work status		
Unemployment	82	20.6%
Part-time job	53	13.3%
Full-time job	264	66.2%
Father's highest educational level		
High school or below	234	58.6%
College or undergraduate	152	38.1%
Master or above	13	3.3%
Mother's highest educational level		
High school or below	254	63.7%
College or undergraduate	140	35.1%
Master or above	5	1.3%
Total	399	100%

2.2. *Measures*

2.2.1. Mobile Phone Addiction at T1

We used the Mobile Phone Addiction Index Scale (MPAI) [49] to measure the participants' frequency of using MPs at T1. This scale consists of 17 items rated on a five-point scale (from 1 = never done to 5 = almost always). A mean score can be calculated by averaging all the items, with a higher score indicating more the frequent use of MP. Sample items are "Your friends and family complained about your use of the mobile phone" and "You feel lost without your mobile phone". In the current study, the Cronbach's alpha of this scale was 0.97.

2.2.2. Self-Control at T1 and T2

We used the Chinese version of Tangney et al.'s (2004) Brief Self-Control Scale (BSCS) [50,51] to assess the participants' self-control ability at T1 and T2. This scale consists of 13 items rated on a five-point scale (from 1 = not like me at all to 5 = like me very much). A higher mean score indicates a better self-control ability. The sample items are "I am good at resisting temptation" and "Sometimes I can't stop myself from doing something, even if I know it is wrong". In this research, the Cronbach's alpha of this scale at T1 and T2 was 0.79 and 0.80, respectively.

2.2.3. Risk-Taking Behavior at T1, T2, and T3

Risk-taking behavior was assessed by the 15-item Adolescent Risk-Taking Questionnaire (ARQ) [17] through T1 to T3. Adolescents reported the frequency of performing various risk-taking behavior (e.g., unprotected sex, driving/cycling after drinking) on a five-point Likert scale (from 0 = never done to 4 = done very often). A mean score was calculated by averaging all the items. This measure has been translated into Chinese and demonstrated to be valid and reliable in Chinese samples [18]. In this study, Cronbach's alpha of this scale at T1, T2 and T3 was 0.96, 0.81 and 0.76, respectively.

2.2.4. Covariates at T1

The child's age, only child at home or not (0 = Yes, 1 = No), parents' employment status (1 = freelance, 2 = par-time job, 3 = full-time job) and educational levels (1 = junior middle school and below, 2 = high school degree, 3 = college degree, 4 = bachelor's degree, 5 = master's degree or doctoral degree) were included as covariates since prior studies have found significant associations between these demographic variables with risk-taking behavior [52,53].

2.3. Data Analyses

Initially, descriptive statistics and bivariate correlations were performed using SPSS 22.0 ((IBM, Armonk, NY, USA) to examine the centrality and association among the variables of interest. Second, structural equation modeling (SEM) was performed using Mplus 7.0 (Muthén & Muthén, Los Angeles, CA, USA) to test the hypothesized moderated mediation model. The missing data were handled with the full information maximum likelihood estimation (FIML) [54]. In this model, T1 MP addiction was the independent variable; T2 self-control was the mediator; T3 risk-taking behavior was the outcome; and sex was the moderator. In this model, we also controlled for the baseline levels of self-control at T1 and risk-taking behavior at T1 and T2, as well as the effect of covariates on the outcome (i.e., T3 risk-taking behavior). Given that the bootstrapping technique has several advantages over the traditional approaches in examining mediation models such as higher statistical power [55], we used bootstrapping ($N = 5000$) and its 95% confidence intervals to judge the significance of the mediation. As long as the 95% confidence interval excludes 0, significant mediation effect is tenable. The following indices were used to evaluate the overall model fit [56]: a nonsignificant chi-square statistics (χ^2), the comparative fit index (CFI), the root mean square error of approximation (RMSEA) [57] with its 90% confidence interval (CI), and the standardized root mean square residual (SRMR). However, given that the sample size of the current study is large and the χ^2 statistic is sensitive to sample size, a significant χ^2 statistic was expected.

3. Results

3.1. Descriptive Statistics and Bivariate Correlation

Means, standard deviations, and bivariate associations are shown in Table 2. As can be seen in the table, MP addiction at T1 was negatively related to T1 and T2 self-control ($r = -0.43$ and -0.35, $ps < 0.001$), but positively associated with T1/T2/T3 risk-taking behavior ($r = 0.22$–0.37, $ps < 0.001$). Adolescent self-control and risk-taking behavior were also negatively correlated, within and across time points ($r = -0.22$–-0.30, $ps < 0.001$). According to Cohen's (1992) standard [58], the effect sizes of these correlation coefficients were small-to-medium.

Table 2. Descriptive statistics and bivariate correlations among the study variables and covariates.

Study Variables	1	2	3	4	5	6	7	8	9	10	11	12	13
1. MP addiction (T1)	—												
2. Self-control (T1)	−0.43 ***												
3. Self-control (T2)	−0.35 ***	0.51 ***											
4.Risk-taking behavior (T1)	0.37 ***	−0.28 ***	−0.22 ***										
5.Risk-taking behavior (T2)	0.32 ***	−0.25 ***	−0.30 ***	0.27 ***									
6.Risk-taking behavior (T3)	0.22 ***	−0.22 ***	−0.27 ***	0.19 ***	0.38 ***								
7. Sex (0 = boys, 1 = girls)	−0.17 ***	0.06	0.01	−0.24 ***	−0.19 ***	−0.13 **							
Covariates at T1													
8. Age	0.02	0.01	0.07	−0.03	−0.03	0.04	0.00						
9. Only child at home	−0.16 **	0.03	0.10	−0.02	−0.11 *	−0.04	0.20 ***	−0.01					
10. Father's work status	0.02	0.07	0.01	−0.01	0.06	0.04	−0.09	0.04	−0.03				
11. Mother's work status	0.03	−0.07	−0.06	0.05	0.06	0.01	−0.06	0.11 *	−0.09	0.23 ***			
12. Father's education	0.13 **	−0.05	−0.11 *	0.14 **	0.01	0.02	−0.00	−0.10 *	−0.18 ***	0.07	−0.00		
13. Mother's education	0.05	−0.05	−0.03	0.19 ***	0.08	−0.03	−0.02	−0.09	−0.17 **	0.02	0.11 *	0.56 ***	
M	2.16	3.05	3.19	1.41	0.28	0.27	0.52	15.37	1.50	2.73	2.46	2.53	2.38
SD	0.99	0.55	0.54	0.73	0.37	0.33	0.50	0.52	0.50	0.60	0.81	1.02	0.95

Note: N ranges from 353 to 399. MP addiction = mobile phone addiction; T1 = Time 1; T2 = Time 2; T3 = Time 1. * $p < 0.05$, ** $p < 0.01$, *** $p < 0.001$.

3.2. Examination of the Hypothesized Moderated Mediation Model

The hypothesized moderated mediation model was examined. The fit indices were $\chi^2 = 36.91$, $df = 22$, $p < 0.05$, RMSEA = 0.04 (90% CI = [0.015, 0.064]), CFI = 0.959, and SRMR = 0.039, indicating that the model was a good fit. This model accounted for the 20.5% variance of "risk-taking behavior", and the corresponding effect size was medium to large ($f = 0.26$) [58].

As shown in Figure 2 and Table 3, T1 MP addiction was not directly related to T3 risk-taking behavior at the statistically significant level. Nevertheless, the T1 MP addiction was significantly related to T2 self-control ($B = -0.08$, $SE = 0.03$, $p = 0.009$). Moreover, T2 self-control was significantly related to T3 risk-taking behavior ($B = -0.11$, $SE = 0.04$, $p = 0.003$). More importantly, T2 self-control significantly linked the association between T1 MP addiction and T3 risk-taking behavior ($B = 0.01$, 95% CI = [0.002, 0.021]), but not the effect of baseline levels of self-control, risk-taking behavior, and covariates.

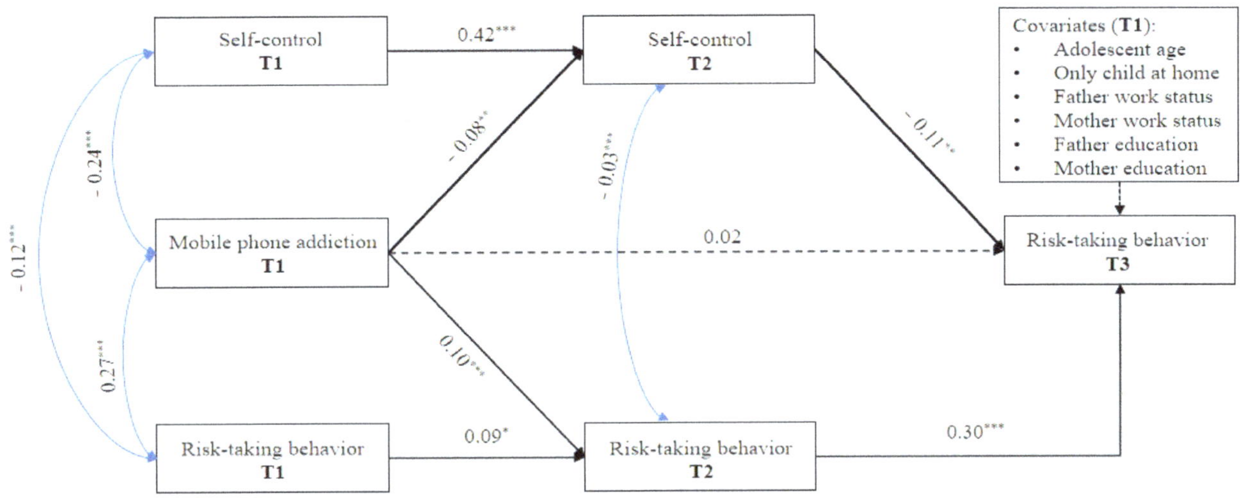

Figure 2. The mediation model of self-control in the association between mobile phone addiction and risk-taking behavior. Note: unstandardized estimates are presented; $\chi^2 = 36.91$, $df = 22$, $p < 0.05$, root mean square error of approximation (RMSEA) = 0.041 with 90% CI [0.015, 0.064], comparative fit index (CFI) = 0.959, standardized root mean square residual (SRMR) = 0.039; * $p < 0.05$, ** $p < 0.01$, *** $p < 0.001$. Dashed line indicates a non-significant coefficient.

Table 3. Regression model for the moderation effect of adolescent sex.

	Self-Control (T2, $R^2 = 0.29$)			Risk-Taking Behavior (T2, $R^2 = 0.13$)			Risk-Taking Behavior (T3, $R^2 = 0.20$)		
	B	*SE*	*p*	*B*	*SE*	*p*	*B*	*SE*	*p*
Covariates at T1									
Age							0.03	0.03	0.41
Only child at home							−0.03	0.02	0.19
Father's work status							0.01	0.02	0.56
Mother's work status							0.01	0.03	0.92
Father's education							0.01	0.04	0.80
Mother's education							−0.01	0.02	0.77
Independent variable									
MP addiction (T1)	−0.03	0.05	0.48	**0.10**	**0.02**	**<0.001**	0.02	0.02	0.37
Mediating variable									
Self-control (T1)	**0.40**	**0.06**	**<0.001**						
Self-control (T2)							**−0.11**	**0.04**	**0.002**
Moderating variable									
Sex	0.23	0.14	0.10						
Interaction term									
MP addiction (T1) × Sex	**−0.13**	**0.06**	**0.02**						

Note: only child at home: 0 = yes, 1 = no; work status: 1 = freelance, 2 = par-time job, 3 = full-time job; education: 1 = junior middle school and below, 2 = high school degree, 3 = college degree, 4 = bachelor's degree, 5 = master's degree or doctoral degree; sex: 0 = boys, 1 = girls; MP addiction = mobile phone addiction; T1 = Time 1; T2 = Time 2; T3 = Time 3. Significant results are in bold.

Regarding the moderation effect of sex, there is a significant interaction effect between MP addiction and adolescent sex on T2 self-control ($B = -0.13$, $SE = 0.06$, $p = 0.02$). As shown in Figure 3 and Table 4, the association between T1 MP addiction and T2 self-control was significant only for girls ($B = -0.14$, $SE = 0.04$, $p < 0.001$), but not for boys ($B = -0.03$, $SE = 0.04$, $p = 0.56$). Moreover, we found that the mediation of T2 self-control was significant for girls ($B = 0.018$, $SE = 0.007$, 95% CI = [0.006, 0.036]) but not for boys ($B = 0.004$, $SE = 0.005$, 95% CI = [−0.006, 0.016]).

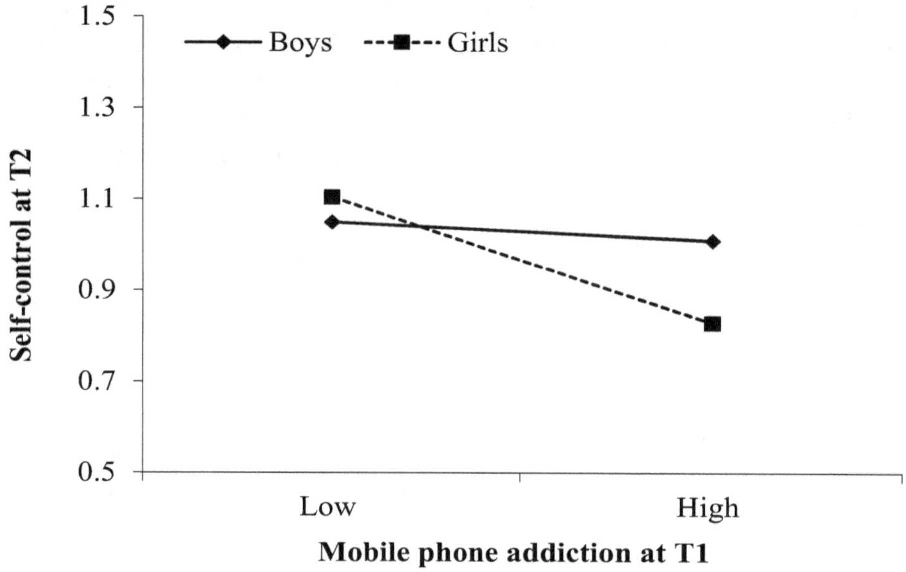

Figure 3. Moderation effect of adolescent sex on the link from T1 mobile phone addiction to T2 self-control.

Table 4. The mediation effect of self-control by sex.

Sex	*B*	*S.E.*	95% CI
Boys	0.004	0.005	[−0.006, 0.016]
Girls	**0.018**	**0.007**	**[0.006, 0.036]**

Note: significant results are in bold.

4. Discussion

MP has become an inseparable part of adolescents' life, but MP addiction can be related to various undesirable outcomes such as high-stake risk-taking behavior. To examine how and for whom MP addiction is related to risk-taking behaviors in adolescents, this three-wave longitudinal study examines the mediation role of self-control and the moderation role of sex in a sample of Chinese high school students. The results reveal that adolescents' MP addiction is related to increased risk-taking behavior via self-control, but this mediation model appears as only significant for girls but not for boys.

4.1. MP Addiction and Adolescents' Risk-Taking Behavior

Prior studies have found that MP addiction is related to risk-driving behavior [25,59]. The current study adds to this line of literature. Supporting our first hypothesis, this study reveals that MP addiction is related to other forms of risk-taking behavior in addition to risk driving. More importantly, using a three-wave longitudinal study and controlling for the baseline levels of risk-taking behavior, our results indicate that MP addiction increases risk-taking behavior over time, although the effect is indirect rather than direct. MPs can be used for multiple content categories, such as gathering information, playing games, and maintaining social networking. Different content categories can be related to different consequences. For example, exposure to risk-taking photos that are posted on the internet may increase adolescents' acceptance and propensity of engaging in risk-taking behavior [60,61]. However, the current study does not examine which content category is most related to risk-taking behavior. This could be a promising avenue for future research to explore.

4.2. The Mediation Effect of Self-Control

Confirming the second hypothesis, the results of the mediation model show that self-control mediates the effect of MP addiction on risk-taking behavior. The first part of the mediation process (i.e., mobile phone addiction → self-control) supports the flow theory. The flow theory suggests that immediate gratification and intrinsic rewards induced by mobile phones render individuals to lose themselves in electronic devices [62]. The perception of the presence of MPs is a temptation, even when people are not using it, because it distracts individuals' attention and increases the difficulty for individuals to focus on a task [9,63]. MP addiction may lead adolescents to develop a bad habit of checking their mobile phone frequently in daily life, which may undermine adolescents' self-control ability [64] and render them vulnerable to immediate rewards [8]. The second part of the mediation process (i.e., self-control → risk-taking behavior) is consistent with previous findings [42,65]. Self-control is a crucial psychological function associated with numerous life outcomes [34,35]. The mediation model suggests that MP addiction may increase risk-taking behavior by limiting one's self-control ability. We call this a "restraining path", such that MP addiction increases risk-taking behavior by restraining protective factors such as self-control. Although the current study does not provide a direct examination, it is worthwhile to note that according to the dual system model, there may be also a "promotive path" that may explain how MP addiction increases risk-taking behavior. For instance, MP addiction may increase adolescents' sensitivity to incentives and rewarding stimuli [10,21], and thus adolescents may meet their desires by engaging in more risk-taking behavior. As this study does not examine this assumption directly, future research may examine other mediators (e.g., increased sensitivity) in the association between MP addiction and risk-taking behavior.

4.3. The Moderation of Sex

Confirming the third and the fourth hypotheses, our results reveal that the mediation of self-control in the association between MP addiction and risk-taking behavior is only significant for girls. This could be because girls' self-control is more sensitive to environmental stimuli (e.g., cell phone) and more malleable [13] compared to boys, and thus MP addiction imposes more negative effect on self-control in girls than boys. As discussed above, the current study provides support to the "restraining path" and finds that this working mechanism only works among girls. Specifically, given that girls' self-control is more malleable and matures earlier [13], girls' self-control can sever as a protective factor of risk-taking behavior. However, MP addiction, as a risk factor, may restrain girls' self-control, thus increasing the likelihood of risk-taking behaviors. In contrast, boys generally have higher sensation-seeking and impulsivity than girls during adolescence, which indicates that boys' self-control cannot play its role well in prohibiting risk-taking behaviors [46]. In this case, the "restraining path" of self-control plays a little role in the association between MP addiction and the increase in risk-taking behaviors in boys. Thus, we suspect whether the "promotive path" works equally well in both sexes. Future research may examine this line of research to further deepen the working mechanisms underlying the "MP addiction–risk-taking behavior" link.

4.4. Implications

This study bears two implications for the prevention and intervention of adolescents' risk-taking behavior. On the one hand, the results show that MP addiction may increase risk-taking behavior over time. This implies that addressing MP addiction may be a crucial way to reduce the occurrence of risk-taking behavior in adolescents. On the other hand, reduced self-control significantly mediates the association between MP addiction and risk-taking behavior in girls. This suggests that using evidence-based programs (e.g., mindfulness) to boost girls' self-control may be useful in reducing girls' risk-taking behavior.

4.5. Limitations

We must acknowledge that this study has several limitations. First, only self-reported data were collected and thus the associations could be inflated because of the common method bias. To enhance the internal validity of the results, future research may use multiple measurement modalities to triangulate each variable. In addition, as discussed above, this study does not reveal which content category of MP addiction is related to risk-taking behavior. Future research may deepen this issue to achieve a fuller understanding of the relationship between MP addiction and risk-taking behavior in adolescents. Finally, family relationship has been found to be associated with adolescents' screen behaviors and risk behaviors [11]. Future research should take family relationship into further consideration.

5. Conclusions

Taken together, this study reveals that MP addiction is a risk factor for risk-taking behavior via reduced self-control in adolescent girls. These findings bear important implications for the prevention and intervention of adolescents' risk-taking behavior and to the promotion of positive youth development.

Author Contributions: Conceptualization, K.D. and J.-B.L.; data curation, K.D. and L.-X.W.; formal analysis, J.-B.L.; funding acquisition, K.D.; investigation, G.-D.W., Y.-Y.L. and Y.-T.H.; methodology, J.-B.L.; project administration, L.-X.W. and Y.-Y.L.; resources, G.-D.W.; software, J.-B.L.; supervision, J.-B.L.; validation, G.-D.W.; visualization, L.-X.W.; writing—original draft, K.D. and L.-X.W.; writing—review and editing, J.-B.L., Y.-Y.L. and Y.-T.H. All authors have read and agreed to the published version of the manuscript.

References

1. China Internet Network Information Center. The 45th China Statistical Report on Internet Development. Available online: http://www.cnnic.net.cn/hlwfzyj/hlwxzbg/hlwtjbg/202004/t20200428_70974.htm (accessed on 27 May 2020).
2. Barczyk, A.N.; Thompson, S.J.; Rew, L. The impact of psychosocial factors on subjective well-being among homeless young adults. *Health Soc. Work* **2014**, *39*, 172–180. [CrossRef] [PubMed]
3. Tyler, K.A.; Schmitz, R.M. Using cell phones for data collection: Benefits, outcomes, and intervention possibilities with homeless youth. *Child. Youth Serv. Rev.* **2017**, *76*, 59–64. [CrossRef] [PubMed]
4. Chahal, H.; Fung, C.; Kuhle, S.; Veugelers, P.J. Availability and night-time use of electronic entertainment and communication devices are associated with short sleep duration and obesity among Canadian children. *Pediatr. Obes.* **2013**, *8*, 42–51. [CrossRef]
5. Demirci, K.; Akgönül, M.; Akpinar, A. Relationship of smartphone use severity with sleep quality, depression, and anxiety in university students. *J. Behav. Addict.* **2015**, *4*, 85–92. [CrossRef]
6. Livingstone, S.; Smith, P.K. Annual Research Review: Harms experienced by child users of online and mobile technologies: The nature, prevalence and management of sexual and aggressive risks in the digital age. *J. Child Psychol. Psychiatry* **2014**, *55*, 635–654. [CrossRef] [PubMed]
7. De-Sola, J.; Talledo, H.; Rubio, G.; de Fonseca, F.R. Development of a mobile phone addiction craving scale and its validation in a Spanish adult population. *Front. Psychiatry* **2017**, *8*, 9. [CrossRef]
8. Tang, Z.; Zhang, H.; Yan, A.; Qu, C. Time is money: The decision making of smartphone high users in gain and loss intertemporal choice. *Front. Psychol.* **2017**, *8*, 363. [CrossRef] [PubMed]
9. Thornton, B.; Faires, A.; Robbins, M.; Rollins, E. The mere presence of a cell phone may be distracting: Implications for attention and task performance. *Soc. Psychol.* **2014**, *45*, 479–488. [CrossRef]
10. Wang, P.C.; Lei, L.; Wang, X.C.; Nie, J.; Chu, X.Y.; Jin, S.N. The exacerbating role of perceived social support and the "buffering" role of depression in the relation between sensation seeking and adolescent smartphone addiction. *Pers. Individ. Differ.* **2018**, *130*, 129–134. [CrossRef]

11. Liu, Q.Q.; Yang, X.J.; Hu, Y.T.; Zhang, C.Y.; Nie, Y.G. How and when is family dysfunction associated with adolescent mobile phone addiction? Testing a moderated mediation model. *Child. Youth Serv. Rev.* **2020**, *111*. [CrossRef]
12. Burt, C.H.; Sweeten, G.; Simons, R.L. Self-control through emerging adulthood: Instability, multidimensionality, and criminological significance. *Criminology* **2014**, *52*, 450–487. [CrossRef]
13. Jo, Y.; Bouffard, L. Stability of self-control and gender. *J. Crim. Justice* **2014**, *42*, 356–365. [CrossRef]
14. Shoenberger, N.; Rocheleau, G.C. Effective parenting and self-control: Difference by gender. *Women Crim. Justice* **2017**, *27*, 271–286. [CrossRef]
15. Jiang, Z.C.; Zhao, X.X. Self-control and problematic mobile phone use in Chinese college students: The mediating role of mobile phone use patterns. *BMC Psychiatry* **2016**, *16*, 416. [CrossRef] [PubMed]
16. Volkmer, S.A.; Lermer, E. Unhappy and addicted to your phone?—Higher mobile phone use is associated with lower well-being. *Comput. Hum. Behav.* **2019**, *93*, 210–218. [CrossRef]
17. Gullone, E.; Moore, S.; Moss, S.; Boyd, C. The adolescent risk-taking questionnaire. *J. Adolesc. Res.* **2000**, *15*, 231–250. [CrossRef]
18. Ju, C.; Wu, R.; Zhang, B.; You, X.; Luo, Y. Parenting style, coping efficacy, and risk-taking behavior in Chinese young adults. *J. Pac. Rim Psychol.* **2020**, *14*, 1–9. [CrossRef]
19. Steinberg, L. A social neuroscience perspective on adolescent risk-taking. *Dev. Rev.* **2008**, *28*, 78–106. [CrossRef]
20. Shulman, E.P.; Smith, A.R.; Silva, K.; Icenogle, G.; Duell, N.; Chein, J.; Steinberg, L. The dual systems model: Review, reappraisal, and reaffirmation. *Dev. Cogn. Neurosci.* **2016**, *17*, 103–117. [CrossRef]
21. van Duijvenvoorde, A.C.; Peters, S.; Braams, B.R.; Crone, E.A. What motivates adolescents? Neural responses to rewards and their influence on adolescents' risk taking, learning, and cognitive control. *Neurosci. Biobehav. Rev.* **2016**, *70*, 135–147. [CrossRef]
22. Oulasvirta, A.; Rattenbury, T.; Ma, L.; Raita, E. Habits make smartphone use more pervasive. *Pers. Ubiquitous Comput.* **2011**, *16*, 105–114. [CrossRef]
23. Lee, Y.K.; Chang, C.T.; Lin, Y.; Cheng, Z.H. The dark side of smartphone usage: Psychological traits, compulsive behavior and technostress. *Comput. Hum. Behav.* **2014**, *31*, 373–383. [CrossRef]
24. Lee, H.; Kim, J.W.; Choi, T.Y. Risk factors for smartphone addiction in Korean adolescents: Smartphone use patterns. *J. Korean Med. Sci.* **2017**, *32*, 1674–1679. [CrossRef]
25. Truong, L.T.; Nguyen, H.T.T.; De Gruyter, C. Correlations between mobile phone use and other risky behaviours while riding a motorcycle. *Accid. Anal. Prev.* **2018**, *118*, 125–130. [CrossRef]
26. Yang, Y.S.; Yen, J.Y.; Ko, C.H.; Cheng, C.P.; Yen, C.F. The association between problematic cellular phone use and risky behaviors and low self-esteem among Taiwanese adolescents. *BMC Public Health* **2010**, *10*, 217. [CrossRef]
27. Hadlington, L.J. Cognitive failures in daily life: Exploring the link with Internet addiction and problematic mobile phone use. *Comput. Hum. Behav.* **2015**, *51*, 75–81. [CrossRef]
28. Hong, W.; Liu, R.D.; Ding, Y.; Sheng, X.; Zhen, R. Mobile phone addiction and cognitive failures in daily life: The mediating roles of sleep duration and quality and the moderating role of trait self-regulation. *Addict. Behav.* **2020**, *107*, 106383. [CrossRef]
29. Acheson, A.; Lake, S.L.; Bray, B.C.; Liang, Y.; Mathias, C.W.; Ryan, S.R.; Charles, N.E.; Dougherty, D.M. Early adolescent trajectories of impulsiveness and sensation seeking in children of fathers with histories of alcohol and other substance use disorders. *Alcoholism* **2016**, *40*, 2622–2630. [CrossRef]
30. Kerin, J.L.; Webb, H.J.; Zimmer-Gembeck, M.J. Intuitive, mindful, emotional, external and regulatory eating behaviours and beliefs: An investigation of the core components. *Appetite* **2019**, *132*, 139–146. [CrossRef]
31. Yang, Y.; Joshi, S.H.; Jahanshad, N.; Thompson, P.M.; Baker, L.A. Neural correlates of proactive and reactive aggression in adolescent twins. *Aggress. Behav.* **2017**, *43*, 230–240. [CrossRef]
32. Moffitt, T.E.; Arseneault, L.; Belsky, D.; Dickson, N.; Hancox, R.J.; Harrington, H.; Houts, R.; Poulton, R.; Roberts, B.W.; Ross, S.; et al. A gradient of childhood self-control predicts health, wealth, and public safety. *Proc. Natl. Acad. Sci. USA* **2011**, *108*, 2693–2698. [CrossRef]
33. De Ridder, D.T.; Lensvelt-Mulders, G.; Finkenauer, C.; Stok, F.M.; Baumeister, R.F. Taking stock of self-control: A meta-analysis of how trait self-control relates to a wide range of behaviors. *Pers. Soc. Psychol. Rev.* **2012**, *16*, 76–99. [CrossRef] [PubMed]

34. Vazsonyi, A.T.; Mikuška, J.; Kelley, E.L. It's time: A meta-analysis on the self-control-deviance link. *J. Crim. Justice* **2017**, *48*, 48–63. [CrossRef]
35. Romero, E.; Go'mez-Fraguela, A.; Luengo, A.; Sobral, J. The self-control construct in the general theory of crime: An investigation in terms of personality psychology. *Psychol. Crime Law* **2003**, *9*, 61–86. [CrossRef]
36. Koning, I.M.; van den Eijnden, R.J.; Engels, R.C.; Verdurmen, J.E.; Vollebergh, W.A. Why target early adolescents and parents in alcohol prevention? The mediating effects of self-control, rules and attitudes about alcohol use. *Addiction* **2011**, *106*, 538–546. [CrossRef]
37. Walters, K.J.; Simons, J.S.; Simons, R.M. Self-control demands and alcohol-related problems: Within- and between-person associations. *Psychol. Addict. Behav.* **2018**, *32*, 573–582. [CrossRef]
38. Flexon, J.L.; Meldrum, R.C.; Young, J.T.N.; Lehmann, P.S. Low self-control and the dark triad: Disentangling the predictive power of personality traits on young adult substance use, offending and victimization. *J. Crim. Justice* **2016**, *46*, 159–169. [CrossRef]
39. Bergen, A.E.; Newby-Clark, I.R.; Brown, A. Low trait self-control in problem gamblers: Evidence from self-report and behavioral measures. *J. Gamb. Stud.* **2012**, *28*, 637–648. [CrossRef] [PubMed]
40. Gavriel-Fried, B.; Ronen, T. Contribution of positivity ratio and self-control to reduced gambling severity among adolescents. *Health Soc. Work* **2015**, *40*, 209–216. [CrossRef] [PubMed]
41. Baumeister, R.F.; Vohs, K.D.; Tice, D.M. The strength model of self-control. *Curr. Dir. Psychol.* **2007**, *16*, 351–355. [CrossRef]
42. Friehe, T.; Schildberg-Hörisch, H. Self-control and crime revisited: Disentangling the effect of self-control on risk taking and antisocial behavior. *Int. Rev. Law Econ.* **2017**, *49*, 23–32. [CrossRef]
43. Barr, N.; Pennycook, G.; Stolz, J.A.; Fugelsang, J.A. The brain in your pocket: Evidence that smartphones are used to supplant thinking. *Comput. Hum. Behav.* **2015**, *48*, 473–480. [CrossRef]
44. Anshari, M.; Alas, Y.; Hardaker, G.; Jaidin, J.H.; Smith, M.; Ahad, A.D. Smartphone habit and behavior in Brunei: Personalization, gender, and generation gap. *Comput. Hum. Behav.* **2016**, *64*, 719–727. [CrossRef]
45. Chen, C.; Zhang, K.Z.K.; Gong, X.; Zhao, S.J.; Lee, M.K.O.; Liang, L. Examining the effects of motives and gender differences on smartphone addiction. *Comput. Hum. Behav.* **2017**, *75*, 891–902. [CrossRef]
46. Shulman, E.P.; Harden, K.P.; Chein, J.M.; Steinberg, L. Sex differences in the developmental trajectories of impulse control and sensation-seeking from early adolescence to early adulthood. *J. Youth Adolesc.* **2015**, *44*, 1–17. [CrossRef]
47. Cross, C.P.; Copping, L.T.; Campbell, A. Supplemental material for sex differences in impulsivity: A meta-analysis. *Psychol. Bull.* **2011**, 97–130. [CrossRef]
48. Cross, C.P.; Cyrenne, D.L.; Brown, G.R. Sex differences in sensation-seeking: A meta-analysis. *Sci. Rep.* **2013**, *3*, 1–5. [CrossRef]
49. Leung, L. Linking psychological attributes to addiction and improper use of the mobile phone among adolescents in Hong Kong. *J. Child. Media* **2008**, *2*, 93–113. [CrossRef]
50. Tangney, J.P.; Baumeister, R.F.; Boone, A.L. High self-control predicts good adjustment, less pathology, better grades, and interpersonal success. *J. Pers.* **2004**, *72*, 271–324. [CrossRef]
51. Situ, Q.M.; Li, J.B.; Dou, K. Reexamining the linear and U-shaped relationships between self-control and emotional and behavioural problems. *Asian J. Soc. Psychol.* **2016**, *19*, 177–185. [CrossRef]
52. Figner, B.; Mackinlay, R.J.; Wilkening, F.; Weber, E.U. Supplemental material for affective and deliberative processes in risky choice: Age differences in risk taking in the Columbia card task. *J. Exp. Psychol.-Learn. Mem. Cogn.* **2009**. [CrossRef]
53. Pentz, M.A.; Shin, H.; Riggs, N.; Unger, J.B.; Collison, K.L.; Chou, C.P. Parent, peer, and executive function relationships to early adolescent e-cigarette use: A substance use pathway? *Addict. Behav.* **2015**, *42*, 73–78. [CrossRef] [PubMed]
54. Acock, A.C. Working with missing values. *J. Marriage Fam.* **2005**, *67*, 1012–1028. [CrossRef]
55. Preacher, K.J.; Hayes, A.F. Asymptotic and resampling strategies for assessing and comparing indirect effects in multiple mediator models. *Behav. Res. Methods* **2008**, *40*, 879–891. [CrossRef] [PubMed]
56. Kline, R.B. *Principles and Practice of Structural Equation Modeling*, 3rd ed.; Guilford Press: New York, NY, USA, 2015.
57. Steiger, J.H. Structural model evaluation and modification: An interval estimation approach. *Multivar. Behav. Res.* **1990**, *25*, 173–180. [CrossRef] [PubMed]

58. Cohen, J. A power primer. *Psychol. Bull.* **1992**, *112*, 155–159. [CrossRef]
59. Sween, M.; Ceschi, A.; Tommasi, F.; Sartori, R.; Weller, J. Who is a distracted driver? Associations between mobile phone use while driving, domain-specific risk taking, and personality. *Risk Anal.* **2017**, *37*, 2119–2131. [CrossRef]
60. Sherman, L.E.; Greenfield, P.M.; Hernandez, L.M.; Dapretto, M. Peer influence via Instagram: Effects on brain and behavior in adolescence and young adulthood. *Child Dev.* **2018**, *89*, 37–47. [CrossRef]
61. Sherman, L.E.; Payton, A.A.; Hernandez, L.M.; Greenfield, P.M.; Dapretto, M. The power of the like in adolescence: Effects of peer influence on neural and behavioral responses to social media. *Psychol. Sci.* **2016**, *27*, 1027–1035. [CrossRef]
62. Chen, C.; Zhang, K.Z.K.; Gong, X.; Zhao, S.J.; Lee, M.K.O.; Liang, L. Understanding compulsive smartphone use: An empirical test of a flow-based model. *Int. J. Inf. Manag.* **2017**, *37*, 438–454. [CrossRef]
63. Zheng, F.Z.; Gao, P.; He, M.D.; Li, M.; Wang, C.X.; Zeng, Q.C.; Zhou, Z.; Yu, Z.P.; Zhang, L. Association between mobile phone use and inattention in 7102 Chinese adolescents: A population-based cross-sectional study. *BMC Public Health.* **2014**, *14*. [CrossRef] [PubMed]
64. Soror, A.A.; Hammer, B.I.; Steelman, Z.R.; Davis, F.D.; Limayem, M.M. Good habits gone bad: Explaining negative consequences associated with the use of mobile phones from a dual-systems perspective. *Inf. Syst. J.* **2015**, *25*, 403–427. [CrossRef]
65. Kahn, R.E.; Holmes, C.; Farley, J.P.; Kim-Spoon, J. Delay discounting mediates parent-adolescent relationship quality and risky sexual behavior for low self-control adolescents. *J. Youth Adolesc.* **2015**, *44*, 1674–1687. [CrossRef] [PubMed]

2

Predicting the Time Spent Playing Computer and Mobile Games among Medical Undergraduate Students Using Interpersonal Relations and Social Cognitive Theory: A Cross-Sectional Survey in Chongqing, China

Li Chen [1,2,3,†], Ruiyi Liu [1,2,3,†], Huan Zeng [1,2,3], Xianglong Xu [1,2,3], Rui Zhu [1,2,3], Manoj Sharma [4,5,6] and Yong Zhao [1,2,3,*]

1 School of Public Health and Management, Chongqing Medical University, Chongqing 400016, China; nameclx@foxmail.com (L.C.); lry981118@foxmail.com (R.L.); zenghuan586@aliyun.com (H.Z.); xianglong1989@126.com (X.X.); 2016111041@stu.cqmu.edu.cn (R.Z.)
2 Research Center for Medicine and Social Development, Chongqing Medical University, Chongqing 400016, China
3 The Innovation Center for Social Risk Governance in Health, Chongqing Medical University, Chongqing 400016, China
4 Department of Behavioural and Environmental Health, Jackson State University, Jackson, MS 39213, USA; manoj.sharma@jsums.edu
5 Health for All, Omaha, NE 68144, USA
6 College of Health Sciences, Walden University, Minneapolis, MN 55401, USA
* Correspondence: zhaoyong@cqmu.edu.cn
† These authors contributed equally to this work.

Abstract: *Background*: Computer and mobile games are widely used among undergraduate students worldwide, especially in China. Our objective was to predict the time spent playing computer and mobile games based on interpersonal relations and social cognitive theory constructs (i.e., expectation, self-efficacy, and self-control). *Methods*: The cross-sectional survey was conducted in two medical universities using a sample of 1557 undergraduate students recruited by cluster sampling. The five-point Likert questionnaire was jointly developed by researchers from Chongqing Medical University and Jackson State University. *Results*: Approximately 30% and 70% of the students played computer and mobile games, respectively. The daily times spent by participants on computer games were 25.61 $\pm$ 73.60 min (weekdays) and 49.96 $\pm$ 128.60 min (weekends), and 66.07 $\pm$ 154.65 min (weekdays) and 91.82 $\pm$ 172.94 min (weekends) on mobile games. Students with high scores of interpersonal relations but low scores of self-efficacy spent prolonged time playing computer games on weekdays and weekends ($p < 0.05$ for all). Students with low scores of expectation spent prolonged time playing computer games on weekdays ($p < 0.05$). Students with high scores of interpersonal relations but low scores of self-efficacy and self-control spent prolonged time playing mobile games on weekdays and weekends ($p < 0.05$ for all). *Conclusions*: The prevalence and duration of playing mobile games were higher than those of playing computer games among medical undergraduate students in Chongqing, China. This study determined the interpersonal relations, self-efficacy, self-control, and expectation of the students at the time of playing computer and mobile games. Future studies may consider studying the interaction among game-related behaviours, environments, and personality characteristics.

Keywords: time; gaming disorder; interpersonal relations; self-efficacy; self-control; expectations

1. Introduction

Globally, computer and mobile games are widely played by undergraduate students and have been identified to cause serious public health problems. The use of computer and mobile games is especially prevalent in China. By the end of December 2015, the number of Chinese teenage netizens (18 to 25 years old) reached 287 million, and of these, 66.5% play computer and mobile games [1]. By 2017, China had more than 390 million students playing computer games, accounting for 25.4% of all Internet users [2]. With the development of portable devices, the number of players shifting to mobile phones from computers has increased. Since 2013, 15.6% of users have not played games on their computers [3]. According to a 2015 survey, 90% of teenagers used mobile phones to surf the Internet, and 51.0% of them played mobile games online [1]. Playing computer games for a long period increases the screen viewing time of undergraduate students, causes dry eye syndrome and visual fatigue [4,5] and raises the risk of sedentary behaviour and obesity [6–8]. Smartphone overuse can lead to neck, wrist and back pains [9]. Excessive smartphone use at night can also shorten sleep time and lead to stress and depression [10]. In addition, a positive correlation was noted between the severity of Internet addiction and depression in adolescents, but no such relationship was found between time spent using social networks and depression [11]. Moreover, being in a state of negative tension, such as anxiety and depression, can promote the use of smartphones and the Internet and even lead to addiction [12,13].

In the study on Internet or smartphone addiction (computer and mobile games), several models of Internet and smartphone addiction are developed, like the IPACE model of Brand or the model concerning problematic smartphone use of Bilieux [12,14,15]. These models suggest that personality characteristics or psychopathological phenomena (depression and anxiety) significantly influence Internet and smartphone addiction. According to Montag's research in 2017, the personality characteristics of Internet and smartphone addiction overlap, and the relationship between personality and Internet addiction is closer, with self-efficacy or self-control as potential precursors of addiction [16]. Empathy and life satisfaction are also linked to Internet and smartphone addiction [17]. In addition, a 2015 study in South Korea found that psychopathological phenomenon, such as anxiety, is a risk factor for Internet and smartphone addiction [13]. Preoccupation and conflict are risk factors for smartphone addiction [18]. Depression and attention deficit both play a critical role in Internet addiction [19]. Internet addiction can also predict stress, depression, anxiety, and loneliness [20]. Personality characteristics, such as self-esteem and resilience, also regulate depression and Internet and smartphone addiction [21]. Moreover, a considerable overlap exists between Internet and smartphone addiction [16,22]. This overlap may explain why studying the factors that influence Internet-use disorders (e.g., computer and mobile games) is crucial. Game disorder has progressed and is now officially included in the ICD-11. However, the inclusion of game disorder in the manual is controversial. The theoretical link between game disorders and personality traits and their role as factors of resilience or vulnerability (e.g., self-directedness, extraversion, impulsivity, and empathy) needs clarification.

Time spent on computer and mobile games is affected by many factors. In terms of gender, males are more interested in playing computer and mobile games than females [23]. A Chinese study found that teenage females spend more time on other extra-curricular and leisure activities, whereas teenage males spend more time playing video games [24]. Previous research showed that the length of time spent playing video games varies with age [25]. Smoking and drinking are associated with video games [26,27]. Family situation is also linked to playing computer and mobile games [6], whereby game behavior can enhance family cohesion to a certain extent [28]. Although game behavior is exhibited separately, most players prefer to share activities with friends or parents [28]. This preference may relatively extend game time. Many studies identified factors that influence the amount of time students spend playing computer and mobile games, but few studies focused on interpersonal relations and social cognitive theory constructs at the time of playing computer and mobile games, especially among Chinese medical undergraduate students.

Interpersonal relations and social cognitive theory constructs (i.e., expectation, self-efficacy, and self-control) are associated with game-playing behaviour [28–30]. Interpersonal relations measure the relationship between a person and those around him/her. A previous study found that people who play video games possess a good friendship network [28]. The social nature of certain video games can extend playing time whilst allowing players to gain new and other relationships [31]. Social cognition theory is a dynamic and reciprocal model based on the interaction among behaviour, personal factors, and environmental influences [32]. In this theory, expectation, self-efficacy and self-control are the core determinants for achieving a goal [33]. Social cognition theory was applied to study Chinese people for smoking cessation [34] and obesity prevention [35,36]. Expectations include the anticipation of the outcome of a particular action and the importance of the value of these results [37]. Self-efficacy describes a person's confidence in exhibiting a particular behaviour at a given moment [38]. Self-control describes a person's capability to regulate behaviour and includes strategies that encourage proximal and distal goal setting and self-rewards [37,38]. Another study found that self-efficacy is a comparatively robust predictor of involvement in massively multiplayer online role-playing game community [29]. In addition, self-control is negatively correlated with online game addiction [30], and students with high self-control spend lesser playing time on video games than those with low self-control. A study on Iranian students revealed that self-control when playing video games differs between male and female students [39].

Despite these efforts, previous studies paid little attention to medical undergraduate students, especially in China. Medical undergraduate students have more academic pressure and longer education years than other college students. Computer and mobile games provide a way for medical undergraduate students to relax. The video game time of medical students and the factors influencing this time may differ from those influencing students of other majors. To the best of our knowledge, this study is the first to use social cognitive theory in predicting the time spent playing computer and mobile games among medical undergraduate students in China. The objectives of this study are to examine the factors influencing students' behaviours in playing computer and mobile games and the effects of interpersonal relations and social cognitive theory constructs (i.e., expectation, self-efficacy, and self-control) on the time spent by students playing computer and mobile games.

2. Materials and Methods

2.1. Study Design

A cross-sectional study on medical undergraduate students was conducted in Chongqing in March 2018. Each medical university/college in Chongqing consists of a comparable number of students. A total of 1557 students were chosen from Chongqing Medical University and Chongqing Medical and Pharmaceutical College by cluster sampling. Cluster sampling was used to select the classes in school, and 27 classes (6 classes from Chongqing Medical and Pharmaceutical College and 19 from Chongqing Medical University) were selected from the two medical schools in Chongqing. The 27 classes were from Grades 1 to 3 (10 classes from Grade 1, 9 classes from Grade 2, and 8 classes from Grade 3). Prior to the investigation, we conducted a pilot survey in March 2018, involving 50 students from Chongqing Medical University and Chongqing Medical and Pharmaceutical College. With the pilot survey as basis, the questionnaire was distributed by a trained student helper to students who gave written consent to participate. For the questionnaire distribution, the student helper was trained on the purpose and method of the research and was the one who explained the research objectives to the students. The students who signed the informed consent filled out the questionnaire 'Study on the video games behaviour of undergraduate students in Chongqing, China', and the participants did not receive incentives. The students were asked to answer the questionnaire in the classroom within 15–20 min. This study was approved by Chongqing Medical University (Reference Number: 2016001), and the ethical approval includes allowing anonymous surveys of minors and adults with the consent of the class counsellor. Written informed consent for processing personal data was obtained from each participant.

2.2. Instruments

Questionnaire refers specifically to the measurement instrument used to obtain games related information in this study. The questionnaire was designed by Chongqing Medical University and Jackson State University researchers. The part on interpersonal relations was developed by research analysts from Chongqing Medical University. The part on social cognitive theory was developed by research analysts from Jackson State University. The questionnaire was translated from English into Chinese. We also checked the readability of the translated questionnaire in the pilot survey. The internal consistency of the total questionnaire was 0.954 (Cronbach's alpha). The games in this study refer to all multiplayer cooperative or independent games that operate on electronic device platforms, including online and offline variants.

The demographic information in this survey included gender, age (15–18, 19–20, 21–28 years old), ethnic group (Han nationals or Minority), grade level (Grade 1, Grade 2, Grade 3) and without siblings (Yes or No). Questions about living habits were also asked, including smoking (Smoker or Non-smoker) and drinking (Drinker or Non-drinker) preferences. This study measured the daily time spent playing computer and mobile games (on weekdays or weekends) with four questions. The participants were asked to answer the questions in min. We considered the score as a game time value which was zero, instead of not playing games when the self-reported game time was zero. The questions about interpersonal relations and social cognitive theory constructs were as follows: 6 items were used to measure interpersonal relations, 4 items were used to measure self-efficacy, 4 items were used to measure the self-control, and 10 items were used to measure the expectation (see Table 1). The internal consistency of the interpersonal relations was 0.929 (see Table 2). The internal consistencies of the self-efficacy, self-control, and expectation subscales were 0.887, 0.915, and 0.944, respectively.

Table 1. Specific problems in interpersonal relationships and social cognitive theory constructs.

Constructs	Specific Problems
Interpersonal relations [1]	How much do you agree with the following statement? I have good relationship with . . .
	(1) my classmates, (2) my roommates, (3) everyone around me, (4) my parents, (5) my teachers, (6) anyone. I don't often have conflicts with people.
Self-efficacy [2]	How sure are you that you will . . .
	(1) play computer or mobile games for less than 3 h daily? (2) reduce the time spent playing computer or mobile games, even if you enjoy playing games? (3) reduce the time spent playing computer or mobile games if you have to hand in your homework? (4) reduce the time spent playing computer or mobile games if you have to do something important?
Self-control [3]	How sure are you that you will . . .
	(1) set a goal to play computer or mobile games for less than 3 h daily? (2) reward yourself for insisting on reducing the time spent playing computer or mobile games daily? (3) remind yourself to insist on playing computer or mobile games for less than 3 h daily? (4) constantly check progress to make sure you play computer or mobile games for less than 3 h daily?
Expectation	If I play computer games or mobile games for less than 3 h daily, I will . . . [4]
	(1) have additional friends, (2) have more spare time, (3) enjoy more, (4) feel more relaxed, (5) be able to study well.
	Which of the following changes are important to you? [5]
	(6) have additional friends, (7) have more spare time, (8) enjoy more, (9) feel more relaxed, (10) be able to study well

[1] Response options were "Not At All Agree", "Slightly Agree", "Moderately Agree", "Very Agree"," Completely Agree". [2] Response options were "Not At All Sure", "Slightly Sure", "Moderately Sure", "Very Sure", "Completely Sure". [3] Response options were "Not At All Sure", "Slightly Sure", "Moderately Sure", "Very Sure", "Completely Sure". [4] Response options were "Never", "Hardly Ever", "Sometimes", "Almost Always", "Always". [5] Response options were "Not At All Important", "Slightly Important", "Moderately Important", "Very Important", "Extremely Important".

Table 2. Times spent playing games by undergraduate students in Chongqing, China (N, %).

Total Time (min)	Time Spent Playing Computer Game on Weekdays	Time Spent Playing Computer Game on Weekends	Time Spent Playing Mobile Game on Weekdays	Time Spent Playing Mobile Game on Weekends
Mean ± SD	25.61 ± 73.60	49.96 ± 128.60	66.07 ± 154.65	91.82 ± 172.94
0 [1]	898 (72.4)	853 (68.7)	387 (31.2)	400 (32.3)
(0–30] [2]	98 (7.9)	52 (4.2)	282 (22.7)	159 (12.8)
(30–60]	108 (8.7)	92 (7.4)	264 (21.3)	201 (16.2)
(60–90]	21 (1.7)	19 (1.5)	21 (1.7)	36 (2.9)
(90–120]	72 (5.8)	101 (8.1)	181 (14.6)	208 (16.8)
(120–150]	2 (0.2)	3 (0.2)	2 (0.2)	14 (1.1)
(150–180]	11 (0.9)	36 (2.9)	38 (3.1)	71 (5.7)
>180	31 (2.5)	85 (6.8)	66 (5.3)	151 (12.2)

[1] 0 min; [2] greater than 0 min is less than or equal to 30 min.

2.3. Data Analysis

Frequencies and percentages were calculated to summarize the distributions of the categorical variables. A *t*-test was employed to compare the differences in the continuous variables between males and females. Generalized linear models were developed using social cognitive theory constructs (i.e., expectations, self-efficacy and self-control), interpersonal relations, healthy habits (smoking and drinking status), gender, age group, grade level, lack of siblings, and nationality as independent variables and time spent playing computer and mobile games on weekdays and weekends as dependent variables. Statistical tests included a two-sided test, and statistical significance was at $p < 0.05$. All data were analyzed using SPSS22.0 for Windows (SPSS Inc., Chicago, IL, USA).

3. Results

3.1. Characteristics of the Sample

This survey involved 1557 undergraduate students. Of the 1241 persons who answered all the questions, 458 (36.9%) were males and 783 (63.0%) were females. All the participants were 15–28 years old, and the average age of the participants was 19.76 ± 1.30 years old. A total of 89.2% were Han nationals; 10.8%, minorities. Of the 1241 participants, 35.1% were Grade 1, 27.0% were Grade 2, and 38.0% were Grade 3. A total of 43.4% had no siblings, and 56.6% had siblings. Moreover, 6% and 11% were smokers and drinkers, respectively, and 94.0% and 89% did not smoke and drink (see Table 3).

Table 3. Demographic characteristics of undergraduate students in Chongqing, China.

Variables	Daily Time Playing Computer Games				Daily Time Playing Mobile Games				Total
	On Weekdays		On Weekends		On Weekdays		On Weekends		
	0 min	>0 min	0 min	>0 min	0 min	>0 min	0 min	>0 min	
	N (%)	N (%)	N (%)	N (%)	N (%)	N (%)	N (%)	N (%)	N (%)
Gender									
Male	109 (8.8)	349(28.1)	114 (9.2)	344 (27.7)	202 (16.3)	256 (20.6)	172 (13.9)	286 (23.0)	458 (36.9)
Female	278 (22.4)	505 (40.7)	287 (23.1)	496 (40.0)	696 (56.1)	87 (7.0)	681 (54.9)	102 (8.2)	783 (63.0)
Age									
15–18 years old	63 (5.1)	460 (12.9)	67 (5.4)	156 (12.6)	158 (12.7)	65 (5.2)	140 (11.3)	83 (6.7)	223 (18.0)
19–20 years old	207 (16.7)	458 (36.9)	215 (17.3)	450 (36.3)	493 (39.7)	172 (13.9)	467 (37.6)	198 (16.0)	665 (53.6)
21–28 years old	117 (9.4)	236 (19.0)	119 (9.6)	234 (18.9)	247 (19.9)	106 (8.5)	246 (19.8)	107 (8.6)	353 (28.4)
Nationality									
Han nationals	334 (23.9)	773 (62.3)	348 (28.0)	759 (61.2)	793 (63.9)	314 (25.3)	753 (60.7)	354 (28.5)	1107 (89.2)
Minority	53 (4.3)	81 (6.5)	53 (4.3)	81 (6.5)	105 (8.5)	29 (2.3)	100 (8.1)	34 (2.7)	134 (10.8)

Table 3. *Cont.*

Variables	Daily Time Playing Computer Games				Daily Time Playing Mobile Games				Total
	On Weekdays		On Weekends		On Weekdays		On Weekends		
	0 min	>0 min	0 min	>0 min	0 min	>0 min	0 min	>0 min	
	N (%)	N (%)	N (%)	N (%)	N (%)	N (%)	N (%)	N (%)	N (%)
Grade levels									
Grade 1	139 (11.2)	332 (26.8)	144 (11.6)	327 (26.3)	349 (28.1)	122 (9.8)	327 (26.3)	144 (11.6)	435 (35.1)
Grade 2	109 (8.8)	226 (18.2)	111 (8.9)	224 (18.0)	245 (19.7)	90 (7.3)	222 (17.9)	113 (9.1)	335 (27.0)
Grade 3	139 (11.2)	296 (23.9)	146 (11.8)	289 (23.3)	304 (24.5)	131 (10.6)	304 (24.5)	131 (10.6)	471 (38.0)
Without siblings									
Yes	162 (13.1)	376 (30.3)	175 (14.1)	363 (29.3)	364 (29.3)	174 (14.0)	342 (27.6)	196 (15.8)	538 (43.4)
No	225 (18.1)	478 (38.5)	226 (18.2)	477 (38.4)	534 (43.0)	169 (13.6)	511 (41.2)	192 (15.5)	703 (56.6)
Smoking status									
Smoker	21 (1.7)	54 (4.4)	20 (1.6)	55 (4.4)	31 (2.5)	44 (3.5)	27 (2.2)	48 (3.9)	75 (6.0)
Non-smoker	366 (29.5)	800 (64.5)	381 (30.7)	785 (63.3)	867 (69.9)	299 (24.1)	826 (66.6)	340 (27.4)	1166 (94.0)
Drinking status									
Drinker	36 (2.9)	100 (8.1)	41 (3.3)	95 (7.7)	78 (6.3)	58 (4.7)	70 (5.6)	66 (5.3)	136 (11.0)
Non-drinker	351 (28.3)	754 (60.8)	360 (29.0)	745 (60.0)	820 (66.1)	285 (23.0)	783 (63.1)	322 (25.9)	1105 (89.0)

3.2. *Daily Time Spent Playing Computer and Mobile Games among Undergraduate Students*

Participants reported spending an average of 25.61 ± 73.60 min playing computer games per day on weekdays. A total of 898 (72.4%) reported spending 0 min playing computer games on weekdays, and 31 participants reported spending over 180 min playing computer games on weekdays. A total of 206 participants played computer games from 0 to 60 min on weekdays daily.

Participants reported an average of 49.96 ± 128.60 min playing computer games per day on weekends. A total of 853 (68.7%) reported spending 0 min playing computer games on weekends, and 85 participants reported spending over 180 min playing computer games on weekends. A total of 144 participants played computer games from 0 to 60 min, and 101 participants played computer games from 90 to 120 min on weekends daily.

Participants reported spending an average of 66.07 ± 154.65 min playing mobile games per day on weekdays. A total of 387 (31.2%) reported spending 0 min playing mobile games on weekdays, and 66 participants reported spending over 180 min playing mobile games on weekdays. The majority of participants spent between 0 to 60 min (546 participants) and 90 to 120 min (181 participants) playing mobile games on weekdays daily.

Participants reported spending an average of 91.82 ± 172.94 min playing mobile games per day on weekends. A total of 400 (32.3%) reported spending 0 min playing mobile games on weekends, and 151 participants reported spending over 180 min on playing mobile games on weekends. The majority of participants spent between 0 to 60 min (360 participants) and 90 to 120 min (208 participants) playing mobile games on weekends daily (see Table 2).

3.3. *Descriptive Statistics of Interpersonal Relations and Social Cognitive Theory Constructs*

Compared with males, females had a significantly higher mean score of interpersonal relations for playing video games ($p = 0.041$). However, no significant differences between males and females were observed in the mean scores of self-efficacy, self-control, and expectation for playing video games (see Table 4).

Table 4. Interpersonal relations and social cognitive theory constructs among undergraduate students in Chongqing, China.

Interpersonal Relations and Social Cognitive Theory Constructs	Min	Max	Mean (SD)	Standardized Cronbach Alpha	Males	Females	p-Value
Interpersonal relations	0.00	24.00	15.56 (5.40)	0.929	15.98 (5.81)	15.31 (5.14)	0.041 *
Self-efficacy	0.00	16.00	10.36 (4.59)	0.887	10.16 (4.36)	10.49 (4.71)	0.208
Self-control	0.00	16.00	9.13 (4.72)	0.915	8.82 (4.57)	9.31 (4.81)	0.068
Expectation	0.00	40.00	25.00 (9.58)	0.944	24.58 (9.32)	25.24 (9.72)	0.238
Total	-	-	-	0.954			

* Statistically significant ($p < 0.05$).

3.4. Generalised Linear Model Analysis for Factors Affecting the Time Spent Playing Video Games

In multivariable analyses, interpersonal relations, self-efficacy, and expectation were associated with the time spent playing computer games (see Table 4). Male students spent considerable time playing computer games on weekdays ($p < 0.001$) and weekends ($p < 0.001$). Students with a high score in interpersonal relations spent a long time playing computer games on weekdays ($p < 0.001$) and weekends ($p < 0.001$). Students with a high score in self-efficacy spent limited time playing computer games on weekdays ($p = 0.010$) and weekends ($p = 0.011$). Students with a high score in expectation spent limited time playing computer games on weekdays ($p = 0.003$).

3.5. Generalised Linear Model Analysis for Factors Affecting the Time Spent Playing Mobile Games

In multivariable analyses, interpersonal relations, self-efficacy, expectations, and self-control were associated with the time spent playing mobile games (see Tables 5 and 6). Students with a high score in interpersonal relations spent a long time playing mobile games on weekdays ($p < 0.001$) and weekends ($p < 0.001$). Students with a high score in self-efficacy spent limited time playing mobile games on weekdays ($p = 0.002$) and weekends ($p < 0.001$). Students with a high score of self-control spent limited time playing mobile games on weekdays ($p = 0.017$) and weekends ($p = 0.029$).

Table 5. Generalised linear model analysis of factors that affect interpersonal relations and social cognitive theory constructs of time spent playing computer games among all participants in Chongqing, China.

Parameter	Time Spent Playing Computer Games on Weekdays			Time Spent Playing Computer Games on Weekends		
	B	SE	p-Value	B	SE	p-Value
Males vs. Females	39.100	4.186	<0.001 **	79.798	7.214	<0.001 **
19–20 years old vs. 15–18 years old	−15.115	5.728	0.008 *	−27.646	9.872	0.005 *
21–28 years old vs. 15–18 years old	−30.535	7.816	<0.001 **	−56.256	13.471	<0.001 **
Han nationals vs. Minority	5.129	6.293	0.415	−3.666	10.847	0.735
Grade 2 vs. Grade 1	5.68	5.307	0.277	4.514	9.147	0.622
Grade 3 vs. Grade 1	20.917	6.266	0.001 *	17.876	10.801	0.098
Without siblings vs. with siblings	−3.149	3.999	0.431	3.711	6.892	0.590
Smoker vs. Non-smoker	1.288	8.532	0.880	51.145	14.706	0.001 *
Drinker vs. Non-drinker	17.201	6.543	0.009 *	14.158	11.277	0.209
Interpersonal relations and Social Cognitive Theory constructs						
Interpersonal relations	2.358	0.465	<0.001 **	3.211	0.801	<0.001 **
Self-efficacy	−1.619	0.627	0.010 *	−2.756	1.081	0.011 *
Self-control	−0.658	0.560	0.239	−0.878	0.964	0.362
Expectation	−0.892	0.296	0.003 *	−0.881	0.510	0.084

* Statistically significant ($p < 0.05$); ** Statistically significant ($p < 0.001$).

Table 6. Generalised linear model analysis of factors that affect interpersonal relations and social cognitive theory constructs of time spent playing mobile games among all participants in Chongqing, China.

Parameter	Time Spent Playing Computer Games on Weekdays			Time Spent Playing Computer Games on Weekends		
	B	SE	*p*-Value	B	SE	*p*-Value
Males vs. Females	6.569	9.264	0.478	19.573	10.314	0.058
19–20 years old vs. 15–18 years old	−8.581	12.676	0.498	−11.780	14.114	0.404
21–28 years old vs. 15–18 years old	−15.332	17.298	0.375	−12.047	19.260	0.532
Han nationals vs. Minority	17.008	13.928	0.222	16.723	15.507	0.281
Grade 2 vs. Grade 1	−8.537	11.746	0.467	−0.442	13.078	0.973
Grade 3 vs. Grade 1	−1.095	13.869	0.937	−1.762	15.442	0.909
Without siblings vs. with siblings	2.453	8.850	0.782	−4.443	9.854	0.652
Smoker vs. Non-smoker	−12.803	18.883	0.498	−5.613	21.025	0.789
Drinker vs. Non-drinker	21.086	14.480	0.145	9.465	16.123	0.557
Interpersonal relations and Social Cognitive Theory constructs						
Interpersonal relations	3.783	1.028	<0.001 **	4.671	1.145	<0.001 **
Self-efficacy	−4.208	1.388	0.002 *	−6.157	1.546	<0.001 **
Self-control	−2.954	1.238	0.017 *	−3.011	1.379	0.029 *
Expectation	−0.490	0.655	0.454	−0.477	0.729	0.513

* Statistically significant ($p < 0.05$); ** Statistically significant ($p < 0.001$).

4. Discussion

The aim of this study is to determine the interpersonal relations, self-efficacy, self-control, and expectation of the students at the time of playing computer and mobile games among Chinese medical undergraduates. Our results indicate that high interpersonal relations, low self-efficacy, and low expectations lead to longer computer games. We find also that high interpersonal relationship, low self-efficacy, and low self-control lead to longer mobile game time.

Approximately 30% and 70% of the participants played computer and mobile games, respectively. According to a previous study, roughly 63.7% participants are active players of computer and mobile games [40]. Our study reported high gaming rates among medical undergraduate students. In addition, mobile games are more popular than computer games among these undergraduate students. This finding implies that an increasing number of medical undergraduate students are replacing computer games with mobile games. A Chinese study found that 22% of medical undergraduates play mobile games or read online novels in class. The use of mobile phones is not limited by space and time and can even penetrate the classroom. The heavy and tedious courses in medical colleges may lead to high mobile game usage in class. This situation may be one reason why mobile gamers outnumber computer gamers in this setting. Medical schools should strengthen classroom management and enhance interest in the curriculum. Attracting students' attention in class should be done as much as possible to improve quality of teaching and reduce use of mobile games.

Medical undergraduate students with high interpersonal relations and low self-efficacy showed increased times spent playing computer games on weekdays and weekends. A previous study found that gamers who spent more time playing computer games display more prosocial behavior [41] and wider friendship networks [28]. Games have gradually become a way of maintaining interpersonal relationships in real life among college students. Extended game time may be due to games' ability to enhance users' social attributes in real life. Extending game time may help maintain a good relationship and enhance users' social attributes in real life. Good social conditions may also further increase game time. If students' interpersonal communication is low, then they tend to avoid social interaction, and the use of games as a popular social way will be reduced. However, people with social difficulties play games for social comfort [42]. Students with poor relationships may also immerse themselves in a game, which is related to the type of game. People with good relationships may be inclined to choose social games, such as massively multiplayer games. People with poor relationships may be inclined to choose games that make them comfortable to ease social difficulties.

A previous study found that self-efficacy in the real world is negatively related to game addiction [43], which is similar to our finding. Self-efficacy may be enhanced or amplified by environmental encouragement. However, our study marks the first time the relationship between social cognition theory and playing time is tested among a specific segment of the Chinese population. Health education workers can enhance self-efficacy for playing a computer game to reduce screen time among undergraduate students, especially students from higher grade levels. A previous study showed that motivational interviewing to enhance self-efficacy through repetition, reinforcement, and encouragement can strengthen the intrinsic motivations of subjects [44]. Short-term goals and rewards can also improve self-efficacy [45].

Students with low expectation reported spending long times spent playing computer games on weekdays. A previous study found that adolescents' expectation for health behaviour can influence the establishment of individual trajectories of health [46]. Therefore, teenagers can achieve healthy goals by raising expectations and controlling playing time. Students with high expectations are more health conscious and willing to take the initiative to reduce their playing time and gain health. Their parents or peers can encourage healthy behaviours, and such an action can lead to higher expectations. Building high expectations for playing video games for less than 3 h a day is important for adolescents. Health educators can enhance the expectation for playing video games to less than 3 h a day to decrease the time spent playing computer games. Medical undergraduate students who are also drinkers and smokers reported spending long time playing computer games on weekdays. This finding is supported by previous studies [27,47,48]. Previous studies have linked interpersonal relations with social behaviours such as smoking and drinking, and we have found that interpersonal relations are also linked to gaming behaviours, which may suggest that games are a social tool in some way [49,50].

For mobile games, medical undergraduate students with high interpersonal relations, low self-efficacy, and low self-control reported spending long time playing mobile games on weekdays and weekends. Playing mobile games can enhance friendships among peers. A study based on massively multiplayer online role-playing games showed that social interaction is essential in gaming experience. A mobile phone-based social network is a major tool for college students to socialize with others. This feature may extend the time spent by undergraduate students on mobile games. A previous study found that mental health self-efficacy influences the symptom outcomes of a mobile phone user. This study also linked self-efficacy with reduced depression, anxiety, and stress symptoms and reported that this improved work and social functioning [51]. We found that students with high self-control spent lesser time on mobile games than on computer games. Self-control is negatively correlated with mobile phone use [52], which supports our finding. The current study determined that self-control is negatively associated with mobile games. Students with low self-control are unable to control themselves from playing mobile games. Health education workers can enhance the self-efficacy and self-control of undergraduate students for playing mobile games to reduce time spent playing mobile games.

However, gender, age, ethic group, and grade levels are not significantly associated with the time spent playing mobile games. No space or time limit is found for mobile games, and mobile games are more popular than computer ones for males and females. A 2014 research found that when surfing and playing games become the main functions of mobile phones, males are more likely to use mobile phones than females [24]. In recent years, an increasing number of mobile games aimed at female groups have been developed, such as 'Love and Producer', which is popular among young Chinese women. This activity may be the reason why no significant difference was observed between genders in mobile games in this study. Moreover, age is not significantly associated with the time spent playing mobile games. The participants in this study were mostly 18–22 years old. Age is insignificant, possibly due to the concentration of participants in the age group. More age groups should be included to determine the relationship between age and mobile games.

This study has notable limitations. Firstly, the cross-sectional survey data cannot determine the direction of causality. We cannot clarify if constructs precede behaviour. Secondly, the time spent playing games was self-reported by the participants, which may not be accurate for game time. Self-reported game time of zero is probably the average time of the last month of zero, and this finding does not mean the participant has never played a game. This study also does not distinguish between excessive games because no clear standard for excessive game time is available. The self-reported game times may have introduced information and measurement bias. Future studies can collect the time spent playing games with Internet technologies. Thirdly, the questionnaire on interpersonal relations was developed by researchers in Chongqing Medical University. The interpersonal relationship scale was only tested for internal consistency and readability. It lacks wide recognition and use. Fourthly, our study was conducted on medical universities, which do not accurately represent all the undergraduates in China. Future research requires a larger sample size to cover more students with different majors. Fifthly, self-efficacy, self-control, and expectation are strictly focused on computer and mobile games, and this focus may have inflated correlations with self-reported gaming. Future studies may consider studying the relationship between self-efficacy, which is not strictly focused on computer and mobile games, and the time spent playing computer and mobile games. Finally, the types of games are not distinguished in this study, and different types of games may have different playing times.

5. Conclusions

The prevalence and duration of playing mobile games are higher than those of playing computer games among medical undergraduate students in Chongqing, China. This study determined the interpersonal relations, self-efficacy, self-control, and expectation on the time spent playing computer and mobile games. This study reported on students' gender, age, grade level, and drinking and smoking status at the time of playing computer and mobile games. Future studies may consider studying the interaction among game-related behaviours, environments, and personality characteristics.

Author Contributions: All authors contributed to the design of the survey. L.C. designed the study, interpreted and analysed the data and drafted the manuscript. R.L. contributed to data analysis and data interpretation as well as drafted the manuscript. H.Z., X.X., R.Z., M.S. and Y.Z. helped draft the manuscript. All authors have read and approved the final manuscript. All authors have seen and approved the final version of the manuscript.

Acknowledgments: We wish to thank the research students from Chongqing Medical University for their help in the data collection.

References

1. China Internet Network Information Center. Research Report on Internet Behavior of Chinese Teenagers in 2015. Available online: http://www.cnnic.cn/hlwfzyj/hlwxzbg/qsnbg/201608/P020160812393489128332.pdf (accessed on 10 July 2018).
2. China Culture and Entertainment Industry Association. China Game Industry Development Report in 2017. Available online: http://www.cnccea.com/index.php?m=newscon&id=408&aid=770 (accessed on 10 July 2018).
3. China Internet Network Information Center. 2013 China Mobile Game User Research Report. Available online: http://www.cnnic.cn/hlwfzyj/hlwxzbg/wybg/201409/P020140911538720279158.pdf (accessed on 10 July 2018).
4. Dumery, B.; Grounauer, P.A.; van Toi, V. *Eyestrain, Blink Rate and Dry Eye Syndromes of Video Display Terminal Users*; Springer: Berlin/Heidelberg, Germany, 2010; pp. 270–273.
5. Rajeev, A.; Gupta, A.; Sharma, M. Visual Fatigue and Computer Use Among College Students. *Indian J. Community Med.* **2006**, *31*, 192–193.

6. He, M.Z.; Piché, L.; Beynon, C.; Harris, S. Screen-related sedentary behaviors: Children's and parents' attitudes, motivations, and practices. *J. Nutr. Educ. Behav.* **2010**, *42*, 17–25. [CrossRef] [PubMed]
7. Bhadoria, A.S.; Kapil, U.; Kaur, S. Association of Duration of Time Spent on Television, Computer and Video Games with Obesity amongst Children in National Capital Territory of Delhi. *Int. J. Prev. Med.* **2015**, *6*, 80. [CrossRef] [PubMed]
8. Xu, X.; Pu, Y.; Sharma, M.; Rao, Y.; Cai, Y.; Zhao, Y. Predicting Physical Activity and Healthy Nutrition Behaviors Using Social Cognitive Theory: Cross-Sectional Survey among Undergraduate Students in Chongqing, China. *Int. J. Environ. Res. Public Health* **2017**, *14*. [CrossRef] [PubMed]
9. Cha, S.S.; Seo, B.K. Smartphone use and smartphone addiction in middle school students in Korea: Prevalence, social networking service, and game use. *Health Psychol. Open* **2018**, *5*. [CrossRef] [PubMed]
10. Lemola, S.; Perkinson-Gloor, N.; Brand, S.; Dewald-Kaufmann, J.F.; Grob, A. Adolescents' electronic media use at night, sleep disturbance, and depressive symptoms in the smartphone age. *J. Youth Adolesc.* **2015**, *44*, 405–418. [CrossRef] [PubMed]
11. Banjanin, N.; Banjanin, N.; Dimitrijevic, I.; Panticd, I. Relationship between internet use and depression: Focus on physiological mood oscillations, social networking and online addictive behavior. *Comput. Hum. Behav.* **2015**, *43*, 308–312. [CrossRef]
12. Billieux, J. Problematic Use of the Mobile Phone: A Literature Review and a Pathways Model. *Curr. Psychiatry Rev.* **2012**, *8*, 299–306. [CrossRef]
13. Choi, S.W.; Kim, D.J.; Choi, J.S.; Ahn, H.; Choi, E.J.; Song, W.Y.; Kim, S.; Youn, H. Comparison of risk and protective factors associated with smartphone addiction and Internet addiction. *J. Behav. Addict.* **2015**, *4*, 308–314. [CrossRef] [PubMed]
14. Brand, M. *Theoretical Models of the Development and Maintenance of Internet Addiction*; Springer International Publishing: Cham, Switzerland, 2017; pp. 19–34.
15. Brand, M.; Young, K.S.; Laier, C.; Wölfling, K.; Potenza, M.N. Integrating psychological and neurobiological considerations regarding the development and maintenance of specific Internet-use disorders: An Interaction of Person-Affect-Cognition-Execution (I-PACE) model. *Neurosci. Biobehav. Rev.* **2016**, *71*, 252–266. [CrossRef] [PubMed]
16. Lachmann, B.; Duke, É.; Sariyska, R.; Montag, C. Who's Addicted to the Smartphone and/or the Internet? *Psychol. Pop. Media Cult.* **2017**. [CrossRef]
17. Lachmann, B.; Sindermann, C.; Sariyska, R.Y.; Luo, R.; Melchers, M.C.; Becker, B.; Cooper, A.J.; Montag, C. The Role of Empathy and Life Satisfaction in Internet and Smartphone Use Disorder. *Front. Psychol.* **2018**, *9*, 398. [CrossRef] [PubMed]
18. Lee, H.; Kim, J.W.; Choi, T.Y. Risk Factors for Smartphone Addiction in Korean Adolescents: Smartphone Use Patterns. *J. Korean Med. Sci.* **2017**, *32*, 1674–1679. [CrossRef] [PubMed]
19. Sariyska, R.; Reuter, M.; Lachmann, B.; Montag, C. Attention Deficit/Hyperactivity Disorder is a Better Predictor for Problematic Internet use than Depression: Evidence from Germany. *J. Addict. Res. Ther.* **2015**, *6*, 209. [CrossRef]
20. Ostovar, S.; Allahyar, N.; Aminpoor, H.; Moafian, F.; Nor, M.B.M.; Griffiths, M.D. Internet Addiction and its Psychosocial Risks (Depression, Anxiety, Stress and Loneliness) among Iranian Adolescents and Young Adults: A Structural Equation Model in a Cross-Sectional Study. *Int. J. Mental Health Addict.* **2016**, *14*, 257–267. [CrossRef]
21. Park, H.; Choi, E. Smartphone Addiction and Depression: The Mediating Effects of Self-esteem and Resilience among Middle School Students. *J. Korean Acad. Community Health Nurs.* **2017**, *28*, 280–290. [CrossRef]
22. Min, K.; Kim, D.-J.; Cho, H.; Yang, S. The Smartphone Addiction Scale: Development and Validation of a Short Version for Adolescents. *PLoS ONE* **2013**, *8*, e83558. [CrossRef]
23. Yang, D.-J.; Chiu, J.-Z.; Chen, Y.-K. Examining the Social Influence on College Students for Playing Online Game: Gender Differences and Implications. *Turk. Online J. Educ. Technol.* **2011**, *10*, 115–122.
24. Jiang, X.X.; Hardy, L.L.; Ding, D.; Baur, L.A.; Shi, H.-J. Recreational screen-time among Chinese adolescents: A cross-sectional study. *J. Epidemiol.* **2014**, *24*, 397–403. [CrossRef] [PubMed]
25. Greenberg, B.S.; Sherry, J.; Lachlan, K.; Lucas, K.; Holmstrom, A. Orientations to Video Games Among Gender and Age Groups. *Simul. Gaming* **2010**, *41*, 238–259. [CrossRef]
26. Forsyth, S.R.; Malone, R.E. Smoking in Video Games: A Systematic Review. *Nicotine Tob. Res. Off. J. Soc. Res. Nicotine Tob.* **2016**, *18*, 1390–1398. [CrossRef] [PubMed]

27. Bőthe, B.; Tóth-Király, I.; Orosz, G. Clarifying the Links among Online Gaming, Internet Use, Drinking Motives, and Online Pornography Use. *Games Health J.* **2015**, *4*, 107–112. [CrossRef] [PubMed]
28. Durkin, K.; Barber, B. Not so doomed: Computer game play and positive adolescent development. *J. Appl. Dev. Psychol.* **2002**, *23*, 373–392. [CrossRef]
29. Hopp, T.; Barker, V.; Schmitz, A.W. Interdependent Self-Construal, Self-Efficacy, and Community Involvement as Predictors of Perceived Knowledge Gain among MMORPG Players. *Cyberpsychol. Behav. Soc. Netw.* **2015**, *18*, 468–473. [CrossRef] [PubMed]
30. Kim, E.J.; Namkoong, K.; Ku, T.; Kim, S.J. The relationship between online game addiction and aggression, self-control and narcissistic personality traits. *Eur. Psychiatry* **2008**, *23*, 212–218. [CrossRef] [PubMed]
31. Smyth, J.M. Beyond self-selection in video game play: An experimental examination of the consequences of massively multiplayer online role-playing game play. *Cyberpsychol. Behav.* **2007**, *10*, 717–721. [CrossRef] [PubMed]
32. Bandura, A. *Social Foundations of Thought and Action: A Social Cognitive Theory/Albert Bandura*; American Psychological Association: Washington, DC, USA, 1986.
33. Glanz, K.; Lewis, F.M.; Rimer, B.K. *Health Behavior and Health Education: Theory, Research, and Practice*; Jossey-Bass: San Francisco, CA, USA, 1997; pp. 344–353.
34. Zheng, P.; Guo, F.; Chen, Y.; Fu, Y.; Ye, T.; Fu, H. A randomized controlled trial of group intervention based on social cognitive theory for smoking cessation in China. *J. Epidemiol.* **2007**, *17*, 147–155. [CrossRef] [PubMed]
35. Murnan, J.; Sharma, M.; Lin, D. Predicting childhood obesity prevention behaviors using social cognitive theory: Children in China. *Int. Q. Community Health Educ.* **2006**, *26*, 73–84. [CrossRef] [PubMed]
36. Chen, Y.; Ma, L.; Ma, Y.; Wang, H.; Luo, J.; Zhang, X.; Luo, C.; Wang, H.; Zhao, H.; Pan, D.; et al. A national school-based health lifestyles interventions among Chinese children and adolescents against obesity: Rationale, design and methodology of a randomized controlled trial in China. *BMC Public Health* **2015**, *15*, 210. [CrossRef] [PubMed]
37. Bandura, A. Health Promotion by Social Cognitive Means. *Health Educ. Behav.* **2004**, *31*, 143–164. [CrossRef] [PubMed]
38. Tougas, M.E.; Hayden, J.A.; McGrath, P.J.; Huguet, A.; Rozario, S. A Systematic Review Exploring the Social Cognitive Theory of Self-Regulation as a Framework for Chronic Health Condition Interventions. *PLoS ONE* **2015**, *10*, e0134977. [CrossRef] [PubMed]
39. Haghbin, M.; Shaterian, F.; Hosseinzadeh, D.; Griffiths, M.D. A brief report on the relationship between self-control, video game addiction and academic achievement in normal and ADHD students. *J. Behav. Addict.* **2013**, *2*, 239–243. [CrossRef] [PubMed]
40. Mohamud, S. Effect of Video Games on Medical Students' Academic Performance: A Two-Institutions, Cross-Sectional Study. *Int. J. Sci. Eng. Res.* **2017**, *8*, 653–658.
41. Mengel, F. Computer games and prosocial behavior. *PLoS ONE* **2014**, *9*, e94099. [CrossRef] [PubMed]
42. Kowert, R.; Oldmeadow, J.A. Playing for social comfort: Online video game play as a social accommodator for the insecurely attached. *Comput. Hum. Behav.* **2015**, *53*, 556–566. [CrossRef]
43. Jeong, E.J.; Kim, D.H. Social activities, self-efficacy, game attitudes, and game addiction. *Cyberpsychol. Behav. Soc. Netw.* **2011**, *14*, 213–221. [CrossRef] [PubMed]
44. Walpole, B.; Dettmer, E.; Morrongiello, B.A.; McCrindle, B.W.; Hamilton, J. Motivational interviewing to enhance self-efficacy and promote weight loss in overweight and obese adolescents: A randomized controlled trial. *J. Pediatr. Psychol.* **2013**, *38*, 944–953. [CrossRef] [PubMed]
45. Schunk, D.H. Enhancing Self-Efficacy and Achievement through Rewards and Goals: Motivational and Informational Effects. *J. Educ. Res.* **1984**, *78*, 29–34. [CrossRef]
46. Mcdade, T.W.; Chyu, L.; Duncan, G.J.; Hoyt, L.T.; Doane, L.D.; Adam, E.K. Adolescents' expectations for the future predict health behaviors in early adulthood. *Soc. Sci. Med.* **2011**, *73*, 391–398. [CrossRef] [PubMed]
47. Frangos, C.C.; Frangos, C.C.; Sotiropoulos, I. Problematic Internet Use among Greek university students: An ordinal logistic regression with risk factors of negative psychological beliefs, pornographic sites, and online games. *Cyberpsychol. Behav. Soc. Netw.* **2011**, *14*, 51. [CrossRef] [PubMed]
48. Ko, C.H.; Yen, J.Y.; Yen, C.F.; Chen, C.S.; Weng, C.C.; Chen, C.C. The association between Internet addiction and problematic alcohol use in adolescents: The problem behavior model. *Cyberpsychol. Behav.* **2008**, *11*, 571–576. [CrossRef] [PubMed]

49. Liang, Y.; Zheng, X.; Zeng, D.D.; Zhou, X.; Leischow, S.J.; Chung, W. Characterizing Social Interaction in Tobacco-Oriented Social Networks: An Empirical Analysis. *Sci. Rep.* **2015**, *5*, 1–11. [CrossRef] [PubMed]
50. Monahan, J.L.; Lannutti, P.J. Alcohol as social lubricant. *Hum. Commun. Res.* **2000**, *26*, 175–202. [CrossRef]
51. Jiang, Z.; Zhao, X. Self-control and problematic mobile phone use in Chinese college students: The mediating role of mobile phone use patterns. *BMC Psychiatry* **2016**, *16*, 416. [CrossRef] [PubMed]
52. Clarke, J.; Proudfoot, J.; Birch, M.R.; Whitton, A.E.; Parker, G.; Manicavasagar, V.; Harrison, V.; Christensen, H.; Hadzi-Pavlovic, D. Effects of mental health self-efficacy on outcomes of a mobile phone and web intervention for mild-to-moderate depression, anxiety and stress: Secondary analysis of a randomised controlled trial. *BMC Psychiatry* **2014**, *14*, 272. [CrossRef] [PubMed]

3

Adolescents' Addictive Phone Use: Associations with Eating Behaviors and Adiposity

Sarah E. Domoff [1], Emma Q. Sutherland [2], Sonja Yokum [3] and Ashley N. Gearhardt [4,*]

1 Department of Psychology, Central Michigan University, Mount Pleasant, MI 48859, USA; domof1se@cmich.edu
2 School of Public Health, University of Michigan, Ann Arbor, MI 48109, USA; emmasuth@umich.edu
3 Oregon Research Institute, Eugene, OR 97403, USA; sonjas@ori.org
4 Department of Psychology, University of Michigan, Ann Arbor, MI 48109, USA
* Correspondence: agearhar@umich.edu;

Abstract: Concerns have been raised about excessive or "addictive" phone use among adolescents, and the impact that addictive phone use (APU) can have on adolescent development and health. Most research on the physical health correlates of smartphone use has been limited to sleep health, whereas other outcomes, such as eating behaviors and obesity risk have not received as much attention. To address this gap in the literature, we examined the association between APU and emotion regulation difficulties, impulsivity, maladaptive eating behaviors, and adiposity in a sample of 111 adolescents. We found that APU is associated with greater emotion regulation difficulties, dysregulated eating, restrained eating, food addiction, and higher percent body fat. Further, we found that emotion regulation difficulties mediated the association between APU and dysregulated eating, restrained eating, and food addiction. Findings suggest that addictive phone use may confer increased risk for obesogenic eating behaviors and food addiction via challenges in regulating emotions.

Keywords: phone; adolescents; addiction; BMI percentile; food addiction; emotional eating; impulsivity; emotion regulation

---

1. Introduction

Smartphone access and ownership continues to increase among adolescents in the United States. Indeed, a majority of youth (53%) own a smartphone by age 11—this increases to over 80% of youth by age 14 [1]. In addition to gaining access to smartphones at younger ages, shifts have also occurred in frequency of smartphone use. Social media applications (apps) are more frequently used by teens, with 38% of teens stating they use social media multiple times per hour, and 16% indicating they use social media nearly constantly [2].

Given the massive shift in adolescents' consumption of social media and other apps on mobile devices, concern has been expressed regarding whether adolescents can become "addicted" to screens, particularly smartphones. Nearly half of parents in the United States report that their children are addicted to mobile devices [3]. Although the term "addiction" may be used colloquially to describe too much use, the construct of addictive phone use is conceptualized in the scientific literature as a behavioral addiction, wherein excessive use leads to dysfunction or impairment [4]. Similar to the measurement of specific types of screen media addiction (e.g., problematic media use in children: [5]; social media dependence: [6]), symptoms of addictive phone use are based on the DSM-5 criteria for Internet Gaming Disorder (IGD [7]), but applied to smartphone use [4]. The nine criteria include indicators of both excessive use and dysfunction related to use, such as tolerance (needing to use phone for longer amounts of time), withdrawal (i.e., feeling irritable when unable to use or access phone), use to manage/modulate mood, and psychosocial impairment due to use.

Most research on addictive phone use has been conducted in college student and other adult populations [8]. Although a growing body of research has examined addictive phone use in adolescents in Europe and Asia [9], very limited research has examined addictive phone use among adolescents in the United States. One recent exception described the development of the Addictive Patterns of Use measure (APU measure) and its association with academic functioning in US adolescents. Domoff, Foley, and Ferkel (2019) found that greater addictive phone use (using the aforementioned DSM-5 criteria) is associated with poorer academic functioning, over and above the amount of time spent using social media on school days [4]. This study suggests that how adolescents use smartphones, and not necessarily the time they spend on smartphones, confers risks to adolescent development.

Traditional screen time (i.e., time spent watching TV) has long been associated with physical health outcomes, such as obesity and poorer sleep, in children and adolescents [10]. A recent review on the literature on physical health correlates of mobile devices noted major gaps in our understanding of the impact of excessive smart phone use on the physical health of youth [11]. Although research has most consistently linked smartphone use with disrupted sleep and shorter sleep duration [12], we are unaware of research examining addictive phone use with other health concerns, such as problematic eating behaviors, food addiction, and adiposity. The limited research that has considered smartphone use and health risks examines overall time spent on smartphones [13–15], but not addictive phone use. Given the high rates of phone use and concerns about phone addiction, it is critical to clarify whether addictive phone use may contribute to problematic eating behaviors and adiposity in US adolescents.

Furthermore, consideration of the underlying mechanisms accounting for the relationship between addictive phone use and physical health should be explored to clarify potential targets for clinical intervention. In particular, theoretical and empirical support exists for the role of impulsivity and emotion regulation difficulties on problematic phone use (see the Billieux et al. (2015) pathway model for the emergence of problematic mobile phone use [16]). Specifically, Billieux et al. (2015) outline three pathways that lead to problematic phone use. Two of these pathways, the excessive reassurance pathway and the impulsive pathway, describe both emotion regulation challenges (i.e., emotional instability) and poor impulse control (i.e., lack of premeditation, low self-control, and ADHD symptoms), as risk factors for addictive patterns of phone use. Billieux et al., (2015)'s theoretical pathways have been supported in studies of adolescents in Turkey and South Korea [17]. Similar correlates have also been defined as likely contributors to maladaptive eating behaviors, food addiction, and obesity in adolescents [18,19]. As such, impulsivity and emotion regulation difficulties will be explored as potential mediators.

In summary, smartphone addiction and its impact on adolescent health is largely understudied [11]. This is a significant area of research as a vast majority of US teens have their own smartphones, and nearly half of US parents are concerned about their adolescents' addiction to mobile devices [3]. Although countless studies have examined additive phone use and adolescent mental health [20], no studies have examined addictive phone use and obesity risk in US adolescents. The United States has a high rate of childhood obesity, with one in five adolescents meeting criteria for obesity [21]. To our knowledge, no research has considered whether smartphone addiction confers obesogenic risk among US adolescents. Given that obesity prevention is critical to the health of adolescents, examining whether and how addictive phone use may increase obesity risk fits within the priorities of the National Institute of Child Health and Human Development's Strategic Plan [22]. Preliminary research is necessary to investigate obesity-related health correlates of addictive phone use.

To address the limitations of previous research and set the foundation for future clinical research, our study aims to: (1) examine differences by gender, race/ethnicity, and parental education in addictive phone use; (2) investigate whether adolescents who report greater addictive phone use have greater emotion regulation difficulties, impulsivity, dysregulated eating, restrained eating, food addiction, and adiposity (objectively measured by body mass index (BMI) percentile and percent body fat); and (3) explore whether emotion regulation difficulties and impulsivity mediate the associations between addictive phone use and eating behaviors and adiposity.

2. Materials and Methods

2.1. Participants

This study is drawn from a larger parent study (N = 193) examining adolescents' neural responsiveness to fast food advertisements [23]. Administration of the Addictive Patterns of Use measure (APU measure) occurred part-way through the study, for a final N of 111 adolescents (see Table 1 for demographic characteristics). Data collection occurred between July 2015 and August 2017.

2.2. Procedure

Study procedures were approved by the Institutional Review Board at the University of Michigan (UM IRB board: HUM00095596). After obtaining parent/legal guardian informed consent and adolescent written assent, participants completed two visits to the lab. These visits consisted of survey completion, anthropometric measurement, and a functional magnetic resonance imaging paradigm (see Gearhardt et al., 2020, for additional information) [23]. Participants received compensation for their participation.

2.3. Measures

2.3.1. Demographic Characteristics

Information about the participants' demographics (e.g., age, gender, ethnicity, race, and highest education level of parent in the household) was provided. We categorized race/ethnicity as White or non-White, and parental education was categorized as college degree or higher or no college degree attained.

2.3.2. Addictive Patterns of Use (APU) Scale

Participants were administered the APU scale [4], which consists of nine items assessing excessive use of Smartphones (α = 0.85). Sample items are as follows: "During the last year, how often have you felt restless or tense when you were unable to use your phone?" and "During the last year, how often have there been times when all you could think about was using your phone?" Participants responded to items on a 5-point Likert scale, ranging from 1 (Never) to 5 (Very often). Mean scores were calculated to provide a total score of addictive phone use, with higher scores indicating greater addictive phone use.

2.3.3. Difficulties in Emotion Regulation Scale (DERS)

The DERS is a 36-item scale (α = 0.90) which assesses adolescents' perceptions of difficulties in regulating emotions [24]. Sample items include, "I have difficulty making sense out of my feelings" and "When I'm upset, I have difficulty controlling my behaviors." Adolescents respond on a Likert scale ranging from Almost Never (1) to Almost Always (5). Responses were summed to calculate a total score, with higher scores indicating greater difficulties in emotion regulation.

2.3.4. Barratt Impulsiveness Scale-Brief (BIS-Brief)

The BIS-Brief is a shortened version of the BIS-11, a widely used measure of trait impulsivity [25]. The BIS-Brief consists of eight items (α = 0.76), including "I do things without thinking" and "I am self-controlled." Participants respond to questions on a scale from rarely/never (1) to almost always/always (4). Responses are summed to provide a total score, with higher scores indicating greater trait impulsivity.

2.3.5. Eating Behaviors

The Dutch Eating Behaviour Questionnaire (DEBQ) is a widely used self-report measure of three types of eating behaviors: restrained eating, emotional eating, and external eating [26]. Participants responded to items on a 5-point Likert scale from (1) never to (5) very often (33 items). Restrained eating is measured by 10 items ($\alpha = 0.93$) such as "Do you try to eat less at mealtimes than you would like to eat?" The mean of these items was calculated to provide an overall restrained eating score. Emotional eating is measured by 13 items ($\alpha = 0.91$), such as "Do you get the desire to eat when you are anxious, worried or tense?" and external eating is measured by responses to 10 items ($\alpha = 0.86$), such as "If you see or smell something delicious, do you have a desire to eat it?" Given the high inter-correlation of emotional and external eating scales ($r = 0.58$, $p < 0.01$), the mean of the emotional and external eating items was calculated for a score of dysregulated eating.

2.3.6. The Dimensional Yale Food Addiction Scale for Children 2.0 (dYFAS-C 2.0)

The dYFAS-C 2.0 [27] consists of 16 items ($\alpha = 0.91$), adapted from the adult version of the Yale Food Addiction Scale 2.0 [28]. Items include: "When I started to eat certain foods, I found it hard to stop" and "When I cut down or stopped eating certain foods, I craved them a lot more." Participants responded to questions on a 5-point Likert-scale, ranging from Never (0) to Always (4). The sum of items was calculated to provide a total score. Higher scores indicate higher levels of food addiction.

2.3.7. Body Mass Index (BMI) Percentile

Objectively measured height and weight via standardized anthropometric measurements occurred, with participants instructed to wear light clothing. Height was measured using an O'Leary Acrylic Stadiometer (Ellard Instrumentation LLD, Monroe, Washington, USA) height (in centimeters, to the nearest tenth); weight was measured using a Detecto Portable Scale (Cardet, Webb City, Missouri, USA) (in kilograms, to the nearest tenth). Sex, age, height, and weight were used to calculate BMI percentiles [29].

2.3.8. Percent Body Fat

After participants completed the standard anthropometric measurements, we also objectively measured their percent body fat (PBF) via InBody 570 scale (InBody USA, Cerritos, California, USA), with an 8-point Bioelectrical Impedance Analyzer (Frequencies 5, 50, 500 kHz). Consistent with the measurement of height and weight, participants were instructed to wear light clothing and to remove coats, shoes, and socks for PBF measurement.

2.4. Statistical Analyses

All variables used in this study were investigated for normality. Given that some of the variables were skewed, non-parametric analyses that do not require normal distributions were used. For Aim 1, Mann-Whitney tests were used to compare mean APU scores across demographic categories. For Aim 2, Spearman rho correlations were used to investigate the association of APU with the outcome variables. For Aim 3, Hayes' PROCESS macro (Model 4) was used to explore whether emotion dysregulation and impulsivity mediated the associations examined in Aim 2 [30]. Due to identified sex differences in APU, sex was entered as a covariate in the mediation analyses.

3. Results

3.1. Participant Characteristics:

The mean age of the participants was 14.57 ($SD = 1.08$) years. The average BMI percentile was 78.59 ($SD = 21.84$) and the average percent body fat (PBF) was 26.84 ($SD = 11.60$). The sample was

44.1% male (n = 49); 71.2% identified as White (n = 79), followed by 17.1% identifying as Black/African American (n = 19; see Table 1 for additional characteristics of the sample).

Table 1. Sample Characteristics.

Characteristics	M (*SD*)/*n* (%)
Age	14.57 (1.08)
Gender	
Female	62 (55.9%)
Male	49 (44.1%)
Ethnicity	
Hispanic	9 (8.1%)
Race	
White	79 (71.2%)
Black	19 (17.1%)
Biracial	8 (7.2%)
Other	5 (4.5%)
Parent education level	
Less than high school or less	12 (10.8%)
High school diploma	7 (6.3%)
Some college courses	18 (16.2%)
Associate's degree	10 (9.0%)
Bachelor's degree	30 (27.0%)
Advanced degree	34 (30.6%)
BMI Percentile	78.59 (21.84)
Percent body fat	26.84 (11.60)
Dysregulated eating	1.97 (0.52)
Restrained eating	2.06 (0.87)
DERS	74.52 (17.37)
BIS-Brief	15.96 (3.66)
dYFAS-C 2.0	26.89 (8.89)
APU	1.83 (0.60)

Note: BMI—Body Mass Index; Dysregulated eating was measured with the external and emotional eating subscales of the Dutch Eating Behaviour Questionnaire (range 1–5); DERS—Difficulties in Emotion Regulation Scale (range: 36–180); BIS-Brief—Barratt Impulsiveness Scale, Brief version (range: 8–32); dYFAS-C 2.0—Dimensional Yale Food Addiction Scale for Children, 2.0 (range: 0–64); APU—Addictive Patterns of Use Scale (range: 1–5).

3.2. *Aim 1*

Demographic differences in APU were examined by gender, race/ethnicity, and parent education level. Girls (M = 2.05, SD = 0.49) reported greater APU than boys (M = 1.55, SD = 0.60; t (109) = −4.69, $p < 0.01$). No significant differences emerged by race/ethnicity and parent education level (p's > 0.05).

3.3. *Aim 2*

To investigate whether adolescents who report greater APU have greater emotion regulation difficulties, impulsivity, dysregulated eating, restrained eating, food addiction, and adiposity (as measured by BMI percentile and percent body fat), we conducted Spearman's Rho correlations. We found significant associations between APU and emotion dysregulation, dysregulated eating, restrained eating, food addiction and percent body fat (see Table 2). APU was not significantly associated with impulsivity, and was thus not included in the exploratory mediation analyses. APU did not significantly associate with BMI percentile.

Table 2. Associations of Addictive Phone Use (APU) with Emotion Regulation Difficulties (DERS), Impulsivity (BIS-Brief), Eating Behaviors, Food Addiction (dYFAS-C 2.0), Body mass index (BMI) Percentile, and Percent Body Fat (PBF).

Variables	1	2	3	4	5	6	7	8
1. APU	-							
2. DERS	0.29 **	-						
3. BIS-Brief	0.18 +	0.20 **	-					
4. Dysregulated eating	0.53 **	0.51 **	0.16 *	-				
5. Restrained eating	0.39 **	0.33 **	0.07	0.68 **	-			
6. dYFAS-C 2.0	0.49 **	0.35 **	0.07	0.56 **	0.39 **			
7. BMI percentile	0.08	0.10	0.00	0.25 **	0.43 **	0.32 **	-	
8. PBF	0.22 *	0.04	−0.04	0.27 **	0.37 **	0.40 **	0.76 **	-

Note: APU—Addictive Patterns of Use Scale; DERS—Difficulties in Emotion Regulation Scale; BIS-Brief—Barratt Impulsiveness Scale, Brief version; dYFAS-C 2.0—Dimensional Yale Food Addiction Scale for Children, 2.0; BMI—Body Mass Index; PBF—Percent Body Fat; **. $p < 0.01$; *. $p < 0.05$.; +. $p < 0.10$.

3.4. Aim 3

To explore whether emotion regulation difficulties mediated the associations between addictive phone use and maladaptive eating behaviors and adiposity, we used Hayes' (2017) PROCESS macro (Model 4). We found that emotion regulation difficulties mediated the association between APU and dysregulated eating (see Table 3), restrained eating (see Table 4), and food addiction (see Table 5).

Table 3. Emotion Regulation Difficulties (DERS) as a Mediator of the Relation Between Addictive Phone Use (APU) and Dysregulated Eating.

Model	*B*	*SE*	*t*	*p*, Cis	*F*	R^2
Model summary				0.00	*F* (3, 107) = 24.47	0.41
Direct effects						
APU	0.33	0.07	4.43	0.00		
DERS	0.01	0.00	4.480	0.00		
Sex	0.11	0.08	1.32	0.19		
Indirect effect						
DERS	0.10	0.03 [a]		(0.04, 0.17) [b]		
Completely Standardized Indirect Effect						
DERS	0.11	0.04 [a]		(0.05, 0.19) [b]		

Note: APU—Addictive Patterns of Use Scale; DERS—Difficulties in Emotion Regulation Scale. Estimates are unstandardized. [a] Bootstrap-derived estimate of standard error of indirect effect, 10,000 bootstrapped samples; [b] 95% lower and upper level confidence intervals.

Table 4. Emotion Regulation Difficulties (DERS) as a Mediator of the Relation Between Addictive Phone Use (APU) and Restrained Eating.

Model	*B*	*SE*	*t*	*p*, CIs	*F*	R^2
Model summary				0.00	*F* (3, 107) = 11.69	0.25
Direct effects						
APU	0.45	0.14	3.21	0.00		
DERS	0.01	0.00	3.05	0.00		
Sex	0.12	0.16	0.71	0.48		
Indirect effect						
DERS	0.12	0.05 [a]		(0.03, 0.24) [b]		
Completely Standardized Indirect Effect						
DERS	0.09	0.04 [a]		(0.02, 0.16) [b]		

Note: APU—Addictive Patterns of Use Scale; DERS—Difficulties in Emotion Regulation Scale. Estimates are unstandardized. [a] Bootstrap-derived estimate of standard error of indirect effect, 10,000 bootstrapped samples; [b] 95% lower and upper level confidence intervals.

Table 5. Emotion Regulation Difficulties (DERS) as a Mediator of the Relation Between Addictive Phone Use (APU) and Food Addiction.

Model	*B*	*SE*	*t*	*p*, CIs	*F*	R^2
Model summary				0.00	*F* (3, 86) = 11.25	0.28
Direct effects						
APU	3.97	1.55	2.57	0.01		
DERS	0.13	0.05	2.58	0.01		
Sex	3.29	1.80	1.83	0.07		
Indirect effect						
DERS	1.33	0.62 [a]		(0.18, 2.64) [b]		
Completely Standardized Indirect Effect						
DERS	0.09	0.04 [a]		(0.01, 0.18) [b]		

Note: APU—Addictive Patterns of Use Scale; DERS—Difficulties in Emotion Regulation Scale. Estimates are unstandardized. [a] Bootstrap-derived estimate of standard error of indirect effect, 10,000 bootstrapped samples; [b] 95% lower and upper level confidence intervals.

4. Discussion

A major aim of this study was to examine the physical health correlates of APU that are under-studied in the literature and that are major areas of public health concern in the United States (see Domoff, Borgen, Foley, & Maffett, 2019 [11] for a review). Specifically, we sought to investigate whether addictive phone use associated with objectively measured indicators of obesity (i.e., percent body fat and body mass index, BMI), as well as adolescents' eating behaviors which have consistently been linked to obesity risk [31]. Consistent with prior research on non-mobile media (e.g., TV, computer, gaming [14]), we similarly found that addictive phone use associates with various obesogenic risk factors, including dysregulated eating, food addiction and percent body fat. We, however, did not find an association between addictive phone use and BMI percentile. It is possible that percent body fat might be a more accurate measure of adiposity. BMI percentile scores may be biased for individuals with elevated lean muscle mass.

We also sought to explore whether emotion regulation difficulties mediated the association of addictive phone use with dysregulated eating, restrained eating, food addiction, and adiposity. We found that emotion regulation difficulties mediated the association between addictive phone use and dysregulated eating, restrained eating, and food addiction, but not adiposity. It is possible that emotion regulation difficulties may be an underlying or common factor for both maladaptive eating behaviors (e.g., dysregulated eating, food addiction) and excessive phone use. As has recently been suggested [32], overlap in the experience of multiple addictions (including behavioral addiction) may indicate an underlying phenotype for addiction proneness. Future research may seek to test out other common factors across addictions, as has been conducted specific to screen-based behavioral addictions (e.g., [24]). Though preliminary, these findings suggest that clinicians assisting youth with emotion regulation challenges should assess for the presence of co-occurring addictions, such as phone addiction and food addiction.

Consistent with prior research in countries outside of the US [9,33], we found that girls had higher rates of addictive phone use and no differences emerged by race/ethnicity or parent education level. Given the social features of several popular smartphone apps (e.g., social media, texting or communication apps), the higher utilization of social media by girls [1], and the salience of peer relations in girls during adolescence, it is understandable that they would be at heightened risk for excessive phone use and dysfunction related to phone use. Although prior research on access to mobile devices and amount of screen time differs across various demographic factors [1], we examined addictive phone use and not hours of smartphone use. When prior research has examined problematic smartphone use, similar findings have emerged in adolescents in other Western countries [9].

Limitations

There are limitations of the study that should be addressed in future research. First, our sample size was small; future research should seek to replicate our findings in a larger, more representative sample of adolescents. It is possible that, with a larger, more representative sample, impulsivity may significantly associate with addictive phone use, as has been found in research on young adults in the US [34]. We should also note that a larger sample size would be beneficial to conduct more sensitive analyses to understand how the associations may be moderated by demographic factors (e.g., race, ethnicity, gender). As has been found in prior research on problematic phone use (e.g., [9,33]), girls may be at greater risk for compulsive use. Additional research should consider gender and stage of development (early adolescent versus older adolescent/emerging adult) in future research. Additionally, the current cross-sectional study does not permit unambiguous conclusions regarding temporal precedence and the directions of effects. It is important to emphasize, however, that given this is the first study to examine the links between addictive phone use and obesity, and underlying mechanisms (i.e., emotion regulation) connecting the constructs, it would have been premature to carry out a longitudinal design as preliminary research was lacking. The current study has thus set the foundation for future research on physical health correlates of addictive phone use, which should utilize a longitudinal design, as some of the physical health outcomes (e.g., obesity) may not emerge until later in adolescence or early adulthood, and to demonstrate temporal precedence and direction of effects.

5. Conclusions

This study provides preliminary evidence demonstrating the physical health risks associated with addictive phone use in US adolescents. Further, we found that emotion regulation difficulties appear to be a mechanism through which youths' addictive phone use may associate with dysregulated eating, restrained eating, and food addiction. On the other hand, it may also be possible that youth with greater emotion regulation concerns are at heightened risk for multiple addictions (e.g., food addiction, addictive phone use). Future research should seek to replicate our findings in a larger, more diverse sample of adolescents in order to inform clinical recommendations and intervention targets.

Author Contributions: Conceptualization, S.E.D. and A.N.G.; methodology, S.E.D., S.Y., and A.N.G.; formal analysis, S.E.D., E.Q.S., and A.N.G.; resources, S.Y. and A.N.G.; data curation, S.E.D., E.Q.S., and A.N.G.; writing—original draft preparation, S.E.D., E.Q.S., and A.N.G.; writing—review and editing, S.E.D., E.Q.S., S.Y. and A.N.G.; supervision, S.E.D. and A.N.G.; project administration, A.N.G.; funding acquisition, S.Y. and A.N.G. All authors have read and agreed to the published version of the manuscript.

References

1. Rideout, V.; Robb, M. The Common Sense Census: Media Use By Tweens and Teens. *Common Sense Media* **2019**, 1–104. [CrossRef]
2. Rideout, V.; Robb, M.B. *Social Media, Social Life: Teens Reveal Their Experiences*; Common Sense Media: San Francisco, CA, USA, 2018. [CrossRef]
3. Common Sense Media. Common Sense and SurveyMonkey Poll Parents on YouTube and Technology Addiction. Available online: https://www.surveymonkey.com/newsroom/common-sense-and-surveymonkey-poll-parents-on-youtube-and-technology-addiction/ (accessed on 10 January 2020).
4. Domoff, S.E.; Foley, R.P.; Ferkel, R. Addictive Phone Use and Academic Performance in Adolescents. *Hum. Behav. Emerg. Technol.* **2019**. [CrossRef]
5. Domoff, S.E.; Harrison, K.; Gearhardt, A.N.; Gentile, D.A.; Lumeng, J.C.; Miller, A.L. Development and Validation of the Problematic Media Use Measure: A Parent Report Measure of Screen Media "Addiction" in Children. *Psychol. Pop. Media Cult.* **2019**, *8*, 2–11. [CrossRef]

6. van den Eijnden, R.J.J.M.; Lemmens, J.S.; Valkenburg, P.M. The Social Media Disorder Scale. *Comput. Hum. Behav.* **2016**, *64*, 478–487. [CrossRef]
7. American Psychiatric Association. *Diagnostic and Statistical Manual of Mental Disorders*, 5th ed.; American Psychiatric Association: Washington, DC, USA, 2013.
8. Yu, S.; Sussman, S. Does Smartphone Addiction Fall on a Continuum of Addictive Behaviors? *Int. J. Environ. Res. Public Health* **2020**, *19*, 422. [CrossRef]
9. López Fernández, O.; Losada López, J.; Honrubia Serrano, M. Predictors of Problematic Internet and Mobile Phone Usage in Adolescents. *Aloma Rev. Psicol. ciències l'educació i l'esport* **2015**, *33*, 49–58.
10. Robinson, T.N.; Banda, J.A.; Hale, L.; Lu, A.S.; Fleming-Milici, F.; Calvert, S.L.; Wartella, E. Screen Media Exposure and Obesity in Children and Adolescents. *Pediatrics* **2017**, *140* (Suppl. 2), S97–S101. [CrossRef]
11. Domoff, S.E.; Borgen, A.L.; Foley, R.P.; Maffett, A. Excessive Use of Mobile Devices and Children's Physical Health. *Hum. Behav. Emerg. Technol.* **2019**, *1*, 169–175. [CrossRef]
12. Carter, B.; Rees, P.; Hale, L.; Bhattacharjee, D.; Paradkar, M.S. Association Between Portable Screen-Based Media Device Access or Use and Sleep Outcomes: A Systematic Review and Meta-Analysis. *JAMA Pediatr.* **2016**, *170*, 1202–1208. [CrossRef]
13. Bradbury, K.M.; Turel, O.; Morrison, K.M. Electronic Device Use and Beverage Related Sugar and Caffeine Intake in US Adolescents. *PLoS ONE* **2019**. [CrossRef]
14. Kenney, E.L.; Gortmaker, S.L. United States Adolescents' Television, Computer, Videogame, Smartphone, and Tablet Use: Associations with Sugary Drinks, Sleep, Physical Activity, and Obesity. *J. Pediatr.* **2017**, *182*, 144–149. [CrossRef] [PubMed]
15. Wada, K.; Yamakawa, M.; Konishi, K.; Goto, Y.; Mizuta, F.; Koda, S.; Uji, T.; Tamura, T.; Nakamura, K.; Tsuji, M.; et al. Associations of Cell Phone Use and Screen Viewing with Overweight in Children. *Child. Obes.* **2019**, *15*, 417–425. [CrossRef] [PubMed]
16. Billieux, J.; Maurage, P.; Lopez-Fernandez, O.; Kuss, D.J.; Griffiths, M.D. Can Disordered Mobile Phone Use Be Considered a Behavioral Addiction? An Update on Current Evidence and a Comprehensive Model for Future Research. *Curr. Addict. Reports* **2015**, *2*, 156–162. [CrossRef]
17. Yıldız, M. Emotion Regulation Strategies as Predictors of Internet Addiction and Smartphone Addiction in Adolescents. *J. Educ. Sci. Psychol.* **2017**, *7*, 66–78.
18. Miller, A.L.; Gearhardt, A.N.; Fredericks, E.M.; Katz, B.; Shapiro, L.F.; Holden, K.; Kaciroti, N.; Gonzalez, R.; Hunter, C.; Lumeng, J.C. Targeting Self-Regulation to Promote Health Behaviors in Children. *Behav. Res. Ther.* **2018**, *101*, 71–81. [CrossRef]
19. Eirini, T.; Kamal, A.; Turvill, A.; Holler, R. Emotion Dysregulation and Loneliness as Predictors of Food Addiction. *J. Heal. Soc. Sci.* **2019**, *4*, 43–48. [CrossRef]
20. Odgers, C.L.; Jensen, M.R. Annual Research Review: Adolescent Mental Health in the Digital Age: Facts, Fears, and Future Directions. *J. Child Psychol. Psychiatry Allied Discip.* **2020**, *61*, 336–348. [CrossRef]
21. Hales, C.M.; Carroll, M.D.; Fryar, C.D.; Ogden, C.L. *Prevalence of Obesity Among Adults and Youth: United States, 2015–2016*; NCHS Data Brief; No 288; National center for Health Statistics: Hyattsville, MD, USA, 2017; pp. 2–7.
22. Eunice Kennedy Shriver National Institute of Child Health and Human Development, NIH, D. *NICHD Strategic Plan 2020*; Government Printing Office: Washington, DC, USA, 2019; pp. 1–44.
23. Gearhardt, A.N.; Yokum, S.; Harris, J.L.; Epstein, L.H.; Lumeng, J.C. Neural Response to Fast Food Commercials in Adolescents Predicts Intake. *Am. J. Clin. Nutr.* **2020**, *3*, 493–502. [CrossRef]
24. Gratz, K.L.; Roemer, L. Multidimensional Assessment of Emotion Regulation and Dysregulation: Development, Factor Structure, and Initial Validation of the Difficulties in Emotion Regulation Scale. *J. Psychopathol. Behav. Assess.* **2004**, *26*, 41–54. [CrossRef]
25. Mathias, C.W.; Stanford, M.S.; Liang, Y.; Goros, M.; Charles, N.E.; Sheftall, A.H.; Mullen, J.; Hill-Kapturczak, N.; Acheson, A.; Olvera, R.L.; et al. A Test of the Psychometric Characteristics of the BIS-Brief among Three Groups of Youth. *Psychol. Assess.* **2018**, *30*, 847–856. [CrossRef]
26. van Strien, T.; Frijters, J.E.R.; Bergers, G.P.A.; Defares, P.B. The Dutch Eating Behavior Questionnaire (DEBQ) for Assessment of Restrained, Emotional, and External Eating Behavior. *Int. J. Eat. Disord.* **1986**, *5*, 295–315. [CrossRef]
27. Schiestl, E.T.; Gearhardt, A.N. Preliminary Validation of the Yale Food Addiction Scale for Children 2.0: A Dimensional Approach to Scoring. *Eur. Eat. Disord. Rev.* **2018**, *26*, 605–614. [CrossRef] [PubMed]

28. Gearhardt, A.N.; Corbin, W.R.; Brownell, K.D. Development of the Yale Food Addiction Scale Version 2.0. *Psychol. Addict. Behav.* **2016**, *30*, 113–121. [CrossRef] [PubMed]
29. Centers for Disease Control and Prevention. BMI Percentile Calculator for Child and Teen. Available online: https://www.cdc.gov/healthyweight/bmi/calculator.html. (accessed on 8 August 2017).
30. Hayes, A.F. *Introduction to Mediation, Moderation, and Conditional Process Analysis, Second Edition: A Regression-Based Approach*, 2nd ed.; Little, T.D., Ed.; The Guilford Preess: New York, NY, USA, 2018.
31. Boutelle, K.N.; Braden, A.; Knatz-Peck, S.; Anderson, L.K.; Rhee, K.E. An Open Trial Targeting Emotional Eating among Adolescents with Overweight or Obesity. *Eat. Disord.* **2018**, *26*, 79–91. [CrossRef]
32. Mak, K.K.; Lai, C.M.; Watanabe, H.; Kim, D.I.; Bahar, N.; Ramos, M.; Young, K.S.; Ho, R.C.; Aum, N.R.; Cheng, C. Epidemiology of Internet Behaviors and Addiction among Adolescents in Six Asian Countries. *Cyberpsychol. Behav. Soc. Netw.* **2014**, *17*, 720–728. [CrossRef]
33. Lee, S.Y.; Lee, D.; Nam, C.R.; Kim, D.Y.; Park, S.; Kwon, J.G.; Kweon, Y.S.; Lee, Y.; Kim, D.J.; Choi, J.S. Distinct Patterns of Internet and Smartphone-Related Problems among Adolescents by Gender: Latent Class Analysis. *J. Behav. Addict.* **2018**, *7*, 454–465. [CrossRef]
34. Grant, J.E.; Lust, K.; Chamberlain, S.R. Problematic Smartphone Use Associated with Greater Alcohol Consumption, Mental Health Issues, Poorer Academic Performance, and Impulsivity. *J. Behav. Addict.* **2019**, *8*, 335–342. [CrossRef]

4

Assessing the Psychometric Properties of the Internet Addiction Test in Peruvian University Students

Arnold Alejandro Tafur-Mendoza [1], Julio César Acosta-Prado [2,3,*], Rodrigo Arturo Zárate-Torres [4] and Duván Emilio Ramírez-Ospina [3]

1 Research Center (CIUP), Universidad del Pacífico, Lima 15072, Peru; aa.tafurm@up.edu.pe
2 School of Business Science, Universidad del Pacífico, Lima 15072, Peru
3 School of Accounting, Economic and Business Sciences, Universidad de Manizales, Manizales 170001, Colombia; merca2@umanizales.edu.co
4 Colegio de Estudios Superiores de Administración, Bogota 111071, Colombia; rodrigo.zarate@cesa.edu.co
* Correspondence: jc.acostap@up.edu.pe

Abstract: The use of the Internet has been gradually and unstoppably gaining ground in all areas of life, from recreational activities to how social relations are established. However, the existence of clinical cases indicates that the addictive use of the Internet is a problem that seriously affects some people. Among the instruments that measure this construct, the Internet Addiction Test (IAT) stands out. However, instrumental studies of this test are scarce in Latin America. The present study sought to analyze the psychometric properties of the IAT in a sample of 227 Peruvian undergraduate university students. Confirmatory factor analysis was used to provide validity evidence based on the internal structure, and evidence based on the relationship with other variables was also provided. Reliability was estimated through the ordinal alpha coefficient. The results indicated that the IAT adequately fits a bifactor model (with two specific factors, time/control and stress/compensate), obtaining good levels of reliability. Additionally, the IAT scores correlate significantly with the average number of hours per day on the internet and social skills. The results lead to the conclusion that the scores in the IAT have evidence of validity and reliability for its use.

Keywords: internet addiction test; university students; Peruvian sample; psychometric properties

---

1. Introduction

In the framework of a society in which both communication and the free flow of information are closely related to the development of the network, it is necessary to know to what extent reality and the virtual sphere intermingle. From the lowering of costs, the multiplicity of ways of accessing the network, and the advent of social networks, the Internet grows exponentially every day [1]. As studies in Sweden [2] and Spain [3] seem to indicate, the fierce proliferation of the network as a means of communication has brought negative consequences (cyberbullying, problematic Internet use, sexting, nomophobia, etc.) that have a stronger impact on the young population, having identified a series of problems among which stand out the addiction to this environment and that affect above all the social sphere of the individual.

However, the use of the Internet has expanded gradually and unstoppably in all areas of life [4]. The existence of clinical cases indicates that maladaptive use of the Internet is an existing problem that seriously affects some people, mainly those with special emotional needs and young people and adolescents [5]. The use or abuse of the Internet arises from disciplines, such as psychology or psychiatry [6]. In this sense, it is not surprising that the term Internet addiction was used for the first time by the psychiatrist Ivan Golberg in 1995 [7]. The literature on problematic use of the Internet shows a very varied terminology to describe the problems derived from the use of the Internet, among which are: Computer addiction, excessive use of the Internet, pathological use of the Internet, Internet dependence, compulsive use of the Internet, disorder by impulsive use, and compulsive use of the Internet or Internet addiction [8,9].

Kimberly Young [10], after reviewing a series of investigations, which indicated that some online users became addicted to the Internet in the same way that others became addicted to drugs, alcohol, or gambling, suggests the need to empirically investigate the concept of addictive use of the Internet. In addition to the review, the study sought to identify whether excessive use of the Internet can be considered addictive and to know the magnitude of the problems created by these abuses. However, Young's approaches to Internet addiction sparked a controversial debate among doctors and academics at the time [11].

On the other hand, there are proposals [12] that suggested that Internet addiction is a disorder that should have been considered in the fifth edition of the Diagnostic and Statistical Manual of Mental Disorders (DSM-V) since it is an impulsive-compulsive spectrum disorder [13], which consists of the use of computers. However, these recommendations or proposals were not reflected in the DSM-V, since the term Internet addiction does not appear in the manual [14]. Among the diagnoses referenced in the DSM-V, Internet gaming disorder (IGD) is strongly related to the pathological nature of Internet use. The excessive use of the Internet not only involves the reproduction of online games (for example, it also implies the excessive use of social networks, such as Facebook or Twitter). Therefore, IGD is within the Internet addiction. Thus, research on other excessive uses of the Internet should follow guidelines analogous to those suggested with IGD [14].

Among the theoretical models proposed to understand Internet addiction, Davis' cognitive-behavioral model [15] is the one that has had the most development and has been empirically tested in different contexts [16]. Two parts are distinguished in this model, one specific and the other general. The first involves excessive use of an aspect of the internet, while generalized use encompasses multiple excessive uses of the Internet [15]. Generalized use is associated with social support and social service uses of the Internet, where maladaptive cognitions are a strong predictor of this component and to a lesser extent of specific use [17]. Under this model, symptoms of Internet addiction are primarily affective or behavioral and are usually preceded or caused by cognitive symptoms, mediated by specific and general pathological Internet use [15,16]. The value of the cognitive-behavioral model lies in that it contemplates a continuum of severity regarding Internet use, allowing a better understanding by mental health specialists of the way and degree to which the excessive use of the internet can affect the lives of people [18].

To measure Internet addiction, various tests have been developed, which, mainly, are based on the diagnosis of this disorder, including the Problematic Internet Use Questionnaire (PIUQ) [19], the Compulsive Internet Use Scale (CIUS) [20], Internet-Related Problem Scale [21], and the Internet-Related Experiences Questionnaire (IREQ) [22]. The PIUQ, made up of 18 items, was built for the general population and measures problems related to Internet use through three subscales: Obsession, neglect, and control disorder. The CUIS is made up of 14 items that measure the severity of compulsive Internet use. The Internet-Related Problem Scale has 20 items that address DSM-IV symptoms for substance abuse: Tolerance, escape from other problems, reduced activities, loss of control, negative effects, withdrawal, craving, and introversion. The IREQ was developed in middle-school students and is made up of 10 items that measure possible Internet addiction based on intrapersonal and interpersonal experiences. However, the test that has had the most development and that has been adapted to various contexts is the Internet Addiction Test (IAT) [23]. Thus, the objective of this study was to analyze the psychometric properties of the IAT in a sample of Peruvian undergraduate university students.

2. Literature Review

For this study, in a search conducted in Scopus and Web of Science (WoS) on studies of the psychometric properties of the IAT, 46 studies were found (April 2020). Table 1 presents a summary of 39 of the 46 studies found, which were those that analyzed the internal structure of the IAT, an aspect that does not have a consensus in all the studies carried out. Most of the studies were carried out in Europe and Asia; in North America, only one study was found in the United States and another in Canada, while, in Latin America, the IAT has been studied in Colombia and Chile. Regarding the populations where these studies have been carried out, the majority were in university students, probably due to the accessibility of the sample and that it is the age group that spends the most time on the Internet (young people between 18 and 25 years old).

Table 1. Previous studies on psychometric properties of the Internet Addiction Test (IAT).

Study	Country	Sample Size	Factors	Data Analysis	Items	Reliability (α)
1. Widyanto et al. (2004) [24]	-	86	6	PCA	20	>0.50 [c]
2. Ngai (2007) [25]	Hong Kong	988	4	PCA	20	>0.60 [c]
3. Chang et al. (2008) [26]	Hong Kong	410	3	PCA, CFA [a]	20	>0.80 [d]
4. Khazaal et al. (2008) [27]	France	246	1	EFA, CFA	20	0.93
5. Widyanto et al. (2011) [28]	-	225	3	PCA	20	-
6. Panayides et al. (2012) [29]	Cyprus	604	1	PCA	20	0.89
7. Jelenchick et al. (2012) [30]	United States	215	2	EFA	20	>0.80 [c]
8. Barke et al. (2012) [31]	Germany	841	2	PCA, CFA	20	0.89
9. Puerta-Cortés et al. (2012) [32]	Colombia	1117	3	PCA	20	0.89
10. Faraci et al. (2013) [33]	Italy	485	1, 2	EFA, CFA	20, 18	>0.70 [c]
11. Watters et al. (2013) [34]	Canada	1948	2	CFA [b]	20	0.93
12. Pawlikowski et al. (2013) [35]	Germany	1049	2	PCA, CFA	11	>0.80 [c]
13. Lee et al. (2013) [36]	Korea	279	4	PCA	20	0.91
14. Hawi (2013) [37]	Lebanon	817	1	PCA, CFA	20	0.92
15. Lai et al. (2013) [38]	Hong Kong	844	3	CFA [a]	20	0.93
16. Pontes et al. (2014) [39]	Portugal	593	1	CFA	20	0.90
17. Karim et al. (2014) [40]	Bangladesh	177	4	PCA	18	0.89
18. Tsimtsiou et al. (2014) [41]	Greece	151	3	EFA	20	0.91
19. Chong et al. (2015) [42]	Malaysia	162	5	PCA	20	0.91
20. Fernández-Villa et al. (2015) [43]	Spain	963	2	EFA, CFA	19	0.91
21. Lu et al. (2015) [44]	Malaysia	104	6	EFA	20	0.93 [e]
22. Dhir et al. (2015) [45]	India	1914	1	EFA, CFA	20	0.88
23. Lai et al. (2015) [46]	Hong Kong, Japan and Malaysia	2535	3	CFA	20	-
24. Fioravanti et al. (2015) [47]	Italy	840	2	EFA, CFA	20	>0.80 [c]
25. Hawi (2015) [48]	Poland	1245	2	PCA, CFA	20	0.90
26. Kaya (2016) [49]	Turkey	990	4	EFA, CFA	20	0.92
27. Servidio (2017) [50]	Italy	659	2	PCA, CFA	18	0.89
28. Boysan et al. (2017) [51]	Turkey	455	1	PCA, CFA	20	0.93
29. Samaha et al. (2018) [52]	Lebanon	256	4	EFA, CFA	19	0.91
30. Waqas et al. (2018) [53]	Pakistan	522	1	EFA, CFA	20	0.90
31. Neelapaijit et al. (2018) [54]	Thailand	324	3	EFA, CFA	20	0.89
32. Tsermentseli et al. (2018) [55]	Greece	725	3	EFA, CFA [b]	19	>0.70 [f]
33. Hernández et al. (2018) [56]	Chile	425	2	CFA	10	0.85
34. Černja et al. (2019) [57]	Croatia	352	3	PCA, CFA	20	0.91
35. Tudorel et al. (2019) [58]	Romania	421	2	EFA, CFA	20	0.86
36. Ndasauka et al. (2019) [59]	Pakistan	506	4	EFA	20	0.88
37. Yaffe et al. (2019) [60]	Israel	180	2	PCA, CFA	18	>0.70 [c]
38. Talwar et al. (2019) [61]	Malaysia	307	3	PCA, CFA	19	>0.70 [c]
39. Lu et al. (2019) [62]	Malaysia	1120	4	EFA, CFA	17	-

Note. [a] Hierarchical model; [b] Bifactor model; [c] α coefficients of the factors; [d] Construct reliability; [e] Rasch model (person reliability); [f] ω coefficients of the factors; PCA = Principal Component Analysis; EFA = Exploratory Factor Analysis; CFA = Confirmatory Factor Analysis.

The reliability of the IAT has usually been estimated through the alpha coefficient, obtaining, in most cases, acceptable values above 0.70, and even exceeding 0.90. However, most of these studies have not considered the assumptions that this coefficient has, such as the one-dimensionality of the data, that the measurement model is tau-equivalent, and that there are no correlated errors [63]. Violation of any of these assumptions would distort the values reported in these studies. Additionally, there is no consideration of the ordinality of the items, which must be considered when working with Likert-type scales [64]. A meta-analysis of the internal consistency of the IAT (reliability generalization) indicates a combined alpha of 0.90 for samples of university students [65].

Regarding the internal structure of the IAT, the literature shows factorial models with one to six factors. Although, the diversity of models increases, because two studies may have the same number of factors, but they differ in the number of items used (not all studies end their analyses with the original 20 items but eliminate some of them because they do not fit their proposed model), in the addition of correlated errors (in many cases to improve the adjustment indices in the confirmatory factor analysis, without taking into account the substantive justification of the correlated errors [66]) or in the distribution of the items by the factor (two models can coincide in the number of factors and items, but the grouping of the items is different). This large number of models does not allow for a uniform IAT structure to be available, and for studies seeking to study this aspect in a particular sample, they have to resort to exploratory techniques or to test a large number of existing models.

An aspect linked to the above is the analysis technique used to find the factor structure in these studies. Almost half of the studies reported in Table 1 indicate that the principal component analysis (PCA) has been performed as the first or only technique, which is not suitable for psychological constructs, since it is a variable reduction technique; therefore, it seeks to explain the greater proportion of explained variance, considering both the variance shared by the items and the error variance. On the contrary, the factor analysis only considers the extraction of the factors the variance that the items share among themselves [67]. The use of the PCA could lead to obtaining structures that do not fit the data, especially since the measurement nature of the data is not considered.

In Peru, only one study of the psychometric properties of IAT [68] in middle-school students between the ages of 13 and 19 years was found. Item 1 was removed from the scale because it presented a low discriminatory capacity; therefore, this version had 19 items. Reliability was estimated through the alpha coefficient, obtaining a value of 0.870. On the other hand, the internal structure was evaluated by PCA, finding a factorial solution of four components. This structure was corroborated in the same sample through confirmatory factor analysis (CFA). It is important to note that the use of middle-school students and university students is different. University students use the Internet primarily for information search; also, they spend more time online and have a wider range of Internet uses than middle-school students [69].

Another source of validity evidence that has been explored in these background studies is evidence based on the relationship with other variables, specifically convergent evidence, where the hours of daily Internet use was used as a measure, in addition to the IAT [38,41,45,50]. In these studies, correlation coefficients between 0.29 and 0.48 were found. Additionally, Internet use has an impact on a person's social life, and studies have shown that Internet addiction is negatively related to social skills [70–72].

Considering all the above, the IAT is one of the most used instruments for measuring Internet addiction and that, in Peru, it has only worked with middle-school students in the adolescence stage but not in other samples, such as university students, which is precisely in this group where most adaptations have been made in other countries. Furthermore, the statistical procedures used in previous studies may be questionable and, in some cases, inadequate. Thus, the IAT does not have a version for Peruvian university students, so its psychometric properties are not known in this population and the extrapolation of results in other contexts would not be appropriate, since validity and reliability are not inherent in a test but correspond to the specific interpretations and uses of the scores obtained in a test [73]. Therefore, the objective of this study was to analyze the psychometric properties of the IAT in a sample of Peruvian undergraduate university students.

3. Materials and Methods

3.1. Design

According to the classification system of research designs in psychology [74], the objective of the study corresponds to an instrumental investigation, since the psychometric properties of a psychological instrument are analyzed in a specific sample. For the development of the study, various standards, guidelines, good practices, and recommendations were followed in instrumental studies in the behavioral and health sciences [73,75].

3.2. *Participants*

The selection of the participants was carried out through an intentional non-probability sampling [76], where the individuals in the sample were directly and selectively chosen, seeking to obtain similar proportions in each of the categories of the variables sex, year of study, and academic discipline. Regarding the sample size, a priori statistical power analysis was performed to determine the minimum recommended sample size. Statistical power is the ability of a statistical test (for example, U Mann–Whitney or H Kruskal–Wallis) to reject a null hypothesis when it is false; in other words, it is the probability of not committing the type II error [77]. The input parameters for this analysis were based on a simple two-tailed correlational model (similar to the one that will be carried out in the collection of validity evidence based on the relationship with other variables), the significance level (α) being 0.05, the expected effect size equal to 0.20 (recommended minimum value representing practical significance in social science data [78]), and an expected statistical power of 0.80 (recommended minimum in behavioral science [79]). The recommended minimum sample size was 191 (Figure 1).

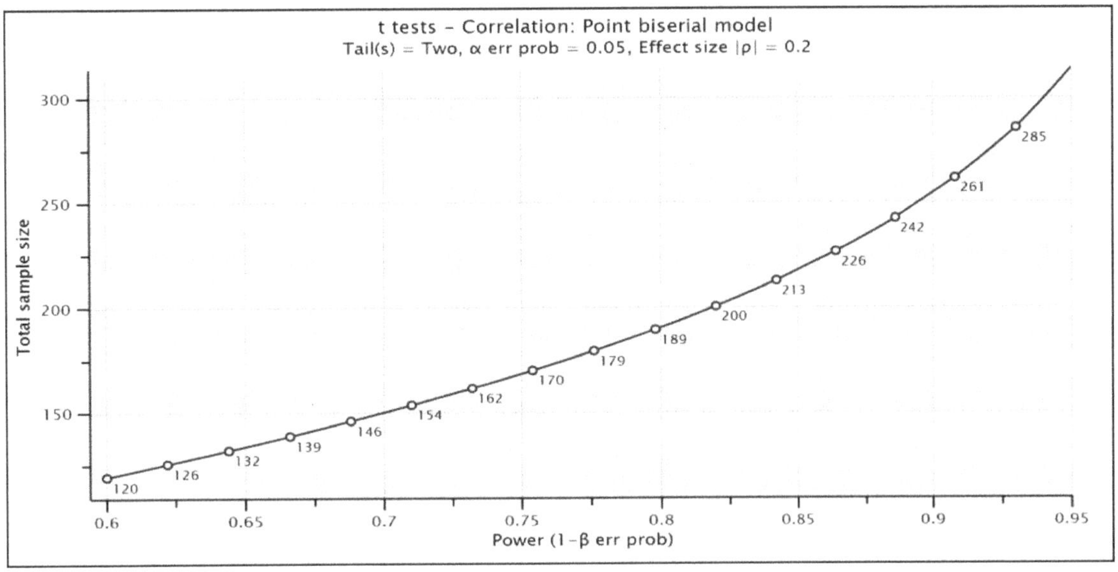

Figure 1. A priori statistical power analysis to determine the minimum recommended sample size.

The final sample was made up of 227 Peruvian undergraduate university students from a public university located in Metropolitan Lima (Peru). The ages of the participants were between 18 and 40 years (M = 20.81, SD = 2.92). The highest proportion of students were females (57.30%), in their second year of studies (30.00%), and belonged to professional careers in the engineering area (19.80%). Table 2 presents a more detailed description of the sample characteristics.

Table 2. Sociodemographic characteristics of participants (n = 227).

Characteristic	n	%
Gender		
Male	97	42.70
Female	130	57.30
Year of study		
First	24	10.60
Second	68	30.00
Third	63	27.80
Fourth	42	18.50
Fifth	30	13.20
Academic discipline		
Health Sciences	41	18.10
Humanities	30	13.20
Social Sciences	27	11.90
Basic sciences	43	18.90
Engineering	45	19.80
Economic-Business	41	18.10

3.3. *Instruments*

3.3.1. IAT—Internet Addiction Test

The Spanish version of the IAT was used (Appendix A), adapted to a sample of Colombian university students [32]. The IAT is made up of 20 items, all in a positive sense, on a five-point Likert-type scale (1 = rarely; 2 = occasionally; 3 = frequently; 4 = usually; 5 = always), the minimum score being 20 and the maximum score 100, where the student was asked to choose the alternative that best suits their reality. The IAT items were reviewed by the authors of this study, pointing out that it was not necessary to adjust their wording. To corroborate this assumption, a pilot study was carried out with 10 university students, who indicated that they had no problems in understanding the items.

In the adaptation study, the total scale had a good level of reliability (α = 0.89). Likewise, through an analysis of the main components, they found an internal structure of three factors (consequences for the use of the Internet, cognitive-emotional dimension, and time control), which together had an explained variance of 47.80%, and correlated positively with the number of hours of daily Internet access, although the magnitudes were low [32].

For the application of this study, in addition to the IAT, a sociodemographic and Internet usage file was added to collect information on the career that the participants studied, as well as the year of studies they were studying, age, gender, and the average daily hours spent on the Internet.

3.3.2. EHS—Social Skills Scale

The Social Skills Scale, developed by Gismero [80], is made up of 33 items. Five items are written in the direct sense, while 28 items are in an inverse sense, seeking to detect the lack of assertion or deficit in social skills. The original instrument is composed of six factors: (1) Self-expression in social situations, eight items; (2) defense of one's rights as a consumer, five items; (3) expression of anger or disagreement, four items; (4) assertiveness, six items; (5) making requests, five items; and (6) starting interactions with the opposite sex, five items. Each item is answered using a four-point response format (A = I do not identify myself at all; B = Rather it does not have to do with me, even if it ever happens to me; C = It describes me approximately, although I do not always act or feel like this; and D = Strongly agree, and I would feel or act like this in most cases). A higher global score indicates that the person has a higher level of social skills and better insertion in various contexts or situations.

This instrument has been studied in various countries, presenting adequate psychometric properties, good levels of reliability, adequate adjustment to the six-factor structure, and discriminant evidence [81]. In the present study, the scores on the items showed good internal consistency at the global level ($\omega = 0.890$). Likewise, in the factors, the omega coefficient (ω) varied from 0.500 to 0.748.

3.4. Procedure

The data collection process began with the request of permits, both to the directors of the schools of each academic discipline and the teachers in charge of some courses for the application of the instrument in classrooms. Before the application of the IAT, the students were given an informed consent form that contained the objective of the evaluation and where they were guaranteed the confidentiality and anonymity of their answers, as well as the possibility of withdrawing from their participation at any time of the evaluation without consequence. Only those students who voluntarily signed the informed consent participated in the study.

The application was collective, with an average duration of 15 min. Data collection lasted approximately five weeks. At the end of each evaluation, the examiners reviewed the application protocols to verify that there are no unanswered items or items with more than one marked answer option. If one or both situations described occurred, the evaluated person was asked to correct and provide their definitive answer. After data collection, each evaluation protocol was coded for the elaboration of the database in a Microsoft Excel 2016 spreadsheet.

During the evaluation process, the ethical guidelines for working with humans outlined in the code of ethics of the American Psychological Association (APA) were followed. Additionally, the ethical principles of the Declaration of Helsinki were respected, including its recent updates and regulations for research on human beings.

3.5. Data Analysis

The statistical analysis was divided into four stages: (1) Item analysis; (2) validity evidence based on the internal structure of the test through CFA; (3) validity evidence based on the relationship with other variables from the convergent evidence; and (4) reliability analysis using the internal consistency method.

The descriptive analysis of the items was performed using the mean and standard deviation, as measures of central tendency and dispersion, respectively. As descriptive measures of the distribution of the items, the skewness and kurtosis coefficients were used, where values between −2.00 and 2.00 indicate that the items follow a normal distribution [82]. Likewise, item discrimination was estimated through the item-rest polyserial correlation, which considers the ordinality of the items, considering values above 0.30 as adequate [83]. Finally, possible floor and ceiling effects in the items were analyzed, that is, to identify the proportion of participants who chose the lowest alternative (floor effect) and the highest (ceiling effect), taking as acceptable effects those that were between 1% and 15% [84].

The CFA was carried out using the 23 models presented in Table 1, considering only those models made up of the 20 original items and whose factors had at least three items. The estimation method used was the weighted least squares with mean and variance adjusted (WLSMV), appropriate for observable ordinal variables and that performs well against slightly non-normal underlying distributions [85]. The WLSMV involves the use of the diagonal weighted least squares (DWLS) estimator with robust standard errors and a statistical test with adjusted mean and variance (using a scale-shifted approach). To assess the level of adequacy of the models, the following fit indices were used [86,87]: $SS\chi^2/df < 2.00$, root mean square error of approximation (RMSEA) < 0.08, comparative fit index (CFI) > 0.90, Tucker–Lewis index (TLI) > 0.90, standardized root mean square residual (SRMR) < 0.08, and weighted root mean square residual (WRMR) < 1.00.

The convergent evidence involved correlating the scores obtained in the IAT with another measure that seeks to evaluate the same construct or other construct with which it is expected is correlated; in this case, these measures were the average of daily hours that the study participants spent on the Internet and a social skills scale. Before selecting the correlation statistic to be used, the presence of outliers in these two variables with which the IAT scores were correlated was examined. Univariate analysis of outliers was visually inspected through boxplots for each variable (including the six dimensions of the social skills scale). A few outliers were found in two factors of the social skills scale and in the average of daily hours that the study participants spent on the Internet. Therefore, a robust statistic was chosen for the correlation between variables, the skipped correlation coefficient. This coefficient is robust to slight changes in any distribution and has the advantage of treating outliers in a way that considers the general structure of a data set [88]. As a measure of the effect size, the coefficient of determination was used, considering its interpretation values of 0.04, 0.25, and 0.64 as the minimum, moderate, and strong effect, respectively [78].

The internal consistency of the items was estimated using the ordinal alpha coefficient [89] since it works with the inter-item polychoric correlation matrix. Values above 0.70 were considered acceptable [90].

A priori statistical power analysis to determine the minimum sample size required for the study was performed using the G*Power 3.1.9.7 software [91]. The other analyses were performed in the R software version 4.0.2 (R Foundation for Statistical Computing, Vienna, Austria, 2016) [92], using the following packages: pacman 0.5.1 [93], readxl 1.3.1 [94], tidyverse 1.3.0 [95], psych 1.9.12.31 [96], lavaan 0.6–6 [97], BifactorIndicesCalculator 0.2.0 [98], semTools 0.5–2.925 [99], and WRS 0.36 [100].

4. Results

4.1. Item Analysis

Table 3 presents the results of the item analysis. The means of the items were between 1.352 (item 20) and 3.084 (items 1 and 7), indicating that the participants' responses were concentrated on the lowest alternatives (rarely, occasionally, and frequently). Likewise, the standard deviation fluctuated between 0.658 (item 20) and 1.211 (item 7), showing low variability in the data. Regarding the skewness and kurtosis measures, most of the items presented values between −2.00 and 2.00. However, items 9, 15, 19, and 20 showed an excess of kurtosis, and these last two also indicated an excess of skewness. Therefore, these four items showed a deviation from a normal distribution.

Table 3. Item analysis for the Internet Addiction Test (IAT).

Item	M	SD	Sk	Ku	Item-Rest Correlation	Floor (%)	Ceiling (%)
Item 1	3.084	1.200	0.115	−0.989	0.378	8	16
Item 2	2.066	0.902	0.734	0.375	0.570	28	1
Item 3	1.885	1.146	1.118	0.203	0.381	53	4
Item 4	1.670	0.826	1.329	1.882	0.381	51	1
Item 5	1.925	1.021	1.092	0.775	0.560	42	3
Item 6	1.828	0.908	1.013	0.437	0.532	43	0
Item 7	3.084	1.211	0.168	−1.016	0.371	7	17
Item 8	1.797	0.889	0.968	0.163	0.591	45	0
Item 9	1.656	0.860	1.506	2.404	0.471	53	1
Item 10	1.753	0.913	1.024	0.245	0.465	51	0
Item 11	1.855	0.898	0.798	−0.072	0.496	43	0
Item 12	1.626	0.900	1.489	1.868	0.451	59	1
Item 13	1.771	0.960	1.275	1.200	0.527	50	2
Item 14	1.877	1.006	1.053	0.442	0.515	45	2
Item 15	1.502	0.772	1.571	2.251	0.684	64	0
Item 16	2.286	1.094	0.833	0.149	0.443	24	6
Item 17	2.093	1.066	0.906	0.138	0.558	33	3
Item 18	1.736	1.000	1.415	1.409	0.538	54	2
Item 19	1.414	0.796	2.275	5.499	0.626	72	1
Item 20	1.352	0.658	2.176	5.640	0.512	73	0

Note. M = Mean; SD = Standard Deviation; Sk = Skewness; Ku = Kurtosis.

Concerning the item-rest polyserial correlation, all the items were above the threshold of 0.30, ranging from 0.371 (item 7) to 0.684 (item 15), indicating good discrimination by the IAT items. On the other hand, in the analysis of the response options, a soil effect was found in all the items, except for items 1 and 7. However, regarding the ceiling effect, most of the items had acceptable values (between 1% and 15%). These effects reflect the tendency of the participants to choose the lowest response options, being the most prominent in items 19 and 20, where more than 70% of the sample chose the response option "rarely". On the contrary, the "always" alternative was selected in a low percentage, even reaching 0% in some items (items 6, 8, 10, 11, 15, and 20).

4.2. *Validity Evidence Based on the Internal Structure*

The models tested were taken from Table 1. However, of the 39 studies presented, the studies selected were those where the factor structure was configured by all the items of the IAT (20 items) and that the proposed factors have at least three items in its composition, which is recommended to achieve an adequate representation of a factor [86]. Twenty-four studies met the two requirements and their factor models were tested. Four studies had the same unifactorial structure [29,45,51,53]. Whereas, five models [26,32,38,46,59] presented problems in the analysis: Covariance matrix of latent variables was not positive definite [59], some estimated latent variable variances were negative [26,38,46], or the model did not converge [32].

Table 4 presents the fit indices of the models tested. The bifactor model of Watters et al. (2013) [34] was the one that obtained the best results ($SS\chi^2/df < 2.00$, RMSEA < 0.08, CFI > 0.90, TLI > 0.90, SRMR < 0.08, and WRMR < 1.00). Figure 2 shows the factor structure of the bifactor model, made up of a general factor that measures Internet addiction through 20 items and two specific factors, time/control and stress/compensate, the first factor consisting of five items (1, 2, 7, 16, and 17) and the second factor of 11 items (3, 4, 9, 10, 11, 12, 13, 15, 18, 19, and 20). Figure 2 also presents the factor loadings of the items in the general factor and the corresponding specific factors.

Table 4. Confirmatory factor analysis for the IAT.

Model	$SS\chi^2$	*df*	$SS\chi^2/df$	RMSEA (90% CI)	CFI	TLI	SRMR	WRMR
1. One-factor [29,45,51,53]	387.285	161	2.405	0.079 (0.069; 0.089)	0.890	0.871	0.092	1.168
2. Khazaal et al. (2008) [27]	449.357	169	2.659	0.086 (0.076; 0.095)	0.864	0.847	0.101	1.288
3. Widyanto et al. (2011) [28]	423.779	167	2.358	0.082 (0.073; 0.092)	0.876	0.859	0.095	1.244
4. Jelenchick et al. (2012) [30]	393.896	169	2.331	0.077 (0.067; 0.087)	0.891	0.878	0.092	1.189
5. Barke et al. (2012) [31]	382.215	167	2.289	0.076 (0.066; 0.086)	0.896	0.881	0.091	1.163
6. Watters et al. (2013) [34]	285.741	154	1.855	0.062 (0.050; 0.073)	0.936	0.921	0.073	0.939
7. Hawi (2013) [37]	462.205	166	2.784	0.089 (0.079; 0.099)	0.857	0.836	0.102	1.311
8. Lee et al. (2013) [36]	340.237	164	2.075	0.069 (0.059; 0.079)	0.915	0.901	0.084	1.086
9. Pontes et al. (2014) [39]	437.216	168	2.602	0.084 (0.075; 0.094)	0.870	0.853	0.099	1.267
10. Tsimtsiou et al. (2014) [41]	375.281	167	2.247	0.074 (0.064; 0.084)	0.899	0.885	0.090	1.156
11. Fioravanti et al. (2015) [47]	390.065	165	2.364	0.078 (0.068; 0.088)	0.891	0.875	0.093	1.182
12. Hawi (2015) [48]	342.871	169	2.029	0.067 (0.057; 0.078)	0.916	0.905	0.085	1.097
13. Dhir et al. (2015) [45]	437.235	166	2.634	0.085 (0.075; 0.095)	0.869	0.850	0.099	1.266
14. Waqas et al. (2018) [53]	475.709	170	2.798	0.089 (0.080; 0.099)	0.852	0.835	0.104	1.336
15. Tudorel et al. (2019) [58]	388.449	167	2.326	0.077 (0.067; 0.087)	0.893	0.878	0.092	1.176
16. Černja et al. (2019) [57]	399.818	167	2.394	0.079 (0.069; 0.088)	0.887	0.872	0.093	1.200

Note. RMSEA = Root Mean Square Error of Approximation; CI = Confidence Interval; CFI = Comparative Fit Index; TLI = Tucker–Lewis Index; SRMR = Standardized Root Mean Square Residual; WRMR = Weighted Root Mean Square Residual.

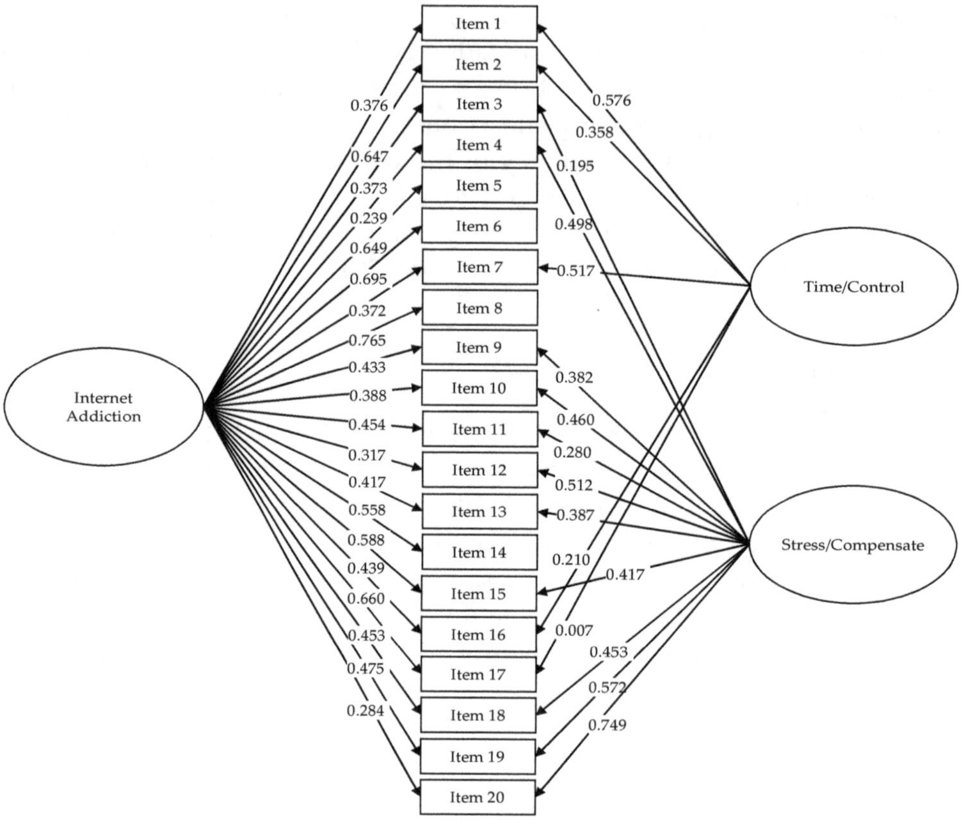

Figure 2. Factorial structure of the bifactor model.

Additionally, complementary statistical indices were calculated that allowed assessment of the robustness of the general factor, as well as the contribution of specific factors [101]. The omega hierarchical was used for the general factor and the specific factors, expecting values above 0.70 (ω_H) for the first and greater than 0.30 (ω_{HS}) for the seconds. The results indicate a value of 0.704 for the general factor, 0.234 for time/control, and 0.478 for stress/compensate. The H coefficient was also calculated, considering values greater than 0.70 to be adequate. The general factor obtained a coefficient of 0.888: For the time/control factor it was 0.785 while, for the stress/compensate factor, the H coefficient was equal to 0.513.

The explained common variance (ECV) for the general factor was 0.612, while the factors (ECV of a specific factor concerning itself) showed an ECV of 0.368 for time/control and 0.562 for stress/compensate. On the other hand, the proportion of uncontaminated correlations (PUCs) was equal to 0.658. At the item level, the ECV index (I-ECV) was between 0.126 and 1.000. Thus, the results allow the use of this bifactor model [102].

4.3. Validity Evidence Based on Relations to Other Variables

The convergent evidence was collected from the correlation between the two specific factors of IAT and the general factor with the average hours per day that study participants spent on the Internet and social skills. The minimum time of hours per day was less than one hour and the maximum 12 h (M = 3.368, SD = 2.277). The skipped correlation coefficients between the average daily hours on the Internet with Internet addiction (and time/control factor) were statistically significant (Table 5). Likewise, the effect size (skipped correlation coefficient squared) in the time/control factor and total Internet addiction was greater than 0.04, indicating a recommended minimum effect size that represents practical significance in social science data [78]. Regarding social skills, the correlations between Internet addiction (and its two factors) with social skills (and the defense of rights factor) were statistically significant (Table 5). Similar results were obtained for correlations between Internet addiction (and stress/compensate factor) with self-expression, disagreement, and assertiveness (Table 5). The size of the effect between Internet addiction and social skills presented practical significance. These findings provide convergent evidence to the IAT.

Table 5. Interfactorial matrix, convergent evidence, and reliability of the IAT.

Variable	Time/Control	Stress/Compensate	Internet Addiction
1. Time/Control	-		
2. Stress/Compensate	0.400 ***	-	
3. Internet Addiction	0.804 ***	0.861 ***	-
4. Self-Expression	−0.117	−0.197 **	−0.331 ***
5. Defense of rights	−0.185 **	−0.189 **	−0.350 ***
6. Disagreement	−0.055	−0.205 **	−0.311 ***
7. Assertiveness	−0.054	−0.189 **	−0.196 **
8. Making requests	0.019	−0.029	−0.118
9. Starting interactions	−0.127	0.058	−0.118
10. Social Skills	−0.137 *	−0.186 **	−0.257 ***
11. Hours on the Internet	0.397 ***	0.112	0.337 ***
12. Ordinal Alpha	0.727	0.856	0.888

Note. * $p < 0.05$; ** $p < 0.01$; *** $p < 0.001$.

On the other hand, the correlation between the specific factors of the IAT presented a minimum effect size (skipped correlation coefficient squared > 0.04). For the correlation between time/control and stress/compensate with Internet addiction, the effect size was strong (skipped correlation coefficient squared > 0.64). In all three cases, the correlations were statistically significant (Table 5).

4.4. Reliability

Reliability was evaluated by the internal consistency method, using for this purpose the ordinal alpha coefficient, which considers the ordinal nature of the items for its calculation. The specific factors and the general factor obtained satisfactory values, above 0.70 (Table 5). Likewise, the coefficients obtained were not remarkably high (0.90 or higher), indicating that the IAT, in the sample studied, does not include redundant items [103].

5. Discussion

The present study analyzed the psychometric properties of the IAT in a sample of Peruvian university students. The 20 items that make up the instrument presented adequate levels of discrimination, although the analysis of the response options indicated the presence of a floor effect in 18 items. Likewise, the levels of skewness and kurtosis were acceptable in most of the items. Regarding the validity evidence based on the internal structure, different models were tested through CFA, being the bifactor model with two specific factors (time/control and stress/compensate), the one that presented the best indexes of adjustment. Another source of validity evidence that was used was that based on the relationship with other variables, specifically the convergent evidence, finding statistically significant correlations between the two specific factors and the general factor with the average number of hours per day on the Internet and social skills. Finally, the reliability, estimated through the ordinal alpha coefficient, was acceptable for the general factor and the specific factors.

The items showed discrimination indexes above 0.30, which implies that each item is related to the other items taken together, which would also justify the presence of an underlying general factor. These results agree with a previous study [43], where all the items were higher than the cut-off point used in this study. However, other studies showed problems only with item 7 ("How often do you check your email before something else that you need to do?"), finding values of 0.170 [42], 0.250 [41], −0.098 [104], and 0.195 [32], while all the other items were greater than 0.30. In this study, item 7 had the lowest item-rest correlation (0.371).

Item 7 is problematic in the literature because it would be mainly relevant for university students or people whose jobs involve communication by this means. In university students, virtual communication occurs mainly with their professors by email, for sending papers, receiving corrected papers, or notifying activities on virtual platforms, as well as with their peers to exchange information (e.g., articles or books) or share working documents. It is important to highlight that, in this study, the item-rest correlation was estimated using the polyserial correlation, unlike previous studies that worked with the Pearson correlation coefficient. The polyserial correlation coefficient considers the ordinality of the items, being more precise in estimating the degree of item discrimination.

The presence of a floor effect in the items, together with low averages in these, shows the low level of Internet addiction of the participants. This result may be due to the characteristics of the study participants, who belong entirely to a public sector university, where most of the population belongs to a medium or medium-low socioeconomic level, having some limitations regarding the Internet accessibility as it involves spending on devices (cell phones, tablets, laptops, etc.) and mobile data for connectivity. On the other hand, Internet addiction is a clinical construct, so its presence in a non-clinical population (university students) should be low under normal conditions.

Regarding the internal structure of the IAT, this study recollected a large part of the models reported in previous studies to test them and find out how the IAT is structured in the Peruvian sample. The bifactor model (one general factor and two specific factors) [34] presented the best fit. In the reviewed literature, the other study that reported a bifactor model found a general factor and three specific factors [56]. Comparing the results obtained in this study with those reported by Watters et al. [34], many points of agreement were observed, both at the level of fit indices and in factor loadings. In both studies, the factor loadings had higher values in the general factor than in the specific factors. In both studies, several items presented factor loadings below 0.30 or 0.40, which are the usual cut-off points in this type of study. However, the results of the present bifactor model indicate that those items that had low factor loadings in the general factor, had higher factor loadings in the specific factors, and vice versa.

The characteristic described above is typical of bifactor models, which allow the simultaneous evaluation of the influence of the general factor and specific factors on the variability of each item. The evaluation of the bifactor model through the omega hierarchical (ω_H and ω_{HS}) and H coefficients (also known as construct reliability), ECV, I-ECV, and PUC, provided evidence regarding the relevance of the model. The remaining 15 models reviewed and tested presented convergence or adjustment problems. The difference in fit between the previous studies and the present study is probably due to the different estimation methods used. In this study, the WLSMV estimator was used that considers the categorical nature of the items. Furthermore, many of the previous studies had problems in choosing the appropriate statistical technique or methods.

The use of the PCA for work with psychological variables is not appropriate since in its conception it considers formative models, useful in other disciplines (economics, marketing, among others), where it seeks to group indicators or reduce the number of variables. By contrast, factor analysis works with reflective models, where an underlying variable (factor) causes certain behaviors (indicators or items). For the factor analysis, the exploratory or non-restrictive version involves making a series of decisions during the analysis, the most critical being the determination of the number of factors. Additionally, the choice of the rotation method should be justified by how the factors are related. In the reviewed antecedents, the use, in most of the studies, of the "Little Jiffy" was observed, which supposes a routine of analysis in the three mentioned aspects: PCA, eigenvalues greater than one (method to choose the number of factors) and Varimax rotation (consider that the factors are not correlated). The use of Little Jiffy has been heavily criticized and its use is not recommended, as it may lead to the acceptance of erroneous factor models [67].

From a theoretical point of view, the time/control factor is related to behavioral symptoms (e.g., neglect household chores to spend more time online), while the stress/compensate factor is made up of cognitive and affective symptoms (e.g., block out disturbing thoughts about your life with soothing thoughts of the Internet or snap, yell, or act annoyed if someone bothers you while you are online). This bifactor model is framed within the cognitive-behavioral perspective, explaining the symptoms of Internet addiction (of varied nature) from specific and generalized uses, which simultaneously influence the symptoms [15]. The model obtained in this study theoretically differs from the models presented in the literature review, because a component (behavioral, cognitive, or affective) is not emphasized, but rather, the components are worked on simultaneously.

Convergent evidence from the IAT was also provided, finding statistically significant correlations with the hours of daily Internet use, and time/control and total Internet addiction presented a recommended minimum effect size that represents practical significance in social science data. These results were like those obtained by other researchers [38,41,45,50]. Additionally, the IAT negatively correlates with social skills measures (total score and self-expression, disagreement, and assertiveness factors). Previous studies also report these relationships with similar degrees of correlation. Internet addiction is associated with greater difficulties in social skills, probably since the emotional burden produced by being connected to the Internet interferes with social aspects. In this way, the development of social skills is left aside due to the few social interactions that the subject experiences, since most of his time is online [2,71].

Regarding the reliability of the scores on the IAT, the ordinal alpha coefficient showed acceptable levels for the general factor and the specific factors. On this point, most of previous studies coincide, including meta-analytical studies [65].

Regarding the limitations of the study, the main one focuses on the size and variety of the sample. Regarding the first aspect, although globally, the sample size is justified in an a priori statistical power analysis, the number of participants within the groups of sociodemographic variables is small, which limits the possibility of carrying out additional analyses in the items. For example, knowing the differential functioning of items or knowing the factorial invariance of the IAT. Regarding the variety of the sample, the students belonged to a public university; therefore, they share various characteristics that make it a homogeneous group, and therefore, the variability in the responses to the items was low.

To know and deepen other characteristics of the IAT, future studies should focus their objectives on analyses that provide evidence of its clinical utility. In this way, the appropriate cut-off points should be determined to be able to classify people addicted to the Internet and, in turn, evaluate the intensity of this addiction. Likewise, it is necessary to previously know how the instrument works in people with a presumption of Internet addiction, as well as to what extent it is related to other tests that measure clinical constructs (e.g., depression or anxiety), being relevant measures to obtain validity evidence based on relations to other variables. Therefore, working with clinical samples is a necessity, since the IAT could have different uses in the diagnosis and treatment of Internet addiction.

Likewise, the study of the IAT in non-academic populations must be accompanied by a review of the content of the items, since some of them may only be valid for the population of university students, for example, item 6 "How often do your grades or school work suffer because of the amount of time you spend online? ", being, in this case, the rewriting of the item or its exclusion from the test. Additionally, given the complexity of the IAT structure, other multivariate techniques could be tried to corroborate what was found here or to propose more stable structures. Techniques, such as network analysis, exploratory structural equation modeling (ESEM), or Bayesian approaches to factor analysis, would help in this regard. Regarding reliability, it is relevant to obtain evidence on temporal stability (test-retest reliability), particularly useful in the IAT, due to the high variability that scores in this type of test can have.

6. Conclusions

This study represents a contribution to the study of the IAT in Latin America, where it has been little studied, unlike other contexts, such as Europe or Asia. The findings indicate that the IAT, in the sample of Peruvian university students, is made up of a general factor and two specific factors (time/control and stress/compensate), or a bifactor model. Likewise, added to the validity evidence based on the internal structure, the IAT showed evidence based on the relationship with other variables (average hours per day on the Internet). On the other hand, the reliability of the scores was acceptable.

The results lead to the conclusion that the scores in the IAT have evidence of validity and reliability for its use. This has implications for both researchers and those who are primarily involved in the patient practice. For researchers, the IAT constitutes an instrument that would allow studies on Internet addiction to be carried out, for example, knowing its prevalence in certain groups, identifying the factors associated with its genesis and evolution in people, or knowing the degree of sensitivity and specificity with which one can diagnose a person with Internet addiction. For professionals, the IAT is a tool that would help diagnose Internet addiction, and it would also allow evaluation of the effects produced by a treatment or therapy that seeks to decrease the level of Internet addiction.

Author Contributions: Conceptualization, A.A.T.-M., J.C.A.-P., R.A.Z.-T. and D.E.R.-O.; methodology, A.A.T.-M., J.C.A.-P., R.A.Z.-T. and D.E.R.-O.; software, A.A.T.-M., J.C.A.-P., R.A.Z.-T. and D.E.R.-O.; validation, A.A.T.-M., J.C.A.-P., R.A.Z.-T. and D.E.R.-O.; formal analysis, A.A.T.-M., J.C.A.-P., R.A.Z.-T. and D.E.R.-O.; investigation, A.A.T.-M., J.C.A.-P., R.A.Z.-T. and D.E.R.-O.; resources, A.A.T.-M., J.C.A.-P., R.A.Z.-T. and D.E.R.-O.; data curation, A.A.T.-M., J.C.A.-P., R.A.Z.-T. and D.E.R.-O.; writing—original draft preparation, A.A.T.-M., J.C.A.-P., R.A.Z.-T. and D.E.R.-O.; writing—review and editing, A.A.T.-M., J.C.A.-P., R.A.Z.-T. and D.E.R.-O.; visualization, A.A.T.-M., J.C.A.-P., R.A.Z.-T. and D.E.R.-O.; supervision, A.A.T.-M., J.C.A.-P., R.A.Z.-T. and D.E.R.-O.; project administration, A.A.T.-M., J.C.A.-P., R.A.Z.-T. and D.E.R.-O. All authors have read and agreed to the published version of the manuscript.

Appendix A

English and Spanish version of the Internet Addiction Test (IAT)

1. How often do you find that you stay online longer than you intended? ¿Con qué frecuencia se conecta a internet más de lo previsto?
2. How often do you neglect household chores to spend more time online? ¿Con qué frecuencia descuida las actividades de la casa para estar más tiempo conectado?
3. How often do you prefer the excitement of the internet to intimacy with your partner? ¿Con qué frecuencia prefiere más la emoción que le produce estar conectado a la intimidad con su pareja o la relación directa con sus amigos?
4. How often do you form new relationships with fellow online users? ¿Con qué frecuencia forma nuevas relaciones con usuarios de Internet?
5. How often do others in your life complain to you about the amount of time you spend online? ¿Con qué frecuencia las personas cercanas a usted se quejan por la cantidad de tiempo que permanece conectado?
6. How often do your grades or school work suffer because of the amount of time you spend online? ¿Con qué frecuencia sus calificaciones o actividades académicas se afectan negativamente por la cantidad de tiempo que permanece en Internet?
7. How often do you check your email before something else that you need to do? ¿Con qué frecuencia revisa su correo electrónico antes de realizar otra tarea que necesita hacer?
8. How often does your job performance or productivity suffer because of the internet? ¿Con qué frecuencia el tiempo que pasa en Internet afecta negativamente su desempeño o productividad en el trabajo?
9. How often do you become defensive or secretive when anyone asks you what you do online? ¿Con qué frecuencia está a la defensiva o se muestra reservado cuando alguien le pregunta qué hace en Internet?
10. How often do you block out disturbing thoughts about your life with soothing thoughts of the internet? ¿Con qué frecuencia bloquea los pensamientos desagradables de su vida con pensamientos agradables relacionados con Internet?

11. How often do you find yourself anticipating when you will go online again? ¿Con qué frecuencia anticipa cuando estará conectado de nuevo?
12. How often do you fear that life without the internet would be boring, empty, and joyless? ¿Con qué frecuencia teme que la vida sin Internet sería aburrida, vacía o triste?
13. How often do you snap, yell, or act annoyed if someone bothers you while you are online? ¿Con qué frecuencia se enoja si alguien lo molesta mientras está conectado?
14. How often do you lose sleep due to being online? ¿Con qué frecuencia se queda sin dormir por conectarse durante la noche?
15. How often do you feel preoccupied with the internet when off-line, or fantasize about being online? ¿Con qué frecuencia se siente preocupado por no estar conectado o imagina estarlo?
16. How often do you find yourself saying "just a few more minutes" when online? ¿Con qué frecuencia dice: "unos minutos más", cuando está conectado?
17. How often do you try to cut down the amount of time you spend online and fail? ¿Con qué frecuencia trata de disminuir el tiempo que pasa en Internet y no lo logra?
18. How often do you try to hide how long you've been online? ¿Con qué frecuencia intenta ocultar el tiempo que permanece conectado?
19. How often do you choose to spend more time online over going out with others? ¿Con qué frecuencia prefiere pasar más tiempo en Internet que salir con otras personas?
20. How often do you feel depressed, moody, or nervous when you are off-line, which goes away once you are back online? ¿Con qué frecuencia se siente deprimido, malhumorado o nervioso cuando no está conectado, pero se siente mejor cuando se conecta de nuevo?

References

1. Freeman, C.G. The implications of online connectivity for world heritage in a digital platform society. *Hist. Environ.* **2018**, *30*, 84–95.
2. Engelberg, E.; Sjöberg, L. Internet use, social skills, and adjustment. *Cyberpsychol. Behav.* **2004**, *7*, 41–47. [CrossRef] [PubMed]
3. Gracia Blanco, M.D.; Vigo Anglada, M.; Fernández Perez, M.J.; Marcó Arbones, M. Problemas conductuales relacionados con el uso de Internet: Un estudio exploratorio. *Psicologia* **2002**, *18*, 273–292.
4. Mayer, M.A. The use of the Internet among adolescents; Risks and benefits. *Aten. Primaria* **2011**, *43*, 287–288. [CrossRef] [PubMed]
5. Sánchez-Carbonell, X.; Beranuy, M.; Castellana, M.; Chamarro, A.; Oberst, U. La adicción a Internet y al móvil: ¿moda o trastorno? *Adicciones* **2008**, *20*, 149–160. [CrossRef] [PubMed]
6. Garcia del Castillo, J.A.; Terol, M.D.C.; Nieto, M.; Lledó, A.; Sánchez, S.; Martín-Aragón, M.; Sitges, E. Uso y abuso de Internet en jóvenes universitarios. *Adicciones* **2008**, *20*, 131–142. [CrossRef] [PubMed]
7. Domínguez, C.; Geijo, S.; Sánchez, I.; Imaz, C.; Cabús, G. Revision of the mechanisms involved in the problematic use of the Internet. *Rev. Asoc. Esp. Neuropsiquiatr.* **2012**, *32*, 691–705.
8. Kuss, D.J.; Lopez-Fernandez, O. Internet addiction and problematic Internet use: A systematic review of clinical research. *World J. Psychiatry* **2016**, *6*, 143. [CrossRef]
9. Starcevic, V.; Aboujaoude, E. Internet addiction: Reappraisal of an increasingly inadequate concept. *CNS Spectr.* **2017**, *22*, 7–13. [CrossRef]
10. Young, K.S. Internet addiction: The emergence of a new clinical disorder. *Cyberpsychol. Behav.* **1998**, *1*, 237–244. [CrossRef]
11. Young, K.S. Internet addiction: A new clinical phenomenon and its consequences. *Am. Behav. Sci.* **2004**, *48*, 402–415. [CrossRef]
12. Block, J.J. Issues for DSM-V: Internet addiction. *Am. J. Psychiatry* **2008**, *165*, 306–307. [CrossRef] [PubMed]
13. Young, K.S.; Nabuco de Abreu, C. *Internet Addiction: A Handbook and Guide to Evaluation and Treatment*; John Wiley & Sons, Ltd.: Hoboken, NJ, USA, 2010; ISBN 978-0-470-55116-5.
14. American Psychiatric Association. *Diagnostic and Statistical Manual of Mental Disorders*, 5th ed.; American Psychiatric Association: Washington, DC, USA, 2013; ISBN 978-0-89042-554-1.

15. Davis, R.A. A cognitive-behavioral model of pathological Internet use. *Comput. Hum. Behav.* **2001**, *17*, 187–195. [CrossRef]
16. Teo, C.P.A.; Lim, K.; Oei, T.P. Problematic Internet Use: Variants of cognitive-behavioural model under path analysis. *Int. J. Psychol. Behav. Anal.* **2017**, *3*, 130. [CrossRef] [PubMed]
17. Díaz-Aguado, M.J.; Martín-Babarro, J.; Falcón, L. Problematic Internet use, maladaptive future time perspective and school context. *Psicothema* **2018**, *30*, 195–200.
18. Fernandes, B.; Rodrigues, B.; Pontes, H.M. Internet addiction or problematic internet use ? Which term should be used ? *Psicol. USP* **2019**, *30*, e190020. [CrossRef]
19. Demetrovics, Z.; Szeredi, B.; Rózsa, S. The three-factor model of Internet addiction: The development of the Problematic Internet Use Questionnaire. *Behav. Res. Methods* **2008**, *40*, 563–574. [CrossRef]
20. Meerkerk, G.-J.; Van Den Eijnden, R.J.J.M.; Vermulst, A.A.; Garretsen, H.F.L. The Compulsive Internet Use Scale (CIUS): Some psychometric properties. *Cyberpsychol. Behav.* **2008**, *12*, 1–6. [CrossRef]
21. Armstrong, L.; Phillips, J.G.; Saling, L.L. Potential determinants of heavier Internet usage. *Int. J. Hum. Comput. Stud.* **2000**, *53*, 537–550. [CrossRef]
22. Casas, J.A.; Ruiz-Olivares, R.; Ortega-Ruiz, R. Validation of the internet and social networking experiences questionnaire in Spanish adolescents. *Int. J. Clin. Health Psychol.* **2013**, *13*, 40–48. [CrossRef]
23. Young, K.S. *Caught in the Net: How to Recognize the Signs of Internet Addiction—And a Winning Strategy for Recovery*; John Wiley & Sons, Ltd.: New York, NY, USA, 1998; ISBN 978-0-471-19159-9.
24. Widyanto, L.; McMurran, M. The psychometric properties of the Internet Addiction Test. *Cyberpsychol. Behav.* **2004**, *7*, 443–450. [CrossRef]
25. Ngai, S.S.Y. Exploring the validity of the Internet Addiction Test for students in grades 5–9 in Hong Kong. *Int. J. Adolesc. Youth* **2007**, *13*, 221–237. [CrossRef]
26. Chang, M.K.; Man, S.P. Factor structure for Young's Internet Addiction Test: A confirmatory study. *Comput. Hum. Behav.* **2008**, *24*, 2597–2619. [CrossRef]
27. Khazaal, Y.; Billieux, J.; Thorens, G.; Khan, R.; Louati, Y.; Scarlatti, E.; Theintz, F.; Lederrey, J.; Van Der Linden, M.; Zullino, D. French validation of the Internet Addiction Test. *Cyberpsychol. Behav.* **2008**, *11*, 703–706. [CrossRef] [PubMed]
28. Widyanto, L.; Griffiths, M.D.; Brunsden, V. A psychometric comparison of the Internet Addiction Test, the Internet-Related Problem Scale, and self-diagnosis. *Cyberpsychol. Behav. Soc. Netw.* **2011**, *14*, 141–149. [CrossRef] [PubMed]
29. Panayides, P.; Walker, M.J. Evaluation of the psychometric properties of the Internet Addiction Test (IAT) in a sample of Cypriot high school students: The Rasch measurement perspective. *Eur. J. Psychol.* **2012**, *8*, 327–351. [CrossRef]
30. Jelenchick, L.A.; Becker, T.; Moreno, M.A. Assessing the psychometric properties of the Internet Addiction Test (IAT) in US college students. *Psychiatry Res.* **2012**, *196*, 296–301. [CrossRef]
31. Barke, A.; Nyenhuis, N.; Kröner-Herwig, B. The German version of the Internet Addiction Test: A validation study. *Cyberpsychol. Behav. Soc. Netw.* **2012**, *15*, 534–542. [CrossRef]
32. Puerta-Cortés, D.X.; Carbonell, X.; Chamarro, A. Análisis de las propiedades psicométricas de la versión en español del Internet Addiction Test. *Trastor. Adict.* **2012**, *14*, 99–104. [CrossRef]
33. Faraci, P.; Craparo, G.; Messina, R.; Severino, S. Internet Addiction Test (IAT): Which is the best factorial solution? *J. Med. Internet Res.* **2013**, *15*, e225. [CrossRef]
34. Watters, C.A.; Keefer, K.V.; Kloosterman, P.H.; Summerfeldt, L.J.; Parker, J.D.A. Examining the structure of the Internet Addiction Test in adolescents: A bifactor approach. *Comput. Hum. Behav.* **2013**, *29*, 2294–2302. [CrossRef]
35. Pawlikowski, M.; Altstötter-Gleich, C.; Brand, M. Validation and psychometric properties of a short version of Young's Internet Addiction Test. *Comput. Hum. Behav.* **2013**, *29*, 1212–1223. [CrossRef]
36. Lee, K.; Gyeong, H.; Yu, B.; Song, Y.M.; Lee, H.K.; Kim, D. Reliability and validity of the Korean version of the Internet Addiction Test among college students. *J. Korean Med. Sci.* **2013**, *28*, 763–768. [CrossRef] [PubMed]
37. Hawi, N.S. Arabic validation of the Internet Addiction Test. *Cyberpsychol. Behav. Soc. Netw.* **2013**, *16*, 200–204. [CrossRef] [PubMed]
38. Lai, C.-M.; Mak, K.-K.; Watanabe, H.; Ang, R.P.; Pang, J.S.; Ho, R.C.M. Psychometric properties of the Internet Addiction Test in Chinese adolescents. *J. Pediatr. Psychol.* **2013**, *38*, 794–807. [CrossRef]

39. Pontes, H.M.; Patrão, I.M.; Griffiths, M.D. Portuguese validation of the Internet Addiction Test: An empirical study. *J. Behav. Addict.* **2014**, *3*, 107–114. [CrossRef]
40. Karim, A.K.M.R.; Nigar, N. The Internet Addiction Test: Assessing its psychometric properties in bangladeshi culture. *Asian J. Psychiatr.* **2014**, *10*, 75–83. [CrossRef]
41. Tsimtsiou, Z.; Haidich, A.B.; Kokkali, S.; Dardavesis, T.; Young, K.S.; Arvanitidou, M. Greek version of the Internet Addiction Test: A validation study. *Psychiatr. Q.* **2014**, *85*, 187–195. [CrossRef]
42. Chong, N.; Isa, S.M.; Hashim, A.H.; Kumar, S.; Harbajan, M.K. Validity of the Malay version of the internet addiction test: A study on a group of medical students in Malaysia. *Asia-Pac. J. Public Heath* **2015**, *27*, NP2210–NP2219. [CrossRef]
43. Fernández-Villa, T.; Molina, A.J.; García-Martín, M.; Llorca, J.; Delgado-Rodríguez, M.; Martín, V. Validation and psychometric analysis of the Internet Addiction Test in Spanish among college students. *BMC Public Health* **2015**, *15*, 953. [CrossRef]
44. Lu, X.; Yeo, K.J. Psychometric properties of the Internet Addiction Test in a sample of Malaysian undergraduate students. *Psicol. Educ.* **2015**, *21*, 17–25. [CrossRef]
45. Dhir, A.; Chen, S.; Nieminen, M. Psychometric validation of Internet Addiction Test with Indian adolescents. *J. Educ. Comput. Res.* **2015**, *53*, 15–31. [CrossRef]
46. Lai, C.M.; Mak, K.K.; Cheng, C.; Watanabe, H.; Nomachi, S.; Bahar, N.; Young, K.S.; Ko, H.C.; Kim, D.; Griffiths, M.D. Measurement invariance of the Internet Addiction Test among Hong Kong, Japanese, and Malaysian adolescents. *Cyberpsychol. Behav. Soc. Netw.* **2015**, *18*, 609–617. [CrossRef] [PubMed]
47. Fioravanti, G.; Casale, S. Evaluation of the psychometric properties of the Italian internet addiction test. *Cyberpsychol. Behav. Soc. Netw.* **2015**, *18*, 120–128. [CrossRef] [PubMed]
48. Hawi, N.S.; Blachnio, A.; Przepiorka, A. Polish validation of the Internet Addiction Test. *Comput. Hum. Behav.* **2015**, *48*, 548–553. [CrossRef]
49. Kaya, F.; Delen, E.; Young, K.S. Psychometric properties of the Internet Addiction Test in Turkish. *J. Behav. Addict.* **2016**, *5*, 130–134. [CrossRef]
50. Servidio, R. Assessing the psychometric properties of the Internet Addiction Test: A study on a sample of Italian university students. *Comput. Hum. Behav.* **2017**, *68*, 17–29. [CrossRef]
51. Boysan, M.; Kuss, D.J.; Barut, Y.; Ayköse, N.; Güleç, M.; Özdemir, O. Psychometric properties of the Turkish version of the Internet Addiction Test (IAT). *Addict. Behav.* **2017**, *64*, 247–252. [CrossRef]
52. Samaha, A.A.; Fawaz, M.; El Yahfoufi, N.; Gebbawi, M.; Abdallah, H.; Baydoun, S.A.; Ghaddar, A.; Eid, A.H. Assessing the psychometric properties of the Internet Addiction Test (IAT) among Lebanese college students. *Front. Public Health* **2018**, *6*, 365. [CrossRef]
53. Waqas, A.; Farooq, F.; Raza, M.; Javed, S.T.; Khan, S.; Ghumman, M.E.; Naveed, S.; Haddad, M. Validation of the Internet Addiction Test in students at a Pakistani medical and dental school. *Psychiatr. Q.* **2018**, *89*, 235–247. [CrossRef]
54. Neelapaijit, A.; Pinyopornpanish, M.; Simcharoen, S.; Kuntawong, P.; Wongpakaran, N.; Wongpakaran, T. Psychometric properties of a Thai version Internet Addiction Test. *BMC Res. Notes* **2018**, *11*, 69. [CrossRef] [PubMed]
55. Tsermentseli, S.; Karipidis, N.; Samaras, P.; Thompson, T. Assessing the factorial structure of the Internet Addiction Test in a sample of Greek adolescents. *Hell. J. Psychol.* **2018**, *15*, 274–288.
56. Hernández, C.; Rivera, D. A Chilean transcultural adaptation and assessment of the Internet Addiction Test's factor structures: Development of a brief version. *Rev. Iberoam. Diag. Eval.* **2018**, *49*, 143–155.
57. Černja, I.; Vejmelka, L.; Rajter, M. Internet Addiction Test: Croatian preliminary study. *BMC Psychiatry* **2019**, *19*, 388. [CrossRef]
58. Tudorel, O.I.; Vintilă, M.; Vlaicu, L.; Bălăuță, D.; Goian, C.; Rusu, A. Romanian version of the Internet Addiction Test: Psychometric properties and cross-gender invariance. *Int. J. Ment. Health Addict.* **2019**, *17*, 234–246. [CrossRef]
59. Ndasauka, Y.; Pitafi, A.; Kayange, G.M. Psychometric properties of Young's Internet Addiction Test (IAT) in Urdu language. *Asian J. Psychiatr.* **2019**, *40*, 39–44. [CrossRef]
60. Yaffe, Y.; Seroussi, D.-E. Further evidence for the psychometric properties of young's Internet Addiction Test (IAT): A study on a sample of Israeli-Arab male adolescents. *Am. J. Health Behav.* **2019**, *43*, 1030–1039. [CrossRef]

61. Talwar, P.; Mohamad, F.S.; Mustaffa, M.S.; Othman, M.K.; Bee, O.Y.; Hian, C.C. Internet addiction among university students: Psychometric properties of three factor model Internet Addiction Test. *Online J. Health Allied Sci.* **2019**, *18*, 1–7.
62. Lu, X.; Yeo, K.J.; Guo, F.; Zhao, Z. Factor structure and a multiple indicators multiple cause model of Internet Addiction Test: The effect of socio-demographic and internet use variables. *Curr. Psychol.* **2019**. [CrossRef]
63. Raykov, T.; Marcoulides, G.A. Thanks coefficient alpha, we still need you! *Educ. Psychol. Meas.* **2019**, *79*, 200–210. [CrossRef]
64. Viladrich, C.; Angulo-Brunet, A.; Doval, E. A journey around alpha and omega to estimate internal consistency reliability. *Psicoogia* **2017**, *33*, 755–782.
65. Moon, S.J.; Hwang, J.S.; Kim, J.Y.; Shin, A.L.; Bae, S.M.; Kim, J.W. Psychometric properties of the Internet Addiction Test: A systematic review and meta-analysis. *Cyberpsychol. Behav. Soc. Netw.* **2018**, *21*, 473–484. [CrossRef] [PubMed]
66. Marcus, C.; Peter, H. Questionable research practices when using confirmatory factor analysis. *J. Manag. Psychol.* **2019**, *34*, 18–30.
67. Sellbom, M.; Tellegen, A. Factor analysis in psychological assessment research: Common pitfalls and recommendations. *Psychol. Assess.* **2019**, *31*, 1428–1441. [CrossRef] [PubMed]
68. Matalinares, M.; Raymundo, O.; Baca, D. Psychometric adaptation of the Test of Internet Addiction. *Rev. Peru. Psicol. Trab. Soc.* **2014**, *3*, 45–66.
69. Wang, L.; Luo, J.; Gao, W.; Kong, J. The effect of Internet use on adolescents' lifestyles: A national survey. *Comput. Hum. Behav.* **2012**, *28*, 2007–2013. [CrossRef]
70. Zegarra, C.O.; Cuba, M.S. Frequency of Internet addiction and development of social skills in adolescents in an urban area of Lima. *Medwave* **2017**, *17*, e6857. [CrossRef]
71. Torrente, E.; Piqueras, J.A.; Orgilés, M.; Espada, J.P. Association of Internet addiction with social anxiety and lack of social skills in spanish adolescents. *Ter. Psicol.* **2014**, *32*, 175–184. [CrossRef]
72. Chou, W.; Huang, M.; Chang, Y.; Chen, Y.; Hu, H.; Yen, C. Social skills deficits and their association with Internet addiction and activities in adolescents with attention-deficit/hyperactivity disorder. *J. Behav. Addict.* **2017**, *6*, 42–50. [CrossRef]
73. American Educational Research Association; American Psychological Association; National Council on Measurement in Education. *Standards for Educational and Psychological Testing*; American Educational Research Association: Washington, DC, USA, 2014; ISBN 978-0935-302-356.
74. Ato, M.; López, J.J.; Benavente, A. A classification system for research designs in psychology. *Psicologia* **2013**, *29*, 1038–1059.
75. Zickar, M.J. Measurement development and evaluation. *Annu. Rev. Organ. Psychol. Organ. Behav.* **2020**, *7*, 213–232. [CrossRef]
76. Kerlinger, F.N.; Lee, H.B. *Foundations of Behavioral Research*, 4th ed.; Harcourt College Publishers: Fort Worth, TX, USA, 2000; ISBN 9780155078970.
77. Turner, D.P.; Houle, T.T. The importance of statistical power calculations. *Headache J. Head Face Pain* **2018**, *58*, 1187–1191. [CrossRef] [PubMed]
78. Ferguson, C.J. An effect size primer: A guide for clinicians and researchers. *Prof. Psychol. Res. Pr.* **2009**, *40*, 532–538. [CrossRef]
79. Cohen, J. *Statistical Power Analysis for the Behavioral Sciences*, 2nd ed.; Lawrence Erlbaum Associates: Hillsdale, NJ, USA, 1988; ISBN 0-8058-0283-5.
80. Gismero, E. *EHS: Escala de Habilidades Sociales*; TEA Ediciones: Madrid, Spain, 2000; ISBN 84-7174-609-3.
81. Miranda-Zapata, E.; Riquelme-Mella, E.; Cifuentes-Cid, H.; Riquelme-Bravo, P. Análisis factorial confrmatorio de la Escala de habilidades sociales en universitarios chilenos. *Rev. Lat. Psicol.* **2014**, *46*, 73–82.
82. Tabachnick, B.G.; Fidell, L.S. *Using Multivariate Statistics*, 7th ed.; Pearson: New York, NY, USA, 2019; ISBN 9780134792866.
83. Meyer, J.P. *Applied Measurement with Jmetrik*; Routledge: New York, NY, USA, 2014; ISBN 978-0-203-11519-0.
84. McHorney, C.A.; Tarlov, A.R. Individual-patient monitoring in clinical practice: Are available health status surveys adequate? *Qual. Life Res.* **1995**, 293–307. [CrossRef] [PubMed]
85. Li, C.-H. Confirmatory factor analysis with ordinal data: Comparing robust maximum likelihood and diagonally weighted least squares. *Behav. Res. Methods* **2016**, *48*, 936–949. [CrossRef]

86. Keith, T.Z. *Multiple Regression and Beyond: An Introduction to Multiple Regression and Structural Equation Modeling*, 3rd ed.; Routledge: New York, NY, USA, 2019; ISBN 9781351667937.
87. DiStefano, C.; Liu, J.; Jiang, N.; Shi, D. Examination of the Weighted Root Mean Square Residual: Evidence for trustworthiness? *Struct. Equ. Model. A Multidiscip. J.* **2018**, *25*, 453–466. [CrossRef]
88. Wilcox, R.R.; Rousselet, G.A.; Pernet, C.R. Improved methods for making inferences about multiple skipped correlations. *J. Stat. Comput. Simul.* **2018**, *88*, 3116–3131. [CrossRef]
89. Zumbo, B.D.; Gadermann, A.M.; Zeisser, C. Ordinal versions of coefficients alpha and theta for Likert rating scales. *J. Mod. Appl. Stat. Method* **2007**, *6*, 21–29. [CrossRef]
90. Nunnally, J.; Bernstein, I. *Psychometric Theory*, 3rd ed.; McGraw-Hill: New York, NY, USA, 1994; ISBN 9780070478497.
91. Erdfelder, E.; Faul, F.; Buchner, A.; Lang, A.-G. Statistical power analyses using G*Power 3.1: Tests for correlation and regression analyses. *Behav. Res. Methods* **2009**, *41*, 1149–1160.
92. R Core Team. *R: A Language and Environment for Statistical Computing*; R Foundation for Statistical Computing: Vienna, Austria, 2020; Available online: https://www.r-project.org (accessed on 9 June 2020).
93. Rinker, T.W.; Kurkiewicz, D. Pacman: Package Management for R. 2018. Available online: http://github.com/trinker/pacman (accessed on 9 June 2020).
94. Hadley, W.; Bryan, J. Readxl: Read Excel Files. 2019. Available online: https://cran.r-project.org/package=readxl (accessed on 9 June 2020).
95. Wickham, H.; Averick, M.; Bryan, J.; Chang, W.; Mcgowan, L.D.A.; François, R.; Grolemund, G.; Hayes, A.; Henry, L.; Hester, J.; et al. Welcome to the tidyverse. *J. Open Source Softw.* **2019**, *4*, 1686. [CrossRef]
96. Revelle, W. Psych: Procedures for Psychological, Psychometric, and Personality Research. 2019. Available online: https://cran.r-project.org/package=psych (accessed on 9 June 2020).
97. Rosseel, Y. Lavaan: An R package for structural equation modeling. *J. Stat. Softw.* **2012**, *48*, 1–36. [CrossRef]
98. Dueber, D. BifactorIndicesCalculator: Bifactor Indices Calculator. 2020. Available online: https://cran.r-project.org/package=BifactorIndicesCalculator (accessed on 9 June 2020).
99. Jorgensen, T.D.; Pornprasertmanit, S.; Schoemann, A.M.; Rosseel, Y. SemTools: Useful tools for structural equation modeling. 2020. Available online: https://cran.r-project.org/package=semTools (accessed on 9 June 2020).
100. Wilcox, R.R.; Schönbrodt, F.D. The WRS Package for Robust Statistics in R. 2019. Available online: https://github.com/nicebread/WRS (accessed on 9 June 2020).
101. Dominguez-Lara, S.; Rodriguez, A. Statistical indices from bifactor models. *Interacciones* **2017**, *3*, 59–65. [CrossRef]
102. Rodriguez, A.; Reise, S.P.; Haviland, M.G. Evaluating bifactor models: Calculating and interpreting statistical indices. *Psychol. Methods* **2016**, *21*, 137–150. [CrossRef]
103. Tavakol, M.; Dennick, R. Making sense of Cronbach's alpha. *Int. J. Med. Educ.* **2011**, *2*, 53–55. [CrossRef]
104. Conti, M.A.; Pelegrino, A.; Hearst, N.; Athanássios, T.; Tavares, H.; Nabuco de Abreu, C. Evaluation of semantic equivalence and internal consistency of a Portuguese version of the Internet Addiction Test (IAT). *Rev. Psiquiatr. Clin.* **2012**, *39*, 106–110. [CrossRef]

5

Problematic Smartphone Use and Mental Health in Chinese Adults: A Population-Based Study

Ningyuan Guo [1], Tzu Tsun Luk [1], Sai Yin Ho [2], Jung Jae Lee [1], Chen Shen [3], John Oliffe [4], Sophia Siu-Chee Chan [1], Tai Hing Lam [2] and Man Ping Wang [1,*]

[1] School of Nursing, University of Hong Kong, Hong Kong, China; nyguo@hku.hk (N.G.); luktt@hku.hk (T.T.L.); leejay@hku.hk (J.J.L.); nssophia@hku.hk (S.S.-C.C.)
[2] School of Public Health, University of Hong Kong, Hong Kong, China; syho@hku.hk (S.Y.H.); hrmrlth@hku.hk (T.H.L.)
[3] Department of Epidemiology and Biostatistics, Imperial College London, London W2 1PG, UK; chen.shen@imperial.ac.uk
[4] School of Nursing, University of British Columbia, Vancouver, BC V6T 2B5, Canada; John.Oliffe@ubc.ca
* Correspondence: mpwang@hku.hk

Abstract: Problematic smartphone use (PSU) has been associated with anxiety and depression, but few explored its mental well-being correlates that could co-occur with or be independent of mental symptoms. We studied the associations of PSU with anxiety, depression, and mental well-being in Hong Kong Chinese adults in a probability-based survey (N = 4054; 55.0% females; mean age ± SD 48.3 ± 18.3 years). PSU was measured using Smartphone Addiction Scale-Short Version. Anxiety and depression symptoms were evaluated using General Anxiety Disorder screener-2 (GAD-2) and Patient Health Questionnaire-2 (PHQ-2). Mental well-being was measured using Subjective Happiness Scale (SHS) and Short Warwick-Edinburgh Mental Well-Being Scale (SWEMWBS). Multivariable regression analyzed associations adjusting for sociodemographic and lifestyle-related variables. Associations of PSU with mental well-being were stratified by symptom severity of anxiety (GAD-2 cutoff of 3) and depression (PHQ-2 cutoff of 3). We found that PSU was associated with higher odds of anxiety and depression symptom severity and lower scores of SHS and SWEMWBS. Associations of PSU with lower SHS and SWEMWBS scores remained in respondents who screened negative for anxiety or depression symptoms. To conclude, PSU was associated with anxiety, depression, and impaired mental well-being. Associations of PSU with impaired mental well-being could be independent of anxiety or depression symptoms.

Keywords: problematic smartphone use; smartphone addiction; anxiety; depression; mental well-being; population-based study

---

1. Introduction

The evolving mobile information and communication technologies (ICTs) have raised debates about the potential effects on mental health. Instant messaging (IM) and social networking sites (SNS) can be used for unpleasant moods avoidance, social contacts, and relationship maintenance especially in females [1], whereas a practical and instrumental use such as for social position advancement was found in males [2]. In contrast, many studies have shown the associations between poor mental health outcomes and excessive or intensive use of phone calls, texts, IM, emails, and SNS [3]. These are privileged applications of problematic smartphone use (PSU), an impaired ability to control smartphone use with core symptoms such as loss of control, tolerance, and withdrawal shared with gaming disorder and substance use disorders [4]. PSU has been associated with an array of health outcomes, including self-reported dependence [5], cyberbullying [5], traffic accidence [5], physical symptoms (e.g., eye strain and fatigue) [6], and sleep disturbances [7,8]. Our previous study also showed the lower levels of family communication and well-being associated with PSU [9].

Research in adolescents and young adults have identified psychopathological correlates with PSU, with affective disorders including anxiety and depression were most studied [1]. Small to medium effect size associations were observed between PSU and the severity of anxiety and depression symptoms [10]. Longitudinal studies further supported the predicting effects of PSU on anxiety and depression in college students [7,8]. Although these age groups were deemed to be at higher risk for PSU because of developing self-control and more access to the ICTs, increasing prevalence of both smartphone ownership and PSU in adults of a wider age range warranted general population studies [11–14].

The definition of mental health has been established as not the mere absence of psychopathological symptoms, which leads researchers to broaden the investigation field to positive psychology [15]. Mental well-being investigates hedonic well-being that includes affective emotions and cognitive assessments of life satisfaction and eudemonic well-being that includes psychological functioning and self-realization [16]. Our previous study showed that people with greater mental well-being tended to have lower risks for anxiety and depression [16]. Despite the correlations, the dual continuum model of mental health proposes that mental illness and well-being are on two distinct dimensions [17]. This notion was supported by studies in adults reporting greater well-being despite concurrent affective disorders or impaired mental well-being but without mental illness [18,19]. One study using data from a sample of college students showed that PSU was negatively correlated with mental well-being outcomes [20]. Little is known about whether such associations could co-occur with or operate independently from affective disorders.

The present study took advantage of a representative population-based survey in Chinese adults in Hong Kong, where the smartphone penetration rate (88.6% in people aged 10 years or above in 2017) has been among the highest worldwide due to advanced cyber-infrastructure and low-cost Internet access [21]. We aimed: (a) to confirm the associations of PSU with anxiety and depression symptom severity in the general population; (b) to examine the associations of PSU with mental health outcomes including hedonic and eudemonic well-being; (c) to examine the associations of PSU with mental well-being outcomes with stratification of symptom severity of anxiety and depression.

2. Materials and Methods

2.1. Participants and Procedure

The Hong Kong Family and Health Information Trends Survey (FHInTS) is a periodic territory-wide telephone survey on the general public's behaviors and views regarding information use, individual health, and family well-being, under the project named "FAMILY: A Jockey Club Initiative for a Harmonious Society." The target population was Cantonese-speaking Hong Kong residents aged 18 years old or above. We have conducted five waves of FHInTS since 2009 and reported details of the study design elsewhere [9,11,16]. The present survey was conducted from February to August 2017, as part of the fifth FHInTS. A two-stage probability-based sampling procedure was used. In the first stage, landline telephone numbers were randomly generated using known prefixes assigned to telecommunication services providers under the numbering plan provided by the Office of the Communication Authority. Invalid numbers were then removed according to the computer and manual dialing records. Numbers of successful cases from previous FHInTS were also filtered. In the second stage, once a household was successfully reached, an eligible family member who would have the nearest next birthday was invited to the survey. Interviews were conducted by trained interviewers from the Public Opinion Programme (POP) at the University of Hong Kong. Of 5773 respondents invited, 4054 were successfully interviewed, yielding a response rate of 70.2%.

2.2. Measurements

The ten-item Smartphone Addiction Scale-Short Version (SAS-SV) measured five addiction-like symptoms of PSU, including daily-life disturbance, withdrawal, cyberspace-oriented relationship, overuse, and tolerance [22]. Each item scores on a Likert scale of 1 (strongly disagree) to 6 (strongly agree), with a higher total score (range 10 to 60) indicating a higher PSU level [22]. The Chinese version of SAS-SV was valid and reliable (Cronbach's alpha 0.84) and indicated acceptable fit for the one-factor model (comparative fit index [CFI] 0.98 [> 0.90 acceptable, > 0.95 excellent]; root mean square error of approximation [RMSEA] 0.08 [< 0.08 acceptable, < 0.05 excellent]; non-normed fit index [NNFI] 0.96 [> 0.95 acceptable]) in our previous study using the same sample of the Hong Kong general population [11]. The convergent validity was adequate, with composite reliability of 0.85 (CR > 0.70 acceptable) and average variance extracted of 0.37 (AVE > 0.40 acceptable if CR > 0.60).

The four-item Patient Health Questionnaire (PHQ-4) includes the two-item General Anxiety Disorder screener (GAD-2) and the two-item Patient Health Questionnaire (PHQ-2) [23]. PHQ-2 has two DSM-IV diagnostic core criteria for major depression disorder, and GAD-2 has two core criteria for generalized anxiety disorder that can also screen for panic and social anxiety disorders [23]. Each item scores on a Likert scale of 0 (not at all) to 3 (nearly every day), with total scores of each subscale ranging 0 to 6 [23]. GAD-2 and PHQ-2 Scores of ≥ 3 are recommended to screen positive for anxiety and depression symptoms, respectively [24]. The Chinese version of PHQ-2 has been validated in our previous study in the Hong Kong general population [25]. In the present sample, confirmatory factor analysis (CFA) indicated an excellent fit for the two-factor model of PHQ-4 (Relative Chi-Square 0.24; $p = 0.63$; incremental fit index [IFI] 1.00 [> 0.95 excellent]; goodness of fit index [GFI] 1.00 [> 0.95 excellent]; adjusted goodness of fit index [AGFI] 1.00 [> 0.95 acceptable]; CFI 1.00; RMSEA 0.01; standardized root mean square residual [SRMR] 0.001 [< 0.08 acceptable, < 0.05 excellent]). GAD-2 had a Cronbach's alpha of 0.74, CR of 0.65, and AVE of 0.48. PHQ-2 had a Cronbach's alpha of 0.73, CR of 0.63, and AVE of 0.46.

The four-item Subjective Happiness Scale (SHS; mean score range 1 to 7) measured the cognitive and affective state characterized by pleasure or satisfaction from hedonic well-being aspect [26]. The Chinese version of SHS has been validated in our previous study in the Hong Kong general population [27]. In the present sample, CFA indicated an excellent fit for the one-factor model (relative Chi-Square 21.68; $p < 0.001$; IFI 0.993; GFI 0.999; AGFI 0.995; CFI 0.993; RMSEA 0.10; SRMR 0.02). SHS had a Cronbach's alpha of 0.75, CR of 0.77, and AVE of 0.47. The seven-item Short Warwick-Edinburgh Mental Well-Being Scale (SWEMWBS; total score range 7 to 35) was adapted by the WEMWBS that covers both hedonic and eudemonic aspects [28]. A randomly selected subset ($n = 1331$, 32.8%) were asked the frequency of feeling optimistic about the future, useful, relaxed, close to other people, dealing with problems well, thinking clearly, making up their own mind about things in past two weeks [28]. The Chinese version of SWEMWBS was valid and reliable (Cronbach's alpha 0.85) and indicated excellent fit for the one-factor model (CFI 0.995; RMSEA 0.03; SRMR 0.04; normed-fit index [NFI] 0.991 [> 0.95 acceptable]) in our previous study using the same sample of the Hong Kong general population [16]. The convergent validity was adequate, with CR of 0.85 and AVE of 0.44.

Sociodemographic and lifestyle-related variables included sex, age, marital status, employment status, educational attainment, monthly household income, smoking, and alcohol drinking. This list of potential confounders was selected based on prior associations with PSU and mental health outcomes [11,29,30].

2.3. Statistical Analysis

We checked the distributions of all variables independently, with a skewness value of $\leq |2.0|$ and a kurtosis value of $\leq |7.0|$ indicating the normality [31]. All data were weighted by age, sex, and educational attainment distribution of the Hong Kong general population using the random iterative method [32]. Missing data were handled by available case analyses as there were minimal missing values for all variables (< 2.6%). We examined the Spearman correlations of anxiety and depression with mental well-being outcomes, as scores of GAD-2 and PHQ-2 were not normally distributed. Moderate correlation coefficients (r) were observed with scores of SHS (r range −0.35 to −0.38; both $p < 0.001$) and SWEMWBS (both $r = -0.42$; both $p < 0.001$). We examined the associations of SAS-SV score with the odds of severity of anxiety and depression symptoms using bivariate and multivariable logistic regression analyses adjusting for sociodemographic and lifestyle-related variables. Bivariate and multivariable linear regression analyses examined the associations of SAS-SV score with scores of SHS and SWEMWBS. We further stratified the associations of SAS-SV score with scores of SHS and SWEMWBS by symptom severity of anxiety (GAD-2 cutoff of 3) and depression (PHQ-2 cutoff of 3). The interaction effects of anxiety and depression symptoms on the associations of SAS-SV score with mental well-being outcomes were examined using adjusted Wald tests. Values of $p < 0.05$ were considered statistically significant. All analyses were conducted using Stata/MP 15.1 (StataCorp LP, College Station, TX, USA), except for CFA that were conducted using LISREL 9.30 with diagonally weighted least square estimation.

2.4. Ethics

The Institutional Review Board of the University of Hong Kong/Hospital Authority Hong Kong West Cluster approved this study. All respondents provided verbal informed consent. Telephone interviews were tape-recorded for quality checking with respondents' consent. Records were then erased six months after completing the survey.

3. Results

The weighted sample comprised 55.0% females, and the mean age ± standard deviation (SD) was 48.3 ± 18.3 years (Table 1). Smartphone owners (80.0%) reported a mean SAS-SV score ± SD of 28.9 ± 10.1. Using cutoff points ≥ 3 of GAD-2 and PHQ-2, 10.9% ($n = 442$) and 8.1% ($n = 327$) respondents screened positive for anxiety and depression symptoms, respectively. Mean scores of SHS and SWEMWBS were 5.2 ± 1.0 and 23.0 ± 4.2, respectively.

Table 1. Sociodemographic and lifestyle-related characteristics of the sample ($N = 4054$).

Sample Characteristics	Non-Weighted n (%)	Weighted [a] n (%)
Sex		
Male	1535 (37.9)	1826 (45.0)
Female	2519 (62.1)	2228 (55.0)
Age, years		
18–24	417 (10.3)	370 (9.1)
25–44	573 (14.1)	1436 (35.4)
45–64	1437 35.5)	1498 (37.0)
≥ 65	1627 (40.1)	750 (18.5)
Marital status		
Unmarried	852 (21.0)	1164 (28.7)
Cohabitated/married	2577 (63.6)	2478 (61.1)
Divorced/separated/widowed	625 (15.4)	413 (10.2)
Employment status		
Unemployment	128 (3.2)	221 (5.5)
In paid employment	1279 (31.6)	1935 (47.7)
Retired	1632 (40.3)	919 (22.7)
Housekeeper	732 (18.1)	722 (17.8)
Full-time student	283 (7.0)	257 (6.3)
Educational attainment		
Primary or below	959 (23.7)	959 (23.7)
Secondary	1730 (42.7)	1949 (48.1)
Tertiary	1365 (33.7)	1145 (28.3)

Table 1. *Cont.*

Sample Characteristics	Non-Weighted n (%)	Weighted [a] n (%)
Monthly household income (HK $ [b])		
≤19999	1671 (41.2)	1465 (36.1)
≥20000	2258 (55.7)	2486 (61.3)
Unsteady	125 (3.1)	103 (2.5)
Smoking		
Never	3368 (83.1)	3211 (79.2)
Former	435 (10.7)	467(11.5)
Current	251 (6.2)	376 (9.3)
Alcohol drinking		
Never	2065 (51.0)	1908 (47.1)
Former	256 (6.3)	228 (5.6)
Current	1731 (42.7)	1916 (47.3)
Smartphone ownership		
No	1126 (27.8)	811 (20.0)
Yes	2928 (72.2)	3243 (80.0)
SAS-SV score (range 10–60; mean ± SD)	28.2 ± 10.0	28.9 ± 10.1
Anxiety		
Negative (GAD-2 < 3)	3655 (90.2)	3611 (89.1)
Positive (GAD-2 ≥ 3)	397 (9.8)	442 (10.9)
Depression		
Negative (PHQ-2 < 3)	3777 (93.4)	3718 (91.9)
Positive (PHQ-2 ≥ 3)	269 (6.7)	327 (8.1)
SHS score (range 1–7; mean ± SD)	5.2 ± 1.0	5.2 ± 1.0
SWEMWBS score [c] (range 7–35; mean ± SD)	23.4 ± 4.5	23.0 ± 4.2

SAS-SV, Smartphone Addiction Scale-Short Version; GAD-2, Generalized Anxiety Disorder Questionnaire-2 (range 0–6); PHQ-2, Patient Health Questionnaire-2 (range 0–6); SHS, Subjective Happiness Scale; SWEMWBS, Short Warwick-Edinburgh Mental Well-Being Scale. [a] Weighted by age, sex, and educational attainment distributions of the Hong Kong general population. [b] US $1 = HK $7.8. [c] Subset sample ($n$ = 1331).

Higher SAS-SV scores were observed for respondents who screened positive for symptoms of anxiety (31.9 ± 9.4 vs. 28.5 ± 10.2; $p < 0.001$) and depression (33.2 ± 10.2 vs. 28.5 ± 10.0; $p < 0.001$) than those with negative screening results (Table 2). Multivariable analyses showed that a 1-unit increase in SAS-SV score (range 10–60) was associated with a 3% increase in odds of severity of anxiety symptoms (adjusted odds ratio [AOR] = 1.03; 95% CI: 1.01, 1.04) and a 4% increase in odds of severity of depression symptoms (AOR = 1.04; 95% CI: 1.03, 1.06) after adjusting for sociodemographic and health-related variables.

Table 2. Odds of anxiety and depression associated with SAS-SV score (N = 4054).

Outcomes Associated with SAS-SV Score	SAS-SV Score (Mean ± SD) [a]	Unadjusted Association		Adjusted [b] Association	
		Odds Ratio (95% CI)	p	Odds Ratio (95% CI)	p
Anxiety					
Negative (GAD-2 < 3)	28.5 ± 10.2	1		1	
Positive (GAD-2 ≥ 3)	31.9 ± 9.4	1.03 (1.02, 1.04)	<0.001	1.03 (1.01, 1.04)	<0.001
Depression					
Negative (PHQ-2 < 3)	28.5 ± 10.0	1		1	
Positive (PHQ-2 ≥ 3)	33.2 ± 10.2	1.04 (1.03, 1.06)	<0.001	1.04 (1.03, 1.06)	<0.001

SAS-SV, Smartphone Addiction Scale-Short Version (range 10-60); CI, Confidence Interval; GAD-2, Generalized Anxiety Disorder Questionnaire-2 (range 0–6); PHQ-2, Patient Health Questionnaire-2 (range 0–6). [a] Weighted by age, sex, and educational attainment distributions of the Hong Kong general population. [b] Adjusted for age, sex, marital status, employment status, educational attainment, monthly household income, smoking, and alcohol drinking.

Multivariable analyses showed that a 1-standard-deviation increase in SAS-SV score was associated with a 0.07-standard-deviation decrease in SHS score (adjusted B = −0.07; SE: 0.002; $p < 0.001$) and a 0.10-standard-deviation decrease in SWEMWBS score (adjusted B = -0.10; SE: 0.01; $p = 0.002$) (Table 3). Reduction in effect size of these associations were observed after stratifications by screening results of anxiety and depression symptoms, except for the stronger association of SAS-SV score with lower SHS score in respondents who screened positive for anxiety symptoms (adjusted B = −0.16; SE: 0.01; $p = 0.013$). The associations of SAS-SV score with lower SHS score remained in respondents who screened negative for anxiety symptoms (adjusted B = −0.04; SE: 0.002; $p = 0.040$) and depression symptoms (adjusted B = −0.05; SE: 0.002; $p = 0.014$). The associations of SAS-SV score with lower SWEMWBS score remained in respondents who screened negative for anxiety symptoms (adjusted B = −0.08; SE: 0.01; $p = 0.022$) and were marginally significant in those who screened negative for depression symptoms (adjusted B = −0.06; SE: 0.01; $p = 0.054$). We observed no interaction effects of anxiety or depression symptoms on the associations of SAS-SV score with lower scores of SHS and SWEMWBS.

Table 3. Standardized beta (B) of SHS and SWEMWBS scores associated with SAS-SV score ($N = 4054$).

Outcomes Associated with SAS-SV Score	Stratification	Unadjusted Association				Adjusted [a] Association				*p* for Interaction [a]
		B (SE)	*p*	F (df = 1)	r^2	B (SE)	*p*	F (df = 21)	R^2	
SHS score (range 1–7)	**Overall**	−0.08 (0.002)	<0.001	16.99	0.01	−0.07 (0.002)	<0.001	9.26	0.06	–
	Anxiety									0.197
	Negative (GAD−2 < 3)	−0.04 (0.002)	0.023	5.15	0.002	−0.04 (0.002)	0.040	7.16	0.06	
	Positive (GAD−2 ≥ 3)	−0.11 (0.01)	0.076	3.17	0.01	−0.16 (0.01)	0.013	0.88	0.07	
	Depression									0.626
	Negative (PHQ−2 < 3)	−0.05 (0.002)	0.008	7.13	0.003	−0.05 (0.002)	0.014	7.89	0.06	
	Positive (PHQ−2 ≥ 3)	−0.01 (0.01)	0.864	0.03	0.0002	−0.03 (0.01)	0.707	0.61	0.07	
SWEMWBS score (range 7–35) [b]	**Overall**	−0.11 (0.01)	0.001	10.84	0.01	−0.10 (0.01)	0.002	5.72	0.12	–
	Anxiety									0.565
	Negative (GAD−2 < 3)	−0.09 (0.01)	0.014	6.10	0.01	−0.08 (0.01)	0.022	4.54	0.11	
	Positive (GAD−2 ≥ 3)	0.01 (0.03)	0.950	0	0	0.02 (0.04)	0.866	1.00	0.19	
	Depression									0.982
	Negative (PHQ−2 < 3)	−0.07 (0.01)	0.028	4.87	0.01	−0.06 (0.01)	0.054	4.85	0.11	
	Positive (PHQ−2 ≥ 3)	−0.03 (0.03)	0.826	0.05	0.001	−0.02 (0.04)	0.895	1.75	0.42	

SAS−SV, Smartphone Addiction Scale−Short Version (range 10–60); SE, Standardized Error; GAD−2, Generalized Anxiety Disorder Questionnaire−2 (range 0–6); PHQ−2, Patient Health Questionnaire−2 (range 0–6); SHS, Subjective Happiness Scale; SWEMWBS, Short Warwick−Edinburgh Mental Well−Being Scale. [a] Adjusted for age, sex, marital status, employment status, educational attainment, monthly household income, smoking, and alcohol drinking. [b] Subset sample ($n = 1331$).

4. Discussion

With a representative sample of Chinese adults in Hong Kong, we confirmed the associations of PSU with anxiety and depression in the general population. Few studies of potential mental health effects of PSU have incorporated both mental illness and mental well−being outcomes. We provided the first evidence of the associations of PSU with impaired hedonic and eudemonic well−being, which remained in respondents who screened negative for anxiety or depression symptoms.

Our study built on young people studies to indicate that the associations of PSU with anxiety and depression could have expanded to adults of all ages. The associations can be explained by the time displacement hypothesis that posits a possible tradeoff between smartphone activities and offline healthier activities such as social interactions [33]. Our previous study supported this explanation by showing that PSU was associated with lower levels of perceived family communication and family well–being [9]. This lack of social support can induce the onset of affective disorders such as anxiety and depression [34]. Other studies showed that PSU symptoms such as overuse and tolerance could risk people to prolong the night–time smartphone usage, which might lead to sleep problems that could mediate the pathway to anxiety and depression [35]. Increasing evidence has suggested that the most problematic application correlated with PSU could be SNS, which could expose people to negative social comparisons with others in perceived more favorable lives and induce affective disorders [36–38]. However, people with symptoms of mental illness might be at higher risk for PSU given the smartphone could be the first and most obvious process to deflect negative cognition and affectivity [39]. Mechanisms in this potential reverse causality can include cognitive– and affective–related maladaptive coping strategies such as repetitive negative thinking and emotion dysregulation [39]. The bidirectional association was hence possible and evident by the reciprocal relations found in prospective cohort studies in young people [7,40].

We observed the association of PSU with lower scores of subjective happiness (i.e., hedonic well–being), which is characterized by affectivity of pleasure and cognition of satisfaction [16]. This finding was consistent with studies of Internet addiction with lower levels of happiness and life satisfaction in young people [41,42]. An intervention restricting night–time smartphone usage also reported the reduced PSU risk and increased levels of subjective happiness at one–week follow–up [43]. PSU was associated with lower scores of SWEMWBS that covers both hedonic and eudemonic aspects of mental well–being in the present study. In contrast, a study showed the improved mental well–being in self–concealers who intentionally withhold personal information in face–to–face settings but engaged more in online communication even driven by PSU [44]. These conflicting findings highlighted the important role of personality traits when evaluating the potential effects of PSU and suggested to balance our findings with potential benefits of ICTs usage such as fostering social inclusion among those who may feel excluded [45].

The magnitude of the association of PSU with impaired subjective happiness increased in respondents who screened positive for anxiety symptoms, which suggested the co–occurrence of lower levels of hedonic well–being with anxiety disorder. This finding can be supported by the cognitive–and affective–related coping processes in the pathway from anxiety symptoms to PSU [39]. Another explanation can be the moderate correlation between scores of SHS and GAD–2 found in the present sample. Previous studies also showed that people with symptoms of affective disorders had lower levels of mental well–being than those without [46]. Despite the correlated relations, the independence of mental well–being from mental illness was supported by the remained associations of PSU with mental well–being in respondents who screened negative for anxiety or depression. This finding provided insights that the absence of psychopathological symptoms might have non–buffering effects on the impaired mental well–being outcomes associated with PSU.

Our findings need to be interpreted with caution. Consistent with a systematic review that reported the small effect size associations of PSU with symptom severity of anxiety and depression (adjusted B range 0.12 to 0.18) [10], a 1–unit increase in SAS–SV score was associated with 3%–4% increase in the odds of positive screening results of anxiety and depression in the present study. The small effect size was also observed for the association of PSU with mental well–being outcomes (adjusted B range 0.07 to 0.10). A study across three large–scale datasets (total N = 355358) showed a much smaller association (median adjusted B = −0.07) of adolescents' digital technologies use with combined mental illness and well–being outcomes [47]. However, unaccounted factors might affect both PSU and mental health in such cross–sectional associations. Longitudinal and experimental studies are warranted to distill causal and predictive models.

One of the study's limitations is that the cross–sectional data restricts the causal inference of the findings. Residual confounding by unmeasured or unknown confounders might exist even after adjusting for many sociodemographic and lifestyle–related variables. We used the landline telephone survey. Sampling bias might exist due to the lack of data on mobile phone–only households that may have different smartphone use patterns. To increase the sample's representativeness, we weighted data according to the age, sex, and educational attainment distributions of the Hong Kong general population. We used self–reported data, which are subject to recall bias and social desirability bias. Future studies of PSU could include behavioral methods for collecting data on smartphone use, such as objectively examining participants' screen time and usage of individual apps. We used screening instruments rather than diagnostic instruments to measure PSU and mental health outcomes. However, more accurate diagnoses by face–to–face assessments in clinical settings would limit the generalizability of findings compared with the population–based study.

5. Conclusions

Our population–based study indicated that PSU was associated with higher odds of severity of anxiety and depression symptoms and lower levels of mental well–being. The associations of PSU with impaired mental well–being outcomes could remain in people who screened negative for anxiety or depression symptoms. Such findings highlighted the importance to investigate other psychological constructs with PSU, particularly from aspects of positive psychology. Longitudinal and experimental studies are warranted to explain causality and possible mechanisms of the associations between PSU and mental health.

Author Contributions: Conceptualization, M.P.W., S.Y.H., C.S., S.S.-C.C., and T.H.L.; Formal analysis, N.G.; Funding acquisition, T.H.L.; Methodology, M.P.W., S.Y.H., C.S., and T.H.L.; Supervision, M.P.W. and S.Y.H.; Writing—original draft, N.G.; Writing—review & editing, N.G., T.T.L., S.Y.H., J.J.L., C.S., J.O., T.H.L., and M.P.W. All authors have read and agreed to the published version of the manuscript.

Acknowledgments: This project was funded by the Hong Kong Jockey Club Charities Trust. We would like to thank the respondents who completed the telephone surveys and the Public Opinion Programme (HKU) for conducting the interviews.

References

1. De-Sola Gutiérrez, J.; Rodríguez de Fonseca, F.; Rubio, G. Cell–phone addiction: A review. *Front. Psychiatry* **2016**, *7*, 175. [CrossRef] [PubMed]
2. Ling, R. Adolescent girls and young adult men: Two sub–cultures of the mobile telephone. *Revista de Estudios de juventud* **2002**, *52*, 33–46.
3. Thomée, S. Mobile phone use and mental health. A review of the research that takes a psychological perspective on exposure. *Int. J. Environ. Res. Public Health* **2018**, *15*, 2692. [CrossRef] [PubMed]
4. Chóliz, M. Mobile phone addiction: A point of issue. *Addiction* **2010**, *105*, 373–374. [PubMed]
5. Billieux, J.; Maurage, P.; Lopez-Fernandez, O.; Kuss, D.J.; Griffiths, M.D. Can disordered mobile phone use be considered a behavioral addiction? An update on current evidence and a comprehensive model for future research. *Curr. Addict. Rep.* **2015**, *2*, 156–162. [CrossRef]
6. Xie, X.; Dong, Y.; Wang, J. Sleep quality as a mediator of problematic smartphone use and clinical health symptoms. *J. Behav. Addict.* **2018**, *7*, 466–472. [CrossRef]
7. Liu, S.; Wing, Y.K.; Hao, Y.; Li, W.; Zhang, J.; Zhang, B. The associations of long–time mobile phone use with sleep disturbances and mental distress in technical college students: A prospective cohort study. *Sleep* **2019**, *42*, 1–10. [CrossRef]
8. Thomée, S.; Eklöf, M.; Gustafsson, E.; Nilsson, R.; Hagberg, M. Prevalence of perceived stress, symptoms of depression and sleep disturbances in relation to information and communication technology (ICT) use among young adults—an explorative prospective study. *Comput. Hum. Behav.* **2007**, *23*, 1300–1321. [CrossRef]

9. Guo, N.; Wang, M.P.; Luk, T.T.; Ho, S.Y.; Fong, D.Y.T.; Chan, S.S.; Lam, T.H. The association of problematic smartphone use with family well–being mediated by family communication in Chinese adults: A population–based study. *J. Behav. Addict.* **2019**, *8*, 412–419. [CrossRef] [PubMed]
10. Elhai, J.D.; Dvorak, R.D.; Levine, J.C.; Hall, B.J. Problematic smartphone use: A conceptual overview and systematic review of relations with anxiety and depression psychopathology. *J. Affect. Disord.* **2017**, *207*, 251–259. [CrossRef] [PubMed]
11. Luk, T.T.; Wang, M.P.; Shen, C.; Wan, A.; Chau, P.H.; Oliffe, J.; Viswanath, K.; Chan, S.S.; Lam, T.H. Short version of the Smartphone Addiction Scale in Chinese adults: Psychometric properties, sociodemographic, and health behavioral correlates. *J. Behav. Addict.* **2018**, *7*, 1157–1165. [CrossRef]
12. De-Sola, J.; Talledo, H.; de Fonseca, F.R.; Rubio, G. Prevalence of problematic cell phone use in an adult population in Spain as assessed by the Mobile Phone Problem Use Scale (MPPUS). *PLoS ONE* **2017**, *12*, e0181184. [CrossRef] [PubMed]
13. Lopez-Fernandez, O. Short version of the Smartphone Addiction Scale adapted to Spanish and French: Towards a cross–cultural research in problematic mobile phone use. *Addict. Behav.* **2017**, *64*, 275–280. [CrossRef] [PubMed]
14. Nahas, M.; Hlais, S.; Saberian, C.; Antoun, J. Problematic smartphone use among Lebanese adults aged 18–65 years using MPPUS–10. *Comput. Hum. Behav.* **2018**, *87*, 348–353. [CrossRef]
15. World Health Organization. Promoting mental health: Concepts, emerging evidence, practice: Summary report. Available online: https://apps.who.int/iris/bitstream/handle/10665/42940/9241591595.pdf (accessed on 11 November 2019).
16. Sun, Y.; Luk, T.T.; Wang, M.P.; Shen, C.; Ho, S.Y.; Viswanath, K.; Chan, S.S.C.; Lam, T.H. The reliability and validity of the Chinese short Warwick–Edinburgh Mental Well–being Scale in the general population of Hong Kong. *Qual. Life Res.* **2019**, *28*, 2813–2820. [CrossRef] [PubMed]
17. Westerhof, G.J.; Keyes, C.L.M. Mental illness and mental health: The two continua model across the lifespan. *J. Adult. Dev.* **2010**, *17*, 110–119. [CrossRef]
18. Seow, L.S.E.; Vaingankar, J.A.; Abdin, E.; Sambasivam, R.; Jeyagurunathan, A.; Pang, S.; Chong, S.A.; Subramaniam, M. Positive mental health in outpatients with affective disorders: Associations with life satisfaction and general functioning. *J. Affect. Disord.* **2016**, *190*, 499–507. [CrossRef]
19. Keyes, C.L.M. Mental illness and/or mental health? Investigating axioms of the complete state model of health. *J. Consult. Clin. Psychol.* **2005**, *73*, 539–548. [CrossRef]
20. Horwood, S.; Anglim, J. Problematic smartphone usage and subjective and psychological well–being. *Comput. Hum. Behav.* **2019**, *97*, 44–50. [CrossRef]
21. Census and Statistics Department. Thematic household survey report No. 64. Available online: https://www.statistics.gov.hk/pub/B11302642018XXXXB0100.pdf (accessed on 11 November 2019).
22. Kwon, M.; Kim, D.-J.; Cho, H.; Yang, S. The Smartphone Addiction Scale: Development and validation of a short version for adolescents. *PLoS ONE* **2013**, *8*, e83558. [CrossRef]
23. Kroenke, K.; Spitzer, R.L.; Williams, J.B.W.; Löwe, B. An ultra–brief screening scale for anxiety and depression: The PHQ–4. *Psychosomatics* **2009**, *50*, 613–621. [PubMed]
24. Löwe, B.; Wahl, I.; Rose, M.; Spitzer, C.; Glaesmer, H.; Wingenfeld, K.; Schneider, A.; Brähler, E. A 4–item measure of depression and anxiety: Validation and standardization of the Patient Health Questionnaire–4 (PHQ–4) In the general population. *J. Affect. Disord.* **2010**, *122*, 86–95. [CrossRef] [PubMed]
25. Yu, X.; Stewart, S.M.; Wong, P.T.K.; Lam, T.H. Screening for depression with the Patient Health Questionnaire–2 (PHQ–2) among the general population in Hong Kong. *J. Affect. Disord.* **2011**, *134*, 444–447. [CrossRef] [PubMed]
26. Lyubomirsky, S.; Lepper, H.S. A measure of subjective happiness: Preliminary reliability and construct validation. *Soc. Indic. Res.* **1999**, *46*, 137–155. [CrossRef]
27. Nan, H.; Ni, M.Y.; Lee, P.H.; Tam, W.W.S.; Lam, T.H.; Leung, G.M.; McDowell, I. Psychometric evaluation of the Chinese version of the Subjective Happiness Scale: Evidence from the Hong Kong FAMILY Cohort. *Int. J. Behav. Med.* **2014**, *21*, 646–652. [CrossRef] [PubMed]
28. Stewart-Brown, S.; Tennant, A.; Tennant, R.; Platt, S.; Parkinson, J.; Weich, S. Internal construct validity of the Warwick-Edinburgh Mental Well–being Scale (WEMWBS): A rasch analysis using data from the Scottish health education population survey. *Health Qual. Life Outcomes* **2009**, *7*, 15. [CrossRef]

29. Haug, S.; Castro, R.P.; Kwon, M.; Filler, A.; Kowatsch, T.; Schaub, M.P. Smartphone use and smartphone addiction among young people in Switzerland. *J. Behav. Addict.* **2015**, *4*, 299–307. [CrossRef]
30. Lee, K.E.; Kim, S.-H.; Ha, T.-Y.; Yoo, Y.-M.; Han, J.-J.; Jung, J.-H.; Jang, J.-Y. Dependency on smartphone use and its association with anxiety in Korea. *Public Health Rep.* **2016**, *131*, 411–419. [CrossRef]
31. West, S.G.; Finch, J.F.; Curran, P.J. *Structural Equation Models with Non-Normal Variables: Problems and Remedies*; SAGE Publishing: Thousand Oaks, CA, USA, 1995.
32. Izrael, D.; Hoaglin, D.C.; Battaglia, M.P. To rake or not to rake is not the question anymore with the enhanced raking macro. In Proceedings of the Twenty–Ninth Annual SAS Users Group International Conference, Montreal, QC, Canada, 9–12 May 2004.
33. Kraut, R.; Patterson, M.; Lundmark, V.; Kiesler, S.; Mukophadhyay, T.; Scherlis, W. Internet paradox: A social technology that reduces social involvement and psychological well-being? *Am. Psychol.* **1998**, *53*, 1017. [CrossRef]
34. Priel, B.; Shamai, D. Attachment style and perceived social support: Effects on affect regulation. *Pers. Individ. Dif.* **1995**, *19*, 235–241. [CrossRef]
35. Adams, S.K.; Kisler, T.S. Sleep quality as a mediator between technology-related sleep quality, depression, and anxiety. *Cyberpsychol. Behav. Soc. Netw.* **2013**, *16*, 25–30. [CrossRef]
36. Shensa, A.; Escobar-Viera, C.G.; Sidani, J.E.; Bowman, N.D.; Marshal, M.P.; Primack, B.A. Problematic social media use and depressive symptoms among U.S. young adults: A nationally–representative study. *Soc. Sci. Med.* **2017**, *182*, 150–157. [PubMed]
37. Vannucci, A.; Flannery, K.M.; Ohannessian, C.M. Social media use and anxiety in emerging adults. *J. Affect. Disord.* **2017**, *207*, 163–166. [CrossRef] [PubMed]
38. Boers, E.; Afzali, M.H.; Newton, N.; Conrod, P. Association of screen time and depression in adolescence. *JAMA Pediatr.* **2019**, *173*, 853–859. [CrossRef] [PubMed]
39. Elhai, J.D.; Yang, H.; Montag, C. Cognitive– and emotion–related dysfunctional coping processes: Transdiagnostic mechanisms explaining depression and anxiety's relations with problematic smartphone use. *Curr. Addict. Rep.* **2019**, *6*, 410–417. [CrossRef]
40. Li, J.-B.; Mo, P.K.H.; Lau, J.T.F.; Su, X.-F.; Zhang, X.; Wu, A.M.S.; Mai, J.-C.; Chen, Y.-X. Online social networking addiction and depression: The results from a large–scale prospective cohort study in Chinese adolescents. *J. Behav. Addict.* **2018**, *7*, 686–696. [CrossRef]
41. Akın, A. The relationships between internet addiction, subjective vitality, and subjective happiness. *Cyberpsychol. Behav. Soc. Netw.* **2012**, *15*, 404–410. [CrossRef]
42. Lachmann, B.; Sindermann, C.; Sariyska, R.Y.; Luo, R.; Melchers, M.C.; Becker, B.; Cooper, A.J.; Montag, C. The role of empathy and life satisfaction in internet and smartphone use disorder. *Front. Psychol.* **2018**, *9*, 398. [CrossRef]
43. Hughes, N.; Burke, J. Sleeping with the frenemy: How restricting 'bedroom use' of smartphones impacts happiness and wellbeing. *Comput. Hum. Behav.* **2018**, *85*, 236–244. [CrossRef]
44. Magsamen-Conrad, K.; Billotte-Verhoff, C.; Greene, K. Technology addiction's contribution to mental wellbeing: The positive effect of online social capital. *Comput. Hum. Behav.* **2014**, *40*, 23–30. [CrossRef]
45. Council on communications and media. Media use in school–aged children and adolescents. *Pediatrics* **2016**, *138*, e20162592. [CrossRef] [PubMed]
46. Sambasivam, R.; Vaingankar, J.A.; Chong, S.A.; Abdin, E.; Jeyagurunathan, A.; Seow, L.S.E.; Pang, S.; Subramaniam, M. Positive mental health in outpatients: Comparison within diagnostic groups. *BMC Psychiatry* **2016**, *16*, 412. [CrossRef] [PubMed]
47. Orben, A.; Przybylski, A.K. The association between adolescent well–being and digital technology use. *Nat. Hum. Behav.* **2019**, *3*, 173–182. [CrossRef] [PubMed]

6

The Matthew Effect in Recovery from Smartphone Addiction in a 6-Month Longitudinal Study of Children and Adolescents †

Seung-Yup Lee [1], Hae Kook Lee [2], Jung-Seok Choi [3], Soo-young Bang [4], Min-Hyeon Park [1], Kyu-In Jung [1] and Yong-Sil Kweon [2,*]

1 Department of Psychiatry, Eunpyeong St. Mary's Hospital, College of Medicine, The Catholic University of Korea, Seoul 03312, Korea; seungyup@catholic.ac.kr (S.-Y.L.); neominnie@hanmail.net (M.-H.P.); cki@catholic.ac.kr (K.-I.J.)
2 Department of Psychiatry, Uijeongbu St. Mary's Hospital, College of Medicine, The Catholic University of Korea, Seoul 06591, Korea; nplhk@catholic.ac.kr
3 Department of Psychiatry, SMG-SNU Boramae Medical Center, Seoul 07061, Korea; psychoresi@hanmail.net
4 Department of Psychiatry, College of Medicine, Eulji University, Seoul 01830, Korea; dresme@daum.net
* Correspondence: yskwn@catholic.ac.kr
† Running title: Predictors to persistent problematic smartphone use.

Abstract: The clinical course of problematic smartphone use (PSU) remains largely unknown due to a lack of longitudinal studies. We recruited 193 subjects with smartphone addiction problems for the present study. After providing informed consent, the subjects completed surveys and underwent comprehensive interviews regarding smartphone usage. A total of 56 subjects among the 193 initially recruited subjects were followed up for six months. We compared baseline characteristics between persistent addicted users and recovered users at the end of the 6-month follow-up. Persistent problematic smartphone users displayed higher baseline smartphone addiction severity and were more prone to develop mental health problems at the follow-up. However, baseline depressive or anxiety status did not significantly influence the course of PSU. PSU behaved more like an addictive disorder rather than a secondary psychiatric disorder. Harm avoidance, impulsivity, higher Internet use, and less conversation time with mothers were identified as poor prognostic factors in PSU. Lower quality of life, low perceived happiness, and goal instability also contributed to persistent PSU, while recovery increased these scores as well as measures of self-esteem. These findings suggest that the Matthew effect is found in the recovery of PSU with better premorbid psychosocial adjustment leading to a more successful recovery. Greater clinical resources are required for interventions in vulnerable populations to modify the course of this increasingly prevalent problematic behavior worldwide.

Keywords: problematic phone use; internet; pain; dry eye; depression; anxiety; quality of life; recovery; prognosis; cohort

---

1. Introduction

Smartphone use has become an integral part of everyday life. While many conveniences are associated with widespread smartphone use, public health concerns regarding problematic smartphone use (PSU) have also increased over the past decade. In particular, lack of knowledge about the long-term consequences of PSU has raised further concerns in developmental studies of children and adolescents.

Even though connectivity is generally believed to be increased by smartphones, people may also snub others by touching their smartphones rather than engaging in person. This novel type of social exclusion phenomenon is called "phubbing" and was reported to be linked to social anxiety [1]. Thus, we can understand that novel problems may arise following novel technologies.

South Korea reported a smartphone penetration rate of 95% in 2018, the highest in the world [2]. In 2019, a nationally representative survey of South Koreans revealed PSU prevalence of 20.0% across all age groups [3], which corresponds to the global prevalence of 23.3% reported in a recent systemic review [4]. While many reports outline general difficulties in controlling excessive smartphone use, the groups at the highest risk in the 2019 Korean national survey were children and adolescents, with PSU prevalence of 22.9% and 30.2%, respectively [3].

There is contradictory evidence in the literature regarding whether smartphone addiction truly exists [5–7]. PSU is generally not regarded as a serious health issue like substance abuse. In a British survey, the majority of parents report that they do not regulate their children's smartphone time [8].

PSU has been associated with depression, anxiety, aggression, decreased sleep duration/quality, and other addictive behaviors [4,9–14]. It is also related to physical health risks such as dry eye symptoms, musculoskeletal pain, and accidents [15–20]. While such physical problems may arise as a direct consequence of uncontrolled excessive smartphone use, the relationship between psychosocial problems and PSU is yet to be established. For instance, PSU was associated with depression and lower subjective happiness; attention deficit hyperactivity disorder (ADHD) and impulsivity; anxiety, and lower quality of life in cross-sectional studies [10,21,22]. However, it is yet unclear whether such negative mental and behavioral variables act mainly as risk factors that contribute to PSU development or such were derived from PSU as adverse outcomes. To complicate matters, factors such as self-esteem, goal instability, or parent–child relationships may also exert influence over the course of PSU among the developing children and adolescents. To verify their temporal order and relative contributions, well designed longitudinal studies are required.

However, longitudinal studies are scarce, and all existing longitudinal studies recruited convenient samples rather than surveying the clinical population [23–26]. The pre-existing longitudinal studies are limited by drawing conclusions exclusively by conducting surveys on non-clinical convenient samples. Non-clinical samples are more likely to have lower PSU severity and fewer related mental or physical health problems compared to clinical samples [27]. Despite being categorized as smartphone addiction, the severity of the subjects recruited from the non-clinical community settings may have not been severe enough to capture the true clinical picture of the population with clinically significant impairment by PSU.

Together with the lack of any longitudinal studies that demonstrate the diagnostic stability of PSU, the lower severity of the pre-existing studies due to their reliance on non-clinical samples may have contributed to the prior argument that PSU lacks health consequences severe enough to make it a legitimate addictive disorder [5]. Therefore, there is a strong need to investigate the clinical course of PSU in clinical settings and its diagnostic stability in the long term.

The lack of evidence regarding the long-term consequences of PSU is especially alarming since PSU is highly prevalent among children and adolescents [3]. The mental and behavioral consequences of PSU may not only deteriorate current function but may linger through the loss of future opportunities and altered psychosocial development. Furthermore, previous studies indicate that excessive Internet use heightens the risk of substance use [28], and problematic gaming elevates the future risk of developing gambling problems. Addictive use of social media was reported to be related to reduced well-being [29]. These findings demand closer attention to whether PSU occurring during this critical developmental period leads to mental health problems later [30].

The information technologies were suggested to potentially reduce social inequalities by increasing the reachability of information and educational resources to a wider population. However, the "digital divide" created by the disparity in access to online information may further broaden the social health inequalities of our society at the same time [31]. With the growing smartphone penetration around the globe, however, the inequalities by the lack of accessibility will likely decrease. In contrast, other forms of inequalities may emerge due to excessive smartphone use and its long-term consequences.

For instance, children from higher socioeconomic status were more likely to use their digital devices safely while punishing parental attitude was associated with increased risk of PSU [32,33]. While education is generally considered as the "great equalizer", PSU was related to drug consumption and poor academic achievement [34]. The undermined educational opportunity in children and adolescents due to PSU may not only impact their lives in schools but lead to a lifelong socioeconomic disparity through employment and income across the generation by the missed opportunities in the crucial period of development.

"For to everyone who has, more will be given and he will grow rich; but from the one who has not, even what he has will be taken away." (Matthew 25:29) [35]. The Matthew effect, a term derived from the Gospel of Matthew by Merton [36], will also be useful to describe the cumulative disadvantage that may potentially occur when PSU is not properly mitigated in children with individual and environmental vulnerabilities.

Therefore, in this study, we explore the course of PSU and prognostic factors that may influence its course. To the best of our knowledge, this is the first longitudinal study of PSU conducted in a clinical sample. In addition to smartphone-related variables, we performed follow-up measurements of psychosocial variables to determine their contributions to PSU. The identification of risk and prognostic factors related to PSU will facilitate the development of preventive and interventional strategies against this worldwide public health risk among children and adolescents.

2. Materials and Methods

2.1. Study Procedure and Participants

This study was conducted as a part of the clinical Cohort for Understanding of Internet addiction Rescue factors in Early life (c-CURE) study. C-CURE is a multi-center study involving three university hospitals in the Seoul metropolitan area of South Korea that explores risk and protective factors regarding harmful digital media use in children and adolescents. The sample includes subjects who visited the outpatient departments of these hospitals for the treatment of excessive Internet, game, or smartphone use.

After obtaining written informed consent from both participants and their parents/guardians, a brief 15–20 min session of parental coaching was conducted with the additional provision of a 12-page pocket reference outlining parental guidance on digital media use at baseline. The content of the pocket guide includes a parental checklist for children's excessive use, explanation of risk factors (neglect, ADHD, depression, impulse control, and social phobia), explanation of game genres and motivations of children, parenting coaching tips, setting rules, fostering alternative recreational activities, and how to act when childrens relapse (checklist for warning signs, converse more with attentive listening, help children to find other activities that may interest them, provide emotional support, and seek expert's help).

Of the initial 188 participants, we included 85 subjects (64.7% males and 35.3% females) aged between 7 and 18 years old (mean age of 13.2 years old). The inclusion criterion was demonstrating scores equal to or greater than 31 on the smartphone addiction scale-short version (SAS-SV) on the baseline assessment. The subjects were evaluated at three and six months of follow-up.

This study was conducted following the Declaration of Helsinki and was reviewed and approved by the Institutional Review Boards of Uijeongbu St. Mary's Hospital, the Catholic University of Korea (UC15ONMI0072), Seoul Metropolitan Government, Seoul National University Boramae Medical Center (16 April 2016), and Eulji University Seoul Eulji Hospital (EMCS2015-05-020-001).

2.2. Measures

2.2.1. Smartphone Addiction Scale-Short Version (SAS-SV)

This ten-item self-measurement was used to evaluate PSU. It is a shortened version of the original Smartphone addiction scale with 33 items that assess six components of addiction model—excessive use, tolerance, withdrawal, disturbance in daily-life, over-valued online relationship, and positive anticipation [37]. While the first four components correspond to diagnostic criteria of substance use disorder by the 5th edition of Diagnostic and Statistical Manual of Mental Disorders, the last two are unique to smartphone addiction scale.

The SAS-SV is rated on a six-point Likert scale (1 = strongly disagree to 6 = strongly agree) with the total scores ranging from 10 to 60. It questions items such as "Missing planned work due to smartphone use." A higher score indicates greater severity of PSU, and a cutoff score of 31 was used in this study as previously suggested [38]. Cronbach's alpha was 0.63 in this study.

2.2.2. Internet Addiction Test (IAT)

We used the IAT to evaluate the severity of problematic Internet use. It questions items such as "How often do you choose to spend more time online over going out with others?" Rated on a 5-point Likert scale (1 = rarely to 5 = always), this 20 item self-measurement indicates more severe problematic Internet use with increasing scores. Cronbach's alpha was 0.88 in this study.

2.2.3. Survey on the Pattern of Digital-Media Use

Comprehensive surveys were conducted to evaluate digital media use. Participants answered questions about smartphone access such as starting age, average daily time spent on smartphones or the Internet, type of media content, and patterns of use such as bedtime smartphone usage. In addition, participants responded to questions about weight and height for calculating body mass index (BMI) and presence of musculoskeletal pain in the neck, shoulders, and hands/wrists/fingers to assess potential physical consequences of PSU.

2.2.4. Dry Eye Symptoms (DES) Checklist

Questions about dry eye symptoms described jointly by the Korean ministry of health and welfare, the Korean Academy of Medical Science, and the Korean Ophthalmological Society were posed separately to the participants (foreign object sensation in the eyes, heaviness of the eyelid, eye-stiffness, blurry eyes, ocular fatigue, ocular soreness, frequent eye redness, dryness, photosensitivity, ocular pain, and string-like ocular discharge) [39]. The total number of positive responses to the DES checklist was used to measure the severity of DES. Cronbach's alpha was 0.82 in this study.

2.2.5. Junior Temperament Character Inventory (JTCI)

We utilized a child and adolescent version of the Temperament and Character Inventory, which was developed based on the biopsychosocial personality model of Cloninger [40]. The JTCI has been previously validated in Korean [41]. JTCI inventory assesses the four temperament types (novelty seeking, harm avoidance, reward dependence, and persistence) with yes/no responses to the 82 items. As high levels of novelty seeking and harm avoidance are well-known risk factors for addictive disorders such as gaming disorder [42], individual scores were anticipated to shift right in our study subjects. To explore the contributions of these variables within our study sample, individual scores were standardized to T-scores for further analyses.

2.2.6. Depression Assessment

While considering participant age, the 27-item children's depression inventory (CDI) was used to screen for depressive symptoms two weeks prior to assessment in children aged 12 or less. Each item is rated on a 3-point Likert scale from zero to two with descriptive statements such as "I feel sad sometimes, most, or always". Participants with total scores of 22 or greater were classified as having depressive status, as previously suggested in a Korean validation study [43]. Cronbach's alpha was 0.86 in this study.

The Beck Depression Inventory-II (BDI-II) was used to screen for depression in adolescents between 13 and 18 years of age. It contains five subscales of negative mood, interpersonal problems, ineffectiveness, anhedonia, and negative self-esteem. Each item is rated on a 4-point Likert scale from zero to three, and answers refer to the two weeks prior to assessment. It uses descriptions such as "I am so sad and unhappy that I cannot stand it" for each scale. Scores of 10 or greater on this 21-item self-questionnaire were used to identify participants with depression according to Beck [44]. Higher scores indicate more severe depressive symptoms in both tests. Cronbach's alpha was 0.93 in this study.

2.2.7. Anxiety Assessment

The Korean version of the State Anxiety Inventory for Children (SAIC), a part of the State-Trait Anxiety Inventory for Children, was used to assess anxiety in children aged 12 or less. This 20-item inventory includes questions regarding how frequently respondents feel worried, bothered, or nervous on a 3-point Likert scale (1 = almost never to 3 = almost always). With total scores ranging from 20 to 60, higher scores indicate greater anxiety. For this study, we used a score of 41 or higher as a cut-off for defining an anxious state, as previously suggested in a Korean validation study [45]. Cronbach's alpha was 0.81 in this study.

The anxiety levels of adolescents between 13 and 18 years of age were examined with the State-Trait Anxiety Inventory-form X (STAI-X). Scores for this 20-item inventory range from 20 to 80 and the previously-defined cut-off point of 52 was used to classify subjects with high anxiety [46]. Cronbach's alpha was 0.90 in this study.

2.2.8. Barratt Impulsiveness Scale-11 (BIS-11)

The Korean version of the BIS-11, which includes three subcomponents of cognitive, motor, and non-planned impulsivity, was utilized to measure impulsivity [47]. This 23-item self-measurement is rated on a 4-point Likert scale (1 = rarely or never to 4 = almost always or always) with higher scores indicating greater impulsivity [48]. It questions items such as "I say things without thinking." Cronbach's alpha was 0.73 in this study.

2.2.9. Conners-Wells' Adolescent Self-Report Scale-Short Form (CASS-S)

We used the Korean version of the CASS-S, which is a 27-item instrument that assesses ADHD [49]. It is answered on a 4-point Likert scale (0 = not true at all to 3 = very often, very frequently). CASS-S has three subcomponents (conduct problems, cognitive problems, and hyperactivity), with higher scores suggesting more severe ADHD symptoms. CASS-S contains questions such as "I have difficulty sitting still." Cronbach's alpha was 0.83 in this study.

2.2.10. Goal Instability

This inventory was developed from concepts derived from the self-psychology of Heinz Kohut that measure goal-directedness, self-competencies, and career decidedness [50]. Participants responded to the Korean version of the goal instability tool, which includes 10 items rated on a 6-point Likert scale [51]. It questions items such as "I have confusion about who I am." Endorsement of each item results in higher scores, which indicate greater goal instability of the respondents. Cronbach's alpha was 0.88 in this study.

2.2.11. Adolescents Happiness Index (AHI)

We used the 30-item AHI to examine levels of positive emotion and well-being. This inventory is rated on a 4-point Likert scale (1 = strongly disagree to 3 = strongly agree) and has four sub-domains including self-concept, family relationship, leisure, and peer relationship [52]. Higher scores indicate higher levels of happiness. AHI asks questions such as "I am satisfied with myself." Cronbach's alpha was 0.92 in this study.

2.2.12. Rosenberg Self-Esteem Scale (RSES)

Self-esteem was measured using a 10-item scale with each item rated on a 5-point Likert scale (1 = strongly disagree to 5 = strongly agree) [53]. With total scores ranging from 10 to 50, the RSES was developed to measure feelings of self-acceptance, self-respect, and positive evaluation of self. A higher score suggests better self-esteem. RSES contains questions such as "I am able to do things as well as most other people." Cronbach's alpha was 0.84 in this study.

2.2.13. Pediatric Quality of Life (pedsQL)

The pedsQL^{TM} Generic Core 4.0 was used to evaluate the quality of life. This is a 23-item tool with responses on a 5-point Likert scale (conversions 0 = 100, 1 = 75, 2 = 50, 3 = 25, and 4 = 0 scores). The pedsQL has four subcomponents including physical, emotional, social, and academic functioning. Better quality of life is suggested by higher scores [54]. It questions items such as "hard to run" Cronbach's alpha was 0.93 in this study.

2.3. Statistical Analyses

Fifty-six participants remained in the study among the 85 subjects included at baseline, for a follow-up rate of 65.9%. We grouped participants into a persistent group and a recovered group according to SAS-SV scores at the endpoint of 6-month follow-up. Participants whose SAS-SV scores were equal to or greater than 31 were classified in the persistent group, while those with SAS-SV scores less than 31 were considered recovered at the endpoint.

To identify prognostic factors of PSU, baseline sociodemographic and clinical variables between the two groups were compared. In addition, PSU-related variables and psychological variables were compared at 3- and 6-month follow-ups.

Chi-square or Fisher's exact tests were performed for categorical variables. Mann–Whitney U-tests were conducted for continuous variables due to the limit of the final sample size at 6 months. To measure the effect size of PSU to variables at the follow-up, Cohen's d, and Cramer's V were calculated for continuous and categorical variables, respectively. All analyses were performed using SPSS Statistics for Windows, Version 24.0 (IBM Corp., Armonk, NY, USA) with two-tailed statistical significance set at $p = 0.05$.

3. Results

The baseline comparison between the PSU recovered and persistent PSU group was performed for the sociodemographic, smartphone-related, psychological, and physical measures to identify the prognostic factors. In addition, we compared the significant variables identified by the analyses at the baseline at the 3- and 6-month follow-ups to explore the clinical course.

There were no significant demographic differences between the recovered group and the persistent group including age, sex, or socioeconomic status (Table 1). However, the persistent group had fewer conversations with their mothers on weekdays ($p = 0.002$). The persistent group also showed significantly higher PSU at baseline as indicated by SAS-SV scores ($p = 0.043$), the average daily amount of time for mobile/smartphone use on both weekdays ($p = 0.026$) and weekends ($p = 0.037$), and Internet use time on weekdays ($p = 0.044$) (Table 1).

Table 1. Baseline comparison of sociodemographic and smartphone-related measures between recovered and persistent groups.

	Recovered Group (n = 21)	Persistent Group (n = 35)	p
Age (years)	12.2 ± 3.0	13.7 ± 2.5	0.083
Sex			0.822
Male	15 (71.4%)	24 (68.6%)	
Female	6 (28.6%)	11 (31.4%)	
Education status of mother			0.288
High school or lower	13 (61.9%)	22 (75.9%)	
College or higher	8 (38.1%)	7 (24.0%)	
Subjective economic status †			0.537
Low	7 (36.8%)	11 (35.5%)	
Middle	6 (31.6%)	6 (19.4%)	
Upper-middle or above	6 (31.6%)	14 (45.2%)	
Living without father	7 (33.3%)	12 (35.3%)	0.882
Living without mother	0 (0%)	5 (14.7%)	0.065
Conversation time with mother (min)			
Weekday (average)	150.7 ± 166.6	71.7 ± 92.7	0.002 **
Weekend (average)	215.5 ± 327.1	142.8 ± 264.0	0.092
Smartphone use start (age)	8.5 ± 1.5	9.2 ± 2.3	0.369
Ownership of smartphone (+) †	20 (95.2%)	34 (97.1%)	>0.999
Smartphone Addiction Scale-Short	37.1 ± 5.6	40.4 ± 6.0	0.043 *
Internet Addiction Test score	56.2 ± 14.9	60.22 ± 14.7	0.371
Mobile/smartphone use time (min)			
Weekday (average)	202.4 ± 111.8	279.43 ± 146.9	0.026 *
Weekend (average)	299.5 ± 137.5	426.00 ± 226.2	0.037 *
Internet use time (min)			
Weekday (average)	211.4 ± 84.0	282.9 ± 132.2	0.044 *
Weekend (average)	352.9 ± 158.7	444.0 ± 200.2	0.108
Internet content use			
News	9 (42.9%)	11 (31.4%)	0.388
Adult material	3 (14.3%)	12 (34.3%)	0.102
Online game	13 (61.9%)	26 (74.3%)	0.329
Blog	9 (42.9%)	6 (17.1%)	0.035
Social networking service	14 (66.7%)	20 (57.1%)	0.480
Bedtime phone use before sleep (min)	31.4 ± 38.2	57.86 ± 61.1	0.143

† Fisher's exact test; * $p < 0.05$, ** $p < 0.01$.

The online content consumed by the groups differed. The persistent group consumed more adult material, but the difference between groups was not statistically significant. The recovered group was more likely to be involved in blogging ($p = 0.035$).

In the comparison of psychological variables, the two groups did not differ significantly regarding the history of psychiatric disorders, current depression, or current anxiety. However, when stratified by age, younger children (less than 13 years of age) in the persistent group showed significantly higher SAIC scores ($p = 0.035$). Furthermore, the persistent group tended to display higher CDI, but the difference between groups was not significant ($p = 0.06$). While the persistent PSU group had significantly higher levels of harm avoidance ($p = 0.014$), BIS-11 ($p = 0.036$), and goal instability ($p = 0.008$), they had significantly lower pedsQL ($p < 0.001$) and AHI ($p = 0.006$) in the whole group comparison (Table 2).

Table 2. Baseline comparison of psychological and physical measures between recovered and persistent groups.

	Recovered Group (*n* = 21)	**Persistent Group (*n* = 35)**	*p*
Psychological Assessment			
Novelty seeking (T-score)	52.1 ± 8.3	52.0 ± 10.3	0.658
Harm avoidance (T-score)	46.8 ± 12.0	55.8 ± 10.2	0.014 *
History of Psychiatric diagnosis †			
Depression (+)	2 (9.5%)	8 (22.9%)	0.290
Attention deficit hyperactivity disorder (+)	4 (19.0%)	7 (20.0%)	>0.999
Depression (+) status	7 (33.3%)	20 (58.8%)	0.066
CDI (n = 14) ∮	10.6 ± 4.8	18.0 ± 6.9	0.060
BDI (n = 41) ∮	17.3 ± 17.9	18.7 ± 12.8	0.306
Anxiety (+) status †	3 (14.3%)	10 (28.6%)	0.330
SAIC (n = 14) ∮	27.0 ± 3.5	35.2 ± 2.9	0.002 **
STAI-X (n = 42) ∮	43.2 ± 14.9	47.4 ± 13.4	0.355
Barratt Impulsiveness Scale-II	56.1 ± 9.1	61.0 ± 6.9	0.036 *
Goal instability	29.9 ± 13.0	38.9 ± 10.8	0.008 **
CASS-Short form	25.9 ± 9.8	28.8 ± 10.6	0.436
Rosenberg Self-Esteem Scale	27.6 ± 6.4	24.4 ± 5.4	0.100
Quality of life	1911.9 ± 350.3	1472.1 ± 420.4	<0.001 **
Happiness scale	60.1 ± 16.1	49.1 ± 12.9	0.006 **
Physical Assessment			
Body mass index	22.6 ± 5.0	21.9 ± 5.9	0.264
Dry Eye Scale	1.6 ± 2.2	2.2 ± 2.1	0.153
Musculoskeletal pain (+)			
Neck	2 (9.5%)	15 (42.9%)	0.009 **
Shoulder †	1 (4.8%)	9 (25.7%)	0.072
Hand/Wrist/Finger †	2 (9.5%)	7 (20.0%)	0.459

† Fisher's exact test, ∮ Stratified by age as CDI and SAIC ≤ 12; BDI and STAI-X > 12; * $p < 0.05$, ** $p < 0.01$. CDI, Children's Depression Inventory; BDI, Beck Depression Inventory; SAIC, State Anxiety Inventory for Children; STAI-X, State-Trait Anxiety Inventory form X; CASS, Conners-Wells' Adolescent Self-Report Scale.

When examining the physical consequences of PSU, baseline variables such as BMI, DES, shoulder, and hand/wrist/finger pain did not differ between the two groups. However, the symptom presentation of neck pain was significantly higher in persistent problematic users ($p = 0.009$) (Table 2).

In follow-up comparisons of variables that showed significant differences at baseline, BIS-11 and weekday conversation time with the mother did not demonstrate significant differences at follow-up visits. However, the recovered group continued to demonstrate higher pedsQL at both 3- and 6-month follow-ups ($p < 0.001$ for both) and also showed greater AHI at 6-month follow-up ($p = 0.003$). In contrast, the persistent PSU group showed higher goal instability ($p = 0.011$) and neck pain ($p = 0.043$) at the endpoint (Table 3).

The two groups continued to display significant differences in SAS-SV and the daily average amount of time for mobile/smartphone use on both weekdays and weekends, with a steeper reduction in the recovered group. IAT scores, which did not differ between groups at baseline ($p = 0.371$), became significantly different at both 3- and 6-month follow-ups ($p = 0.006$, and $p < 0.001$, respectively) (Figure 1).

Table 3. Follow-up findings of the recovered and persistent groups.

		Recovered Group (n = 21)	Persistent Group (n = 35)	p	Cohens' d
Barratt Impulsiveness Scale-II	3 months	54.3 ± 11.1	57.0 ± 9.3	0.373	0.26
	6 months	53.0 ± 10.1	57.0 ± 8.5	0.1	0.43
Goal instability	3 months	28.2 ± 10.6	33.9 ± 11.5	0.073	0.52
	6 months	25.5 ± 12.1	34.7 ± 13.0	0.011 *	0.73
Quality of life	3 months	1994.1 ± 246.7	1591.7 ± 405.9	<0.001 **	1.2
	6 months	2078.6 ± 271.7	1612.1 ± 451.7	<0.001 **	1.25
Happiness scale	3 months	60.9 ± 16.8	52.0 ± 16.1	0.077	0.54
	6 months	60.7 ± 11.1	50.0 ± 14.2	0.003 **	0.84
					Cramer's V
Neck pain	3 months	3 (14.3%)	8 (24.2%)	0.691 †	0.17 (p = 0.46)
	6 months	2 (10.0%)	10 (35.7%)	0.043 *	0.29 (p = 0.04)

† Fisher's exact test; * $p < 0.05$, ** $p < 0.01$.

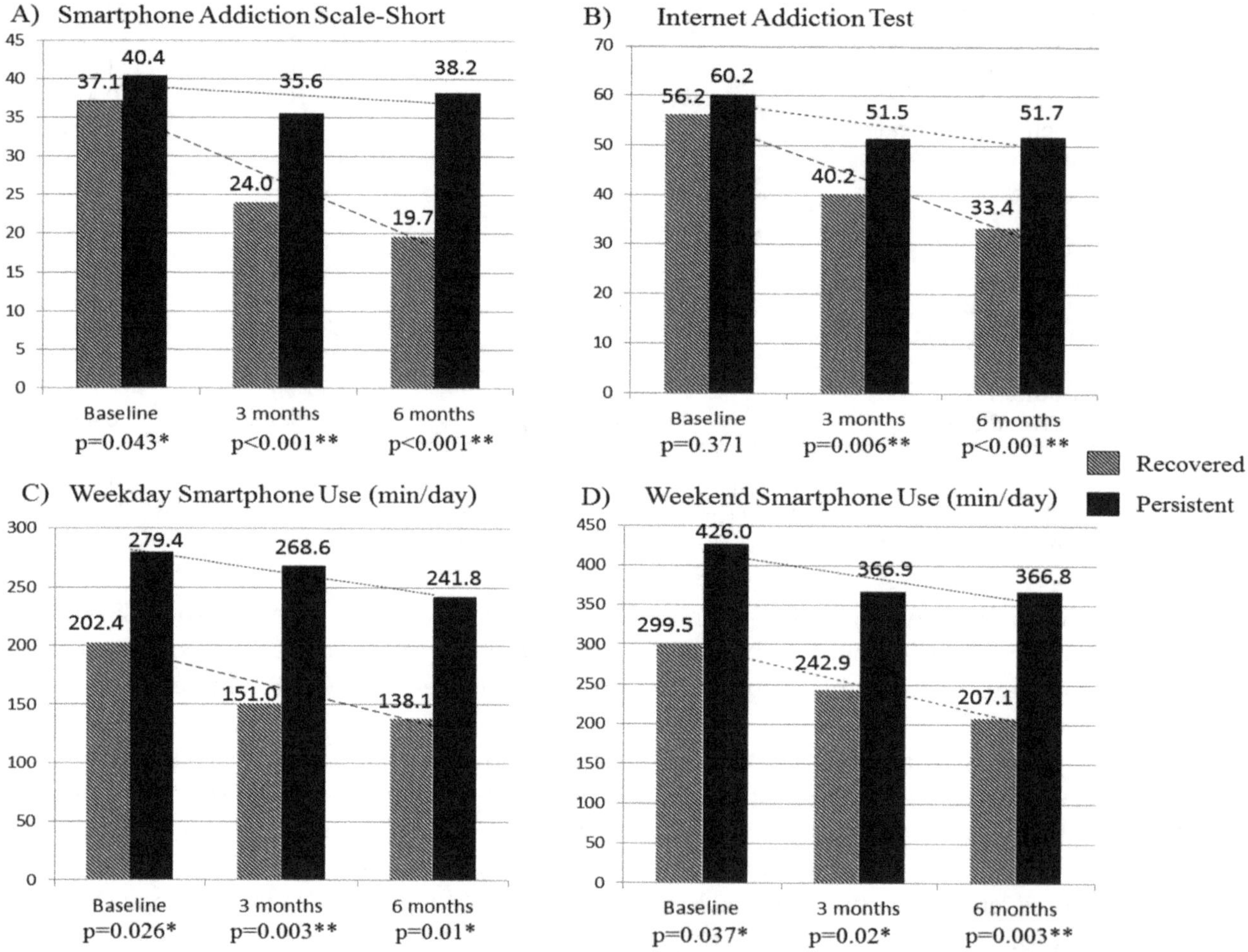

Figure 1. Longitudinal course of smartphone problems by recovery status. * $p < 0.05$, ** $p < 0.01$.

We also conducted analyses at follow-up points of variables that were not significantly different at the baseline. The duration of bedtime phone usage before sleep was significantly lower in the recovered group at both 3- and 6-month follow-ups (p = 0.036, and p = 0.019, respectively). Recovered problematic users were significantly less likely to suffer from DES at 6-month follow-up (p = 0.019). The persistent group, however, was more likely to exhibit depressive and anxious states at 3- and 6-month follow-ups, respectively (Figure 2). RSES, which was not significantly different either at baseline or 3-month follow-up, was significantly different between groups at 6-month follow-up ($p < 0.001$) (Figure 3).

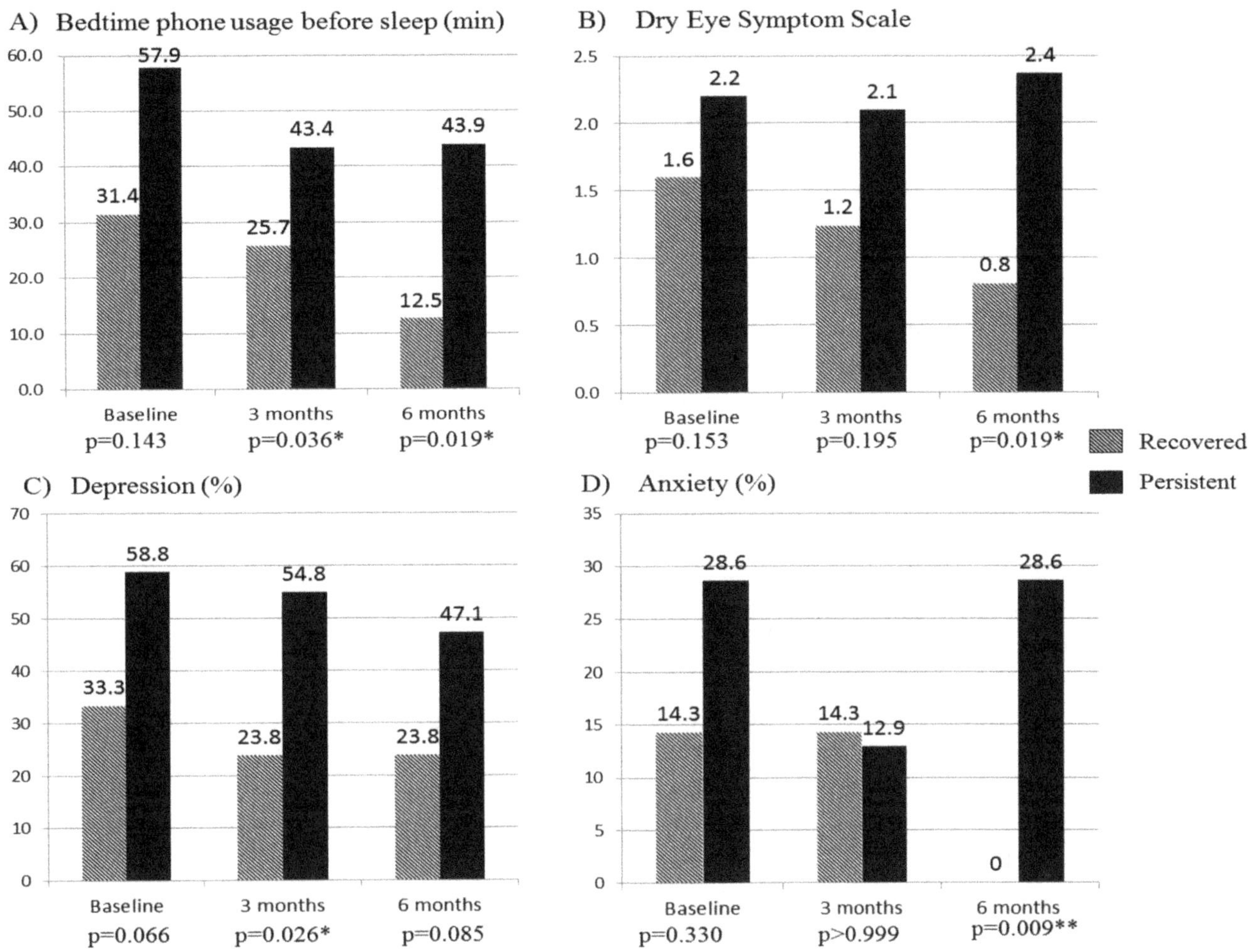

Figure 2. Physical and mental consequences of problematic smartphone use. * $p < 0.05$, ** $p < 0.01$.

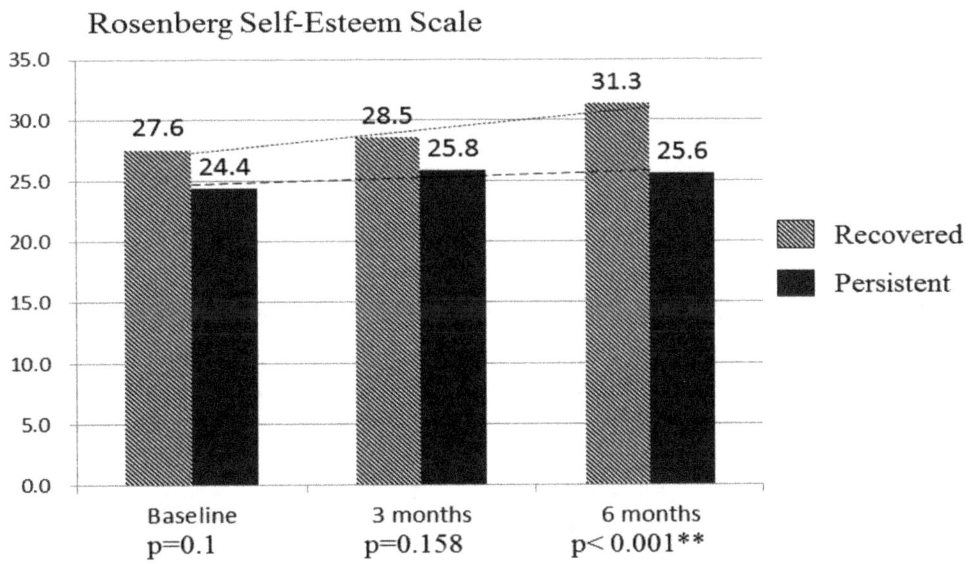

Figure 3. Follow-up comparison of self-esteem between the recovered and the persistent problematic smartphone users. ** $p < 0.01$.

4. Discussion

PSU is increasingly prevalent worldwide. Depression, anxiety, sleep disturbance, poor academic achievement, and physical hazards such as increased risk of accidents, musculoskeletal problems, and ophthalmic problems have been reported in numerous cross-sectional studies [11,12,14–20]. However, the long-term consequences of PSU remain largely unknown. The ever-increasing penetration of smartphones among children and adolescents is particularly alarming since the long-term consequences of PSU on developmental trajectories remain unknown. In addition to direct adverse outcomes on mental or physical health, severely affected children may suffer indirectly by loss of future opportunities through the impoverished acquisition of knowledge or skills during critical periods of development.

The objective of this study was to identify prognostic factors of PSU among children and adolescents. Currently, there are ongoing debates concerning excessive smartphone use, whether it should be considered "addiction" or merely "problematic use" and whether such behavior is "primary" or "secondary". Therefore, we also attempted to explore the temporal relationships between PSU and psychiatric problems, in addition to exploring the clinical course of PSU.

While there were no significant differences between the recovered group and the persistent PSU group in terms of psychiatric diagnosis, depression, or anxiety scores at baseline (Table 2), the persistent problematic smartphone users displayed a significantly higher rate of depression at 3-month follow-up and a significantly higher rate of anxiety at 6-month follow-up (Figure 2). Therefore, our findings support the designation of PSU as a primary disorder rather than a secondary phenomenon following negative emotional experiences in the clinical population. On the contrary, greater depressive or anxiety symptoms displayed by the PSU persistence suggest that adverse psychiatric consequences may develop unless PSU is adequately managed.

Although no significant differences were found in the whole group comparison, the anxiety level was significantly higher in children with persistent PSU aged 12 or less. Furthermore, although the difference was not statistically significant, a similar tendency was observed for depressive status in this younger group. These findings suggest that smartphones may serve as a compensatory measure against negative emotional experiences in younger children. Thus, PSU may also occur as a secondary disorder in young children. However, to confirm such a hypothesis, these findings should be replicated in a larger sample. When PSU is reported in children, considering both age and the context of use may help clinicians to understand the relationship between PSU and mental health.

The psychosocial vulnerabilities associated with persistent PSU at baseline were less conversation time with mothers, goal instability, low quality of life, lower level of perceived happiness, harm avoidance, and impulsivity (Table 2).

Parents exert significant influence over the development of their children. Parental perception of the social media use and parent–child interaction insecure attachment have been suggested as a major risk factors for addictive disorders [55], and punishing parental attitude was previously reported to be related to PSU [33]. Less conversation time with mothers may indicate weaker mother–child relationships. The lack of maternal protective factor was found to significantly increase the risk of continued problematic use of smartphones in this study. Despite not reaching a statistically significant level ($p = 0.065$), the persistent group was more likely to be living without their mothers, and it is in line with the aforementioned finding. Our finding is in line with the previous literature. In a large study of Chinese adolescents, mother–child relationships exerted more significant influence on problematic internet use than father–child relationships, and separated or "left-behind adolescents" were associated with subcomponents of problematic internet use [56].

The persistent PSU group showed lower quality of life and happiness but greater goal instability at baseline as well as at follow-up (Table 3). Further studies are indicated to investigate whether recovery from PSU by active therapeutic intervention also improves the quality of life, perceived happiness, and goal instability.

In short, the likelihood of recovery from PSU was higher among happy children with less goal instability, who interacted more with their mothers and enjoyed a better quality of life. The recovered users also spent significantly less time using smartphones at follow-up. Rosenberg Self-Esteem Scale scores, which demonstrated no significant differences at baseline, significantly increased at the endpoint among recovered participants (Figure 3). This indicates that recovered participants also exhibited increased self-esteem at 6-month follow-up.

The Matthew effect, which describes a psychosocial phenomenon of deepening inequality in which the rich become richer while the poor become even poorer [36], is thereby seen in the recovery process of PSU. The chance of recovery from PSU was lower in children with psychosocial disadvantages. PSU is likely to further widen the gap between children with psychological vulnerabilities or unfavorable family backgrounds and those without. The persistence of PSU may exert a significant influence over the developmental trajectory of self-esteem. While the self-esteem of the recovered children is boosted by the recognition of their success in achieving the recovery and better psychosocial outcomes such as higher quality of life and subjective happiness, the children with persistent PSU are more likely to fall behind in other important areas such as socialization and academic performance. Therefore, greater clinical attention and more intensive resources should be offered to PSU subjects with higher risk factor burdens.

Harm-avoidant temperament and impulsivity are well-known risk factors of PSU and other addictive disorders [12,42,57,58]. These risk factors may act as biological vulnerabilities to PSU. A previous structural imaging study demonstrated a significantly lower gray matter volume of the orbitofrontal cortex, an important structure involved in impulse control, in subjects with PSU compared to normal smartphone users [59]. These findings indicate shared mechanisms underlying PSU and addictive disorders. Further neurobiological studies are required to confirm the potential mechanism. Even though the impulsivity scores were higher in the persistent group throughout the follow-up, statistical significance was not sustained in the follow-up unlike the baseline. Therefore, further studies with a large sample size are required to determine whether impulsivity as a trait has a prognostic value. Another finding suggesting the addictive nature of PSU is the demonstrated prognostic value of PSU severity. Persistent problematic smartphone users demonstrated significantly higher initial PSU severity and spent greater amounts of time using smartphones, findings that are in line with those of a previous longitudinal study [24]. The fact that PSU severity per se at baseline, but not mental health problems, exert significant influence on the clinical course highlights the possibility that addiction plays a key role in PSU.

When participants with PSU were followed for 6 months, the majority (62.5%) continued to demonstrate problematic patterns of smartphone use. This finding suggests that the clinical course of PSU is stable over time and that more active management than parental education is needed to modify its course. The demonstrated diagnostic stability of PSU suggests that it may not be a benign behavioral problem lasting only temporarily.

Comparisons between the recovered group and the persistent group in this study demonstrated various physical consequences of PSU. Those with persistent smartphone problems were more likely to display neck pain not only at baseline but also at 6-month follow-up, which is in line with previous findings in the literature [16,19]. Considering that shoulder and hand/wrist/finger pain did not differ between the two groups, the assessment of neck pain seems to be the most clinically useful musculoskeletal symptom to screen for PSU and to monitor as a sign of PSU recovery.

Although no significant difference was observed at the baseline, the persistent group also showed significantly higher DES at the endpoint (Figure 2). In cross-sectional studies, longer smartphone usage was reported to be associated with DES [15,18]. This study is the first longitudinal study to demonstrate the development of DES as a consequence of persistent PSU.

Another longitudinal study previously showed that smartphone owners sleep significantly less during follow-up than subjects who do not own smartphones [60]. Exposure to blue light from smartphones at night was associated with disruptions of circadian rhythms and decreased performance at attentional tasks [61]. We found that the recovered group spent significantly less time using smartphones at bedtime at 3- and 6-month follow-ups. Therefore, bedtime smartphone usage should be evaluated in subjects with PSU to better manage potential sleep problems or difficulty concentrating in the daytime.

The two groups in this study were compared in the context of online content consumption. The consumption of adult material tended to be higher in the persistent group, but the difference was not statistically significant. However, the recovered group was more likely to engage in blogging. Still, it is too early to conclude that blogging is protective against PSU persistence. Maintaining a blog often involves sharing information such as the bloggers' point of view, and it usually requires more time to write a blog than to write on social networking services such as Instagram. Therefore, bloggers may display lower harm avoidance or impulsivity. Further studies are needed to verify whether recovery is facilitated by such individual traits or actually by the maintenance of blogs.

To summarize, the results of our study support the application of the addiction model to PSU. PSU severity but not psychiatric comorbidity increased the risk of persistent PSU. Moreover, children and adolescents were more likely to develop physical and mental health problems with persistent problematic smartphone use. PSU not only showed characteristics of a primary disorder but also demonstrated diagnostic stability. As PSU shares common risk factors with addictive disorders such as impulsivity and harm avoidance, it manifests characteristics of addiction. However, it was previously argued that PSU is not an addictive disorder [5].

Several factors may have contributed to the traditional view. First, the traditional view was drawn from studies that utilized convenient samples and cross-sectional designs. To the best of our knowledge, the present study is the first longitudinal study conducted in clinical settings. The severity of problematic smartphone use in the non-clinical population is likely to be lower than in the clinical population, with higher self-remission. Therefore, the benign nature of PSU in the non-clinical population may have played a role in the formulation of such a benign view. In addition to differences in severity, the wide use of smartphones in everyday life may also make researchers more reluctant to label PSU as addictive behavior, in a desire to avoid criticism due to pathologizing and medicalizing daily behaviors. Even though we are also against pathologizing the simple overuse of smartphones by referring to it as an addictive disorder, PSU may have a wide spectrum in terms of severity and longitudinal course. Heavy users at the end of the continuum may display clinical characteristics resembling those of addicts. For such users, broader management options should be available, and the allocation of greater therapeutic resources will be required to improve clinical outcomes.

The strength of our study lies in its comprehensive assessment of demographic, psychosocial, and digital media-related risk factors. However, this study also has some limitations. While the majority of participants were followed throughout the study period, a substantial number (34.1%) dropped out at the 6-month follow-up. We conducted secondary analyses comparing the completed group and dropouts. There were no significant differences in demographics between groups. However, the baseline SAS-SV scores of the dropouts were significantly lower compared to the participants that remained in the study. Subjects with lower PSU severity may have been less motivated to continue the study.

Although our sample size is relatively large compared to those of other longitudinal studies, we were unable to perform parametric analyses for continuous variables due to the sample size. Lack of such analyses generally leads to a loss in statistical power, and small potential differences that otherwise might have been detected in parametric analyses may not have been found in the non-parametric analyses. Another limitation is the lack of objective measurements to validate the responses of the participants. Although the participants were reassured regarding the confidentiality of assessments to parents or guardians unless immediate harm was anticipated, the reliance on self-reports may result in an under-estimation of problems or severity. Significant discordance was reported between self-reported and clinician-rated severity of problematic gaming in a previous study [62]. Social desirability is known to contribute to under-reporting of deviant or socially undesirable behaviors [63]. Therefore, the utilization of objective measures such as smartphone applications that analyze patterns of use is required to manage the potential for under-reported PSU in children and adolescents.

5. Conclusions

In this longitudinal study, diagnostic stability was observed for PSU, with the majority of participants displaying persistent PSU six months after the beginning of the study. Prognostic factors of PSU were individual traits such as harm avoidance and impulsivity; psychological vulnerabilities such as high SAS-SV, low quality of life, low perceived happiness, and goal instability; and social risk factors such as shorter weekday conversations with mothers. We suggest that the bio-psychosocial framework could be useful in the evaluation of PSU and in predicting its course. The exploration of causality between PSU and psychiatric problems showed that PSU increased the risk of developing psychiatric problems later, which supports the interpretation of PSU as a primary disorder. While the recovered group demonstrated fewer psychological risk factors at baseline than persistent problematic users, they also benefited from further gains in psychological well-being and were less afflicted by physical consequences. This Matthew effect in the recovery of PSU calls for additional attention to be paid to disadvantaged children or adolescents with PSU, to better facilitate their recovery and reduce the harmful long-term consequences of PSU as a secondary prevention strategy.

Author Contributions: S.-Y.L. analyzed and interpreted the data and drafted the manuscript; J.-S.C., S.-y.B. and Y.-S.K. participated in the recruiting and data collection; H.K.L., and Y.-S.K. developed concepts and supervised; M.-H.P., and K.-I.J. reviewed and edited the manuscript. All authors have read and agree to the published version of the manuscript.

Acknowledgments: This study was supported by a grant of the Korean Mental Health Technology R&D Project, Ministry of Health & Welfare, Republic of Korea (HM14C2603).

References

1. Guazzini, A.; Duradoni, M.; Capelli, A.; Meringolo, P. An Explorative Model to Assess Individuals' Phubbing Risk. *Future Internet* **2019**, *11*, 21. [CrossRef]
2. O'Dea, S. Smartphone Penetration Rate by Country 2018. Available online: https://www.statista.com/statistics/539395/smartphone-penetration-worldwide-by-country/ (accessed on 4 April 2020).
3. Ministry of Science and ICT; National Information Society Agency. 2019 The Survey on Smartphone Overdependence. 2020. Available online: https://www.nia.or.kr/site/nia_kor/ex/bbs/View.do?cbIdx=65914&bcIdx=21939&parentSeq=21939 (accessed on 1 May 2020).
4. Sohn, S.; Rees, P.; Wildridge, B.; Kalk, N.J.; Carter, B. Prevalence of problematic smartphone usage and associated mental health outcomes amongst children and young people: A systematic review, meta-analysis and GRADE of the evidence. *BMC Psychiatry* **2019**, *19*, 356. [CrossRef]
5. Panova, T.; Carbonell, X. Is smartphone addiction really an addiction? *J. Behav. Addict.* **2018**, *7*, 252–259. [CrossRef]
6. Yu, S.; Sussman, S. Does Smartphone Addiction Fall on a Continuum of Addictive Behaviors? *Int. J. Environ. Res. Public Health* **2020**, *17*, 422. [CrossRef] [PubMed]
7. Elhai, J.D.; Levine, J.C.; Hall, B.J. The relationship between anxiety symptom severity and problematic smartphone use: A review of the literature and conceptual frameworks. *J. Anxiety Disord.* **2019**, *62*, 45–52. [CrossRef] [PubMed]
8. Quarter of Children Under Six Have A Smartphone, Study Finds. Agency reporter, 8 April 2018.
9. Beyens, I.; Nathanson, A.I. Electronic Media Use and Sleep Among Preschoolers: Evidence for Time-Shifted and Less Consolidated Sleep. *Health Commun.* **2019**, *34*, 537–544. [CrossRef]
10. Grant, J.E.; Lust, K.; Chamberlain, S.R. Problematic smartphone use associated with greater alcohol consumption, mental health issues, poorer academic performance, and impulsivity. *J. Behav. Addict.* **2019**, *8*, 335–342. [CrossRef]

11. Kim, Y.J.; Jang, H.M.; Lee, Y.; Lee, D.; Kim, D.J. Effects of Internet and Smartphone Addictions on Depression and Anxiety Based on Propensity Score Matching Analysis. *Int. J. Environ. Res. Public Health* **2018**, *15*, 859. [CrossRef]
12. Lee, S.Y.; Lee, D.; Nam, C.R.; Kim, D.Y.; Park, S.; Kwon, J.G.; Kweon, Y.S.; Lee, Y.; Kim, D.J.; Choi, J.S. Distinct patterns of Internet and smartphone-related problems among adolescents by gender: Latent class analysis. *J. Behav. Addict.* **2018**, *7*, 454–465. [CrossRef]
13. Yang, J.; Fu, X.; Liao, X.; Li, Y. Association of problematic smartphone use with poor sleep quality, depression, and anxiety: A systematic review and meta-analysis. *Psychiatry Res.* **2020**, *284*, 112686. [CrossRef]
14. Vahedi, Z.; Saiphoo, A. The association between smartphone use, stress, and anxiety: A meta-analytic review. *Stress Health J. Int. Soc. Investig. Stress* **2018**, *34*, 347–358. [CrossRef] [PubMed]
15. Moon, J.H.; Kim, K.W.; Moon, N.J. Smartphone use is a risk factor for pediatric dry eye disease according to region and age: A case control study. *Bmc Ophthalmol.* **2016**, *16*, 188. [CrossRef]
16. Lee, S.; Choi, Y.H.; Kim, J. Effects of the cervical flexion angle during smartphone use on muscle fatigue and pain in the cervical erector spinae and upper trapezius in normal adults in their 20s. *J. Phys. Ther. Sci.* **2017**, *29*, 921–923. [CrossRef]
17. Eitivipart, A.C.; Viriyarojanakul, S.; Redhead, L. Musculoskeletal disorder and pain associated with smartphone use: A systematic review of biomechanical evidence. *Hong Kong Physiother. J. Off. Publ. Hong Kong Physiother. Assoc. Ltd. Wu Li Chih Liao* **2018**, *38*, 77–90. [CrossRef] [PubMed]
18. Choi, J.H.; Li, Y.; Kim, S.H.; Jin, R.; Kim, Y.H.; Choi, W.; You, I.C.; Yoon, K.C. The influences of smartphone use on the status of the tear film and ocular surface. *PLoS ONE* **2018**, *13*, e0206541. [CrossRef] [PubMed]
19. Alsalameh, A.M.; Harisi, M.J.; Alduayji, M.A.; Almutham, A.A.; Mahmood, F.M. Evaluating the relationship between smartphone addiction/overuse and musculoskeletal pain among medical students at Qassim University. *J. Fam. Med. Prim. Care* **2019**, *8*, 2953–2959. [CrossRef]
20. Kim, H.J.; Min, J.Y.; Kim, H.J.; Min, K.B. Accident risk associated with smartphone addiction: A study on university students in Korea. *J. Behav. Addict.* **2017**, *6*, 699–707. [CrossRef]
21. Guo, N.; Luk, T.T.; Ho, S.Y.; Lee, J.J.; Shen, C.; Oliffe, J.; Chan, S.S.; Lam, T.H.; Wang, M.P. Problematic Smartphone Use and Mental Health in Chinese Adults: A Population-Based Study. *Int. J. Environ. Res. Public Health* **2020**, *17*, 844. [CrossRef] [PubMed]
22. Gao, Q.; Sun, R.; Fu, E.; Jia, G.; Xiang, Y. Parent-child relationship and smartphone use disorder among Chinese adolescents: The mediating role of quality of life and the moderating role of educational level. *Addict. Behav.* **2020**, *101*, 106065. [CrossRef] [PubMed]
23. Karsay, K.; Schmuck, D.; Matthes, J.; Stevic, A. Longitudinal Effects of Excessive Smartphone Use on Stress and Loneliness: The Moderating Role of Self-Disclosure. *Cyberpsychology Behav. Soc. Netw.* **2019**, *22*, 706–713. [CrossRef] [PubMed]
24. Lapierre, M.A.; Zhao, P.; Custer, B.E. Short-Term Longitudinal Relationships Between Smartphone Use/Dependency and Psychological Well-Being Among Late Adolescents. *J. Adolesc. Health Off. Publ. Soc. Adolesc. Med.* **2019**, *65*, 607–612. [CrossRef]
25. Lee, J.E.; Jang, S.-I.; Ju, Y.J.; Kim, W.; Lee, H.J.; Park, E.-C. Relationship between Mobile Phone Addiction and the Incidence of Poor and Short Sleep among Korean Adolescents: A Longitudinal Study of the Korean Children & Youth Panel Survey. *J. Korean Med. Sci.* **2017**, *32*, 1166–1172.
26. Tossell, C.; Kortum, P.; Shepard, C.; Rahmati, A.; Zhong, L. Exploring Smartphone Addiction: Insights from Long-Term Telemetric Behavioral Measures. *Int. J. Interact. Mob. Technol.* **2015**, *9*, 7. [CrossRef]
27. Feliciano, L.; Yochim, B.; Steers, M.E.; Jay, A.A.; Segal, D.L. *Understanding Research in Clinical and Counseling Psychology*, 2nd ed.; Jay, C., Hersen, T.M., Eds.; Routledge Taylor & Francis: New York, NY, USA, 2011.
28. Lee, B.H.; Lee, H.K. Longitudinal study shows that addictive Internet use during adolescence was associated with heavy drinking and smoking cigarettes in early adulthood. *Acta Paediatrica (Oslo Norway 1992)* **2017**, *106*, 497–502. [CrossRef]
29. Duradoni, M.; Innocenti, F.; Guazzini, A. Well-Being and Social Media: A Systematic Review of Bergen Addiction Scales. *Future Internet* **2020**, *12*, 24. [CrossRef]
30. Vadlin, S.; Aslund, C.; Nilsson, K.W. A longitudinal study of the individual—And group-level problematic gaming and associations with problem gambling among Swedish adolescents. *Brain Behav.* **2018**, *8*, e00949. [CrossRef]

31. Latulippe, K.; Hamel, C.; Giroux, D. Social Health Inequalities and eHealth: A Literature Review with Qualitative Synthesis of Theoretical and Empirical Studies. *J. Med. Internet Res.* **2017**, *19*, e136. [CrossRef]
32. Wang, X.; Xing, W. Exploring the Influence of Parental Involvement and Socioeconomic Status on Teen Digital Citizenship: A Path Modeling Approach. *J. Educ. Technol. Soc.* **2018**, *21*, 186–199.
33. Lee, H.; Kim, J.W.; Choi, T.Y. Risk Factors for Smartphone Addiction in Korean Adolescents: Smartphone Use Patterns. *J. Korean Med. Sci.* **2017**, *32*, 1674–1679. [CrossRef]
34. Muñoz-Miralles, R.; Ortega-González, R.; López-Morón, M.R.; Batalla-Martínez, C.; Manresa, J.M.; Montellà-Jordana, N.; Chamarro, A.; Carbonell, X.; Torán-Monserrat, P. The problematic use of Information and Communication Technologies (ICT) in adolescents by the cross sectional JOITIC study. *BMC Pediatr.* **2016**, *16*, 140. [CrossRef]
35. United States Conference of Catholic Bishops Matthew 25:29. Available online: http://www.usccb.org/bible/mt/25:29 (accessed on 5 May 2020).
36. Merton, R.K. The Matthew effect in science: The reward and communication systems of science are considered. *Science* **1968**, *159*, 56–63. [CrossRef] [PubMed]
37. Kwon, M.; Lee, J.-Y.; Won, W.-Y.; Park, J.-W.; Min, J.-A.; Hahn, C.; Gu, X.; Choi, J.-H.; Kim, D.-J. Development and Validation of a Smartphone Addiction Scale (SAS). *PLoS ONE* **2013**, *8*, e56936. [CrossRef] [PubMed]
38. Kwon, M.; Kim, D.J.; Cho, H.; Yang, S. The smartphone addiction scale: Development and validation of a short version for adolescents. *PLoS ONE* **2013**, *8*, e83558. [CrossRef] [PubMed]
39. Ministry of Health & Welfare; Korean Academy of Medical Science; Korean Ophthalmological Society. The Symptoms and Complications of Dry Eye Syndrome. Available online: http://health.cdc.go.kr/health/mobileweb/content/group_view.jsp?CID=F98951A125 (accessed on 1 March 2020).
40. Cloninger, C.R.; Svrakic, D.M.; Przybeck, T.R. A psychobiological model of temperament and character. *Arch. Gen. Psychiatry* **1993**, *50*, 975–990. [CrossRef]
41. Lyoo, I.K.; Han, C.H.; Lee, S.J.; Yune, S.K.; Ha, J.H.; Chung, S.J.; Choi, H.; Seo, C.S.; Hong, K.E. The reliability and validity of the junior temperament and character inventory. *Compr. Psychiatry* **2004**, *45*, 121–128. [CrossRef]
42. Jeong, H.; Lee, H.K.; Kwon, Y.-S.; Yim, H.W.; Lee, S.-Y. Gaming disorder and bidirectional relationships with aggression and impulsivity. *Curr. Opin. Behav. Sci.* **2020**, *31*, 69–75. [CrossRef]
43. Cho, S.C.; Lee, Y.S. Development of the Korean form of the Kovacs' Childeren's Depression Inventory. *J. Korean Neuropsychiatr. Assoc.* **1990**, *29*, 943–956.
44. Beck, A.; Steer, R.; Brown, G. Manual for the Beck depression inventory-II (BDI-II). *Behav. Res. Ther.* **1996**, *37*, 183–190.
45. Cho, S.C.; Choi, C.J. Development of the Korean form of the State-Trait anxiety Inventory for Children. *Seoul J. Psychiatry* **1989**, *14*, 150–157.
46. Kim, J.T. *Relationship between State-Train Anxiety and Socializing*; Korea University: Seoul, Korea, 1978.
47. Patton, J.H.; Stanford, M.S.; Barratt, E.S. Factor structure of the Barratt impulsiveness scale. *J. Clin. Psychol.* **1995**, *51*, 768–774. [CrossRef]
48. HS, L. *Manual for Impulsivity Test*; Guidance Korea: Seong Nam, Korea, 1992.
49. Bahn, G.H.; Shin, M.S.; Cho, S.C.; Hong, K.E. A Preliminary Study For The Development Of The Assessment Scale For Adhd In Adolescents:Reliability And Validity For Cass(S). *J. Korean Acad. Child Adolesc. Psychiatry* **2001**, *12*, 218–224.
50. Robbins, S.B.; Payne, E.C.; Chartrand, J.M. Goal instability and later life adjustment. *Psychol. Aging* **1990**, *5*, 447–450. [CrossRef]
51. Lee, E.H. The role of goal instability and resolving style of problems between nurses' job stressors and emotional exhaustion. *Korean J. Woman Psychol.* **2008**, *13*, 397–413. [CrossRef]
52. Kim, B.H.; Bang, S.Y.; Lee, H.K.; Cho, S.S.; Choi, S.; Ryu, C.S. *Developing and Study of happiness index of Korean Adolescents*; Happy Home Foundation: Seoul, Korea, 2007.
53. Rosenberg, M. *Society and the Adolescent Self-Image*; Princeton University Press: Princeton, NJ, USA, 1965.
54. Choi, E.S. Psychometric test of the PedsQLTM 4.0 Generic Core Scale in Korean adolescents. 2004. Available online: http://dcollection.yonsei.ac.kr/public_resource/pdf/000000125930_20200701160223.pdf (accessed on 3 May 2020).

55. Nakhoul, L.; Obeid, S.; Sacre, H.; Haddad, C.; Soufia, M.; Hallit, R.; Akel, M.; Salameh, P.; Hallit, S. Attachment style and addictions (alcohol, cigarette, waterpipe and internet) among Lebanese adolescents: A national study. *BMC Psychol.* **2020**, *8*, 33. [CrossRef] [PubMed]
56. Xu, J.; Shen, L.X.; Yan, C.H.; Hu, H.; Yang, F.; Wang, L.; Kotha, S.R.; Ouyang, F.; Zhang, L.N.; Liao, X.P.; et al. Parent-adolescent interaction and risk of adolescent internet addiction: A population-based study in Shanghai. *BMC Psychiatry* **2014**, *14*, 112. [CrossRef] [PubMed]
57. Hanafi, E.; Siste, K.; Wiguna, T.; Kusumadewi, I.; Nasrun, M.W. Temperament profile and its association with the vulnerability to smartphone addiction of medical students in Indonesia. *PLoS ONE* **2019**, *14*, e0212244. [CrossRef]
58. Alvarez, A.; Avila, J.J.; Palao, D.J.; Montejo, A.L. Influence of Personality Traits on the Severity of Alcohol Use Disorders. *J. Clin. Med.* **2018**, *7*, 127. [CrossRef]
59. Lee, D.; Namkoong, K.; Lee, J.; Lee, B.O.; Jung, Y.C. Lateral orbitofrontal gray matter abnormalities in subjects with problematic smartphone use. *J. Behav. Addict.* **2019**, *8*, 404–411. [CrossRef]
60. Schweizer, A.; Berchtold, A.; Barrense-Dias, Y.; Akre, C.; Suris, J.C. Adolescents with a smartphone sleep less than their peers. *Eur. J. Pediatr.* **2017**, *176*, 131–136. [CrossRef]
61. Heo, J.Y.; Kim, K.; Fava, M.; Mischoulon, D.; Papakostas, G.I.; Kim, M.J.; Kim, D.J.; Chang, K.J.; Oh, Y.; Yu, B.H.; et al. Effects of smartphone use with and without blue light at night in healthy adults: A randomized, double-blind, cross-over, placebo-controlled comparison. *J. Psychiatr. Res.* **2017**, *87*, 61–70. [CrossRef]
62. Jeong, H.; Yim, H.W.; Lee, S.Y.; Lee, H.K.; Potenza, M.N.; Kwon, J.H.; Koo, H.J.; Kweon, Y.S.; Bhang, S.Y.; Choi, J.S. Discordance between self-report and clinical diagnosis of Internet gaming disorder in adolescents. *Sci. Rep.* **2018**, *8*, 10084. [CrossRef] [PubMed]
63. Johnson, T.; Fendrich, M. Modeling sources of self-report bias in a survey of drug use epidemiology. *Ann. Epidemiol.* **2005**, *15*, 381–389. [CrossRef] [PubMed]

7

Associations Among Resilience, Stress, Depression and Internet Gaming Disorder in Young Adults

Ju-Yu Yen [1,2], Huang-Chi Lin [1,3], Wei-Po Chou [3], Tai-Ling Liu [3] and Chih-Hung Ko [3,4,5,*]

1 Department of Psychiatry, Faculty of Medicine, College of Medicine, Kaohsiung Medical University, Kaohsiung City 807, Taiwan
2 Department of Psychiatry, Kaohsiung Municipal Ta-Tung Hospital, Kaohsiung Medical University, Kaohsiung City 812, Taiwan
3 Department of Psychiatry, Kaohsiung Medical University Hospital, Kaohsiung Medical University, Kaohsiung City 807, Taiwan
4 Department of Psychiatry, Kaohsiung Municipal Siaogang Hospital, Kaohsiung Medical University, Kaohsiung 801, Taiwan
5 Substance and Behavior addiction Research Center, Kaohsiung Medical University, Kaohsiung City 807, Taiwan
* Correspondence: chihhungko@gmail.com or cyberko@seed.net.tw

Abstract: *Background and Aims*: Using gaming to escape emotional difficulty has been suggested to be a candidate mechanism contributing to Internet gaming disorder (IGD). This study evaluated the associations among resilience, perceived stress, depression, and IGD. *Methods*: A total of 87 participants in an IGD group and 87 participants in a control group were recruited into this study. IGD was diagnosed using the Diagnostic and Statistical Manual of Mental Disorders. Stress levels, resilience, and depression were measured by a self-reported questionnaire. *Results*: The IGD group had a lower resilience, higher perceived stress, and depression than the control group. Hierarchical regression analysis demonstrated that resilience was associated with IGD when perceived stress was controlled. After depression was controlled, resilience and perceived stress were not associated with IGD. Among the IGD group, those with low resilience had higher depression. Furthermore, discipline was the resilience characteristic associated with IGD. *Conclusions*: Low resilience was associated with a higher risk of IGD. IGD individuals with low resilience had higher depression. Depression was more associated with IGD than resilience. Depression assessments and stress coping interventions should be provided for individuals with IGD who exhibit low resilience or high stress.

Keywords: internet gaming disorder; stress; resilience; escape; depression

---

1. Introduction

Internet gaming disorder (IGD) has been identified as a potential psychiatric disorder because of its negative effects on multiple domains of functioning [1–3]. The international prevalence ranges from 0.3% to 12%, and it is an increasing public health concern, especially in Asian countries. As well as cognitive and behavioral symptoms similar to those of substance-use disorder, IGD also reportedly has associations with psychiatric symptoms, including attention-deficit hyperactivity disorder, depression, anxiety, and psychosomatic symptoms [4–7]. High comorbidity of emotional symptoms suggests that individuals with IGD might use gaming to escape emotional difficulties [8,9].

Addictive behaviors are often initiated as a maladaptive mechanism for coping with stress [10]. Stress may enhance abstinent individuals' memories of addictive behaviors as stress relievers then increase the risk of relapse to addictive behaviors after abstinence [11]. Tao et al. [12] were first to use the escape from stress through gaming as a criterion for Internet addiction. It was subsequently listed as a diagnostic criterion for IGD in the Diagnostic and Statistical Manual of Mental Disorders (DSM-5) [13]. "Negative escapism" describes gaming being negatively reinforced as a means of avoiding stress and was reported among 77.8% of internalizing patients [14]. Kim et al. [6] found escape from negative emotions to be associated with depression in IGD [9]. Furthermore, high levels of escapism were also reported to be associated with more IGD symptoms [15]. Moreover, the motives for escapism mediate the association between psychiatric distress and problematic online gaming [16]. Thus, negative escapism is associated with the symptoms of Internet addiction, psychological distress, and poor life satisfaction among massively multiplayer online role-playing gamers [17], and escapism under stress could play a major role in excessive gaming behavior.

Convincing evidence indicates that stress is a risk factor for addiction and triggers relapses [18]. The negative reinforcement model of addiction is defined as drug-taking or addictive behavior that alleviates a negative emotional state. According to some hypotheses, the negative emotional state that drives such behaviors as negative reinforcement is derived from dysregulation of brain stress systems involved in addiction processes [19]. Thus, investigating the perceived stress among adults with IGD could contribute to understanding its role in developing addictive online gaming behavior.

Not all individuals who face stress develop addictions. Therefore, resilience factors may protect these mentally healthy individuals [20]. For example, psychosocial resilience, such as positive emotions, optimism, humor, cognitive flexibility, and reappraisal could attenuate stress-induced psychopathology [21]. Thus, resilience was reported to be a buffering factor against Internet addiction [22]. Furthermore, resilience was reportedly lower among adolescents with IGD according to questionnaire assessments [15]. Its moderating role in the association between stress and IGD severity was demonstrated by an online questionnaire survey [23]. However, the difference in resilience was not evaluated among adults with IGD based on diagnostic interviewing. Further, resilience included a variety of personal characteristics, such as acceptance, problem-solving skills, capacity to recover, self-regulation, personal competence, and self-efficacy [23,24]. Which characteristics of resilience plays an important role involving development of IGD and should be intervened firstly has not been well-evaluated.

Depression is one of the most reported correlates of IGD [25]. Although the causal relationship had not been confirmed between depression and IGD, a longitudinal study suggested that depression could be an outcome of pathological gaming [26]. Prolong stressful events contribute to depression and resilience plays an important role in stress-related disorder and depression [27]. Resilience has been also reported to decrease the likelihood of stress-induced depression [21]. Both stress and depression were reported to be associated with IGD [23,25]. However, the associations among stress, depression, and resilience have not been well examined through interview studies among adults with IGD. Further, we might hypothesize that resilience could be associated with IGD and contribute to perceived stress and depression.

According to the aforementioned studies, resilience enables people to adapt successfully to stress or emotional difficulty and to avoid stress-related disorders [28]. Thus, we hypothesized that an individual with lower resilience could have higher perceived stress and depression. As IGD could be a maladjustment behavior to depression or stress, we hypothesized that individuals with low resilience were more likely to have IGD. Further, the higher perceived stress and depression could involve the association between low resilience and IGD. Moreover, among individuals of IGD, we hypothesized that those with lower resilience had higher perceived stress and depression. Thus, the aim of the study was to evaluate: (1) the difference in resilience, perceived stress, and depression between IGD and healthy controls; (2) the difference in depression and perceived stress between individuals with lower resilience and those with adequate resilience; (3) the confounding effect of perceived stress and depression in association between resilience and IGD; (4) the difference in depression and perceived stress between individuals with lower resilience and those with adequate resilience among the IGD group; and (5) the most associated resilience characteristics of IGD.

2. Methods

2.1. Participants

Our participants comprised individuals who had IGD at the time of the study (the IGD group) and individuals who had never had IGD (the control group) based on a design of case-control study. All participants were recruited by advertisement from September 2012 to October 2013. The criteria for the IGD group specified that participants be: (1) young adults aged 20 to 30 years and with more than 9 years of education; (2) individuals spending either ≥40 h per week or ≥4 h per day on weekdays and ≥8 h per day on weekends engaged in Internet gaming; and (3) individuals who maintained a pattern of Internet gaming for more than 2 years. Participants who met all of three criteria underwent an additional interview with a psychiatrist using the criteria of the DSM-5 [13] for IGD diagnosis. Those who had IGD at the time were classified into the IGD group.

For each participant in the IGD group, we matched a participant to be included in the control group by gender, education level, and age (within a range of 1 year). The recruitment criterion of participants in the control group was that their daily nonessential Internet use was less than 4 h. These participants were classified into the control group after a diagnostic interview with a psychiatrist.

All participants underwent the interview, which comprised two steps: (1) a diagnostic interview based on the Mini-International Neuropsychiatric Interview (MINI) to assess psychotic disorders, bipolar I disorder, and substance-use disorders; and (2) a history-taking interview to evaluate psychotropic medication use, mental retardation, severe physical disorder, and brain injury. Those who had psychotic disorders, bipolar I disorder, substance-use disorders, mental retardation, severe physical disorder, or brain injury or used psychotropic medication were excluded.

2.2. Measures

The diagnostic criteria of IGD were those of the DSM-5 [13]. The nine criteria comprised preoccupation, withdrawal, tolerance, unsuccessful attempts to control others, loss of interests other than gaming, continued excessive use despite psychosocial problems, deceit regarding online gaming, escape, and functional impairment [13]. We developed a semi-structured interview schedule to assess the DSM-5 criteria for IGD among our participants. Those who met five or more criteria for IGD were classified into the IGD group.

2.2.1. Chinese Version of the MINI

We conducted a diagnostic interview based on the psychotic disorder, bipolar I disorder, and substance-use disorder modules in the Chinese version of the MINI [29] to detect those excluding psychiatric disorders.

2.2.2. 14-Item Resilience Scale (R14)

The R14, which provides reliable internal consistency and external validity, was developed to evaluate the levels of resilience in the general population. Participants' resilience was assessed using this scale [24], in which scores are calculated through summation of the response values for each item, enabling scores to range from 14 to 98. The internal consistency reliability (Cronbach's alpha) of the total scale is 0.93 in the current study. Scores less than 65 indicate low resilience, scores between 65 and 81 indicate moderate resilience, and scores of more than 81 indicate high levels of resilience [24]. In this study, participants scoring more than 64 were classified into an adequate resilience group, and those scoring 64 or less were classified into a low resilience group.

2.2.3. Perceived Stress Scale

The Perceived Stress Scale (PSS) was designed to measure the extent to which situations in one's life are perceived as stressful. The PSS score was correlated with life-event scores, depression, and physical symptomatology [30]. It is suggested that the scale possesses adequate reliability for as outcome measure for experienced stress level. In this study, the 10-item PSS-10 was used to evaluate the level of stress experienced by participants and its internal consistency reliability (Cronbach's alpha) was 0.86.

2.2.4. Center for Epidemiological Studies' Depression Scale

The 20-item Mandarin Chinese version [31] of the Center for Epidemiological Studies' Depression Scale (CES-D) [32] is a self-administered evaluation of the frequency of depressive symptoms during the past week. This was used to evaluate depression. Its internal consistency reliability (Cronbach's alpha) was 0.92 in the current study.

2.2.5. Clinical Global Impression Scale for IGD

The Clinical Global Impression (CGI) scale [33] asks "Considering your total clinical experience with this particular population, how mentally ill is the patient at this time?" Possible responses were 1 for normal, not at all ill; 2 for borderline mentally ill; 3 for mildly ill; 4 for moderately ill; 5 for markedly ill; 6 for severely ill; and 7 for among the most ill patients. We modified the scale for IGD to 1 for normal, not at all ill; 2 for excessive online gaming without fulfilling the IGD criteria; 3 for fulfilling the IGD criteria with mild functional impairment; 4 for moderate functional impairment in health or one field such as academics, socializing, or profession; 5 for moderate functional impairment in multiple dimensions; 6 for severe impairment in one field; and 7 for severe impairment in multiple dimensions of daily life.

2.3. Statistical Analysis

We evaluated the associations of resilience, perceived stress, and depression with IGD using an independent *t*-test. The associations between gender, lower resilience, and IGD were evaluated through Chi-squared analysis. A hierarchical logistic regression model was used to evaluate associations of resilience, perceived stress, and depression with IGD. Finally, we evaluated the associations of resilience, perceived stress, and depression with CGI score among participants with IGD. A logistic regression evaluated the association between items of R14 and IGD with gender, age, and educational level controlled. A value of $p < 0.05$ was considered significant for all analyses, which were performed using the SPSS package (SPSS Inc., Chicago, IL, USA).

A total of 87 participants in the IGD group and 87 in the control group were enrolled in the study after informed consent was obtained. This study was approved by the Institutional Review Board of Kaohsiung Medical University Hospital (KMUH-IRB-990380).

3. Results

A total of 87 participants from the IGD group and 87 participants from the control group were enrolled in this study. No significant differences were exhibited in gender, age, or education level between the IGD and control groups, as revealed in Table 1. The IGD group scored lower on resilience, scored higher on perceived stress, and received a higher CGI score than the control group. When participants were further classified into the adequate and low resilience groups, participants with low resilience were more likely to be diagnosed with IGD. Furthermore, participants with low resilience exhibited higher perceived stress and depression, as shown in Table 2.

Table 1. Associations of age, educational level, gender, perceived stress, depression, Clinical Global Impression score, and resilience with Internet gaming disorder (IGD).

Variables	IGD Diagnosis		χ^2 Test
	Yes (N = 87) N(%)	No (N = 87) N(%)	
Gender			
Female (N = 34)	17(50.0)	17(50.0)	0.000
Male (N = 140)	70(50.0)	70(50.0)	
Resilience			
Lower (N = 53)	37(69.8)	16(30.2)	11.97 **
Adequate (N = 121)	50(41.3)	71(58.7)	
	Mean ± SD	**Mean ± SD**	***t*-Test**
Age	23.29 ± 2.34	23.38 ± 2.40	0.26
Educational level	15.93 ± 1.15	16.14 ± 1.22	1.15
Perceived stress	21.71 ± 5.54	17.76 ± 5.62	−4.67 ***
Resilience	66.57 ± 12.72	73.06 ± 12.66	3.37 **
Depression	20.44 ± 10.00	12.01 ± 7.90	−6.16 ***
CGI score	4.56 ± 0.94	1.09 ± 0.29	−33.02 ***

: <0.01; *: <0.001. Resilience: score on 14-Item Resilience Scale; participants scoring 64 or less were classified into a low resilience group. Perceived stress: score on Perceived Stress Scale-10. Depression: score on Center for Epidemiological Studies' Depression Scale. CGI: Clinical Global Impressions scale.

Table 2. The difference in perceived stress and depression between individuals with low resilience and those with adequate resilience.

Variables	Resilience		*t*-Test
	Low Mean ± SD	Adequate Mean ± SD	
Among all subjects	(N = 53)	(N = 121)	
Perceived stress	22.38 ± 5.87	18.58 ± 5.56	3.99 ***
Depression	21.77 ± 9.19	13.79 ± 9.28	5.24 ***
Among IGD group	(N = 37)	(N = 50)	
Perceived stress	22.97 ± 5.85	20.78 ± 5.16	1.85 [a]
Depression	23.16 ± 9.30	18.42 ± 10.12	2.23 *

*: <0.05; ***: <0.001. Resilience: score on 14-Item Resilience Scale; participants scoring 64 or less were classified into a low resilience group. Perceived stress: score on Perceived Stress Scale-10. Depression: score on Center for Epidemiological Studies' Depression Scale. [a]: p = 0.07.

3.1. Associations Among Resilience, Perceived Stress, Depression, and IGD

The hierarchical regression analysis in Table 3 demonstrates that low resilience was positively associated with IGD in Model 1 with gender, age, and educational level controlled. Participants with low resilience had a higher odds ratio (OR, 3.46; 95% confidence interval (CI) = 1.72–6.97) for IGD.

Perceived stress was significantly positively associated with IGD in Model 2. As the Wald χ^2 of perceived stress was higher than that of resilience, perceived stress was more associated with IGD than resilience was (Model 2 in Table 3). This result suggests perceived stress was another important factor to IGD. Further, the resilience was significantly associated with IGD with perceived stress controlled for. It suggested that low resilience had an independent association with IGD from perceived stress.

Depression was significantly positively associated with IGD in Model 3 (OR = 1.1, 95% CI = 1.04–1.17). Resilience and perceived stress exhibited no significant associations with IGD when depression was controlled for. This result demonstrated the mediating effect of depression in the associations of resilience and perceived stress with IGD. It also demonstrated that among resilience, stress, and depression, depression was the factor most associated with IGD.

Table 3. Hierarchical logistic regression model of Internet gaming disorder for resilience, perceived stress, and depression controlling for gender, age, and education level.

Variables	Wald	Exp(β)	95% CI
	Model 1		
Age (year)	0.39	1.05	0.91–1.21
Education level (year)	2.09	0.81	0.60–1.08
Gender	0.00	0.98	0.45–2.14
Resilience (Low)	12.08 **	3.46	1.72–6.97
	Model 2		
Age (year)	0.40	1.05	0.90–1.22
Education level (year)	1.02	0.85	0.63–1.16
Gender	0.05	0.92	0.40–2.08
Resilience (Low)	6.08 *	2.53	1.21–5.30
Perceived stress	11.92 **	1.12	1.05–1.19
	Model 3		
Age (year)	0.52	1.05	0.91–1.23
Education level (year)	1.51	0.82	0.60–1.13
Gender	0.00	1.01	0.43–2.35
Resilience	2.70	1.92	0.88–4.16
Perceived stress	0.03	1.00	0.91–1.09
Depression	9.83 **	1.10	1.04–1.17

*: <0.05; **: <0.01. Resilience: score on 14-Item Resilience Scale; participants scoring 64 or less were classified into a low resilience group. Perceived stress: score on Perceived Stress Scale-10. Depression: score on Center for Epidemiological Studies' Depression Scale.

3.2. *The Difference in Perceived Stress and Depression between Individuals with Low Resilience and Adequate Resilience Among IGD Group*

The t-test in Table 2 demonstrates that individuals with low resilience had higher depression among the IGD group ($t = 0.023$; $p = 0.03$). They also had a trend to have higher percieved stress ($t = 1.85$; $p = 0.07$); however, this did not reach significance.

3.3. *Association of Resilience Characteristics with IGD*

We firstly evaluated the difference in each item of R14 between IGD and the control group. It demonstrated that the IGD group had a lower score in ability to copy ($t = 2.15$; $p = 0.03$), acceptance ($t = 2.63$; $p = 0.01$), drive ($t = 2.81$; $p = 0.01$), discipline ($t = 6.94$; $p < 0.001$), interest/engagement ($t = 2.88$; $p = 0.00$), self-efficacy ($t = 2.29$; $p = 0.02$), dependable ($t = 2.59$; $p = 0.01$), meaning ($t = 3.57$; $p < 0.001$), and resourcefulness ($t = 2.55$; $p = 0.01$). Then, we regressed IGD on these significant items in R14 with gender, age, and educational level controlled. The logistic regression in Table 4 demonstrates that "I am self-disciplined" was the only resilience characteristic associated with IGD.

Table 4. Logistic regression model of Internet gaming disorder for items of 14-Item Resilience Scale with controlling for gender, age, and education level.

Variables	Wald	Exp(β)	95% CI
	Model 1		
Age (year)	0.00	0.97	0.90–1.25
Education level (year)	0.45	1.06	0.56–1.11
Gender	1.85	0.79	0.40–2.33
Ability to cope	0.05	1.05	0.69–1.59
Acceptance	0.13	0.93	0.63–1.39
Drive	0.36	1.12	0.79–1.60
Discipline	24.44 ***	0.41	0.29–0.58
Interest/engagement	0.30	1.13	0.74–1.72
Self-efficacy	0.86	1.22	0.80–1.84
Dependable	0.02	1.03	0.67–1.58
Meaning	2.46	0.73	0.49–1.08
Resourcefulness	0.00	1.00	0.60–1.65

***: <0.001. Items of 14-Item Resilience Scale: the items were significantly associated with IGD in *t*-test evaluation.

4. Discussion

4.1. Perceived Stress of Individuals with IGD

This study demonstrated that participants with IGD experienced higher perceived stress. This result corresponds with those of other studies [14,23]. Stress is conceptualized as a risk factor contributing to progressive long-term changes in the brain and a subsequent drug-prone state characterized by craving and increased risk of relapse [34]. Accordingly, our results might support the possible role of perceived stress in developing IGD addiction. IGD may also have negative consequences. Ko et al. [35] reported that 46.5%, 25.4%,19.7%, and 4.2% of participants with IGD experienced impaired social interaction, professional failures, impaired family relationships, and failures on examinations related to career opportunities, respectively. Such negative consequences may stress adults with IGD and explain the increased perceived stress levels in our study. Further prospective studies to investigate the addiction process may illuminate the causal relationship between stress and IGD.

4.2. Associations among Resilience, Perceived Stress, Depression, and IGD

As in the studies of Wu et al. [36] and Canale et al. [23], the interview in the present study demonstrated an association between resilience and IGD. Furthermore, we demonstrated that those with low resilience have a 3.46 times odds ratio of being diagnosed with IGD. This suggests that low resilience plays a risk role in online gaming addiction. In the R14, resilience is represented as a stable personal resource and a positive personality trait, such as discipline, that can contribute to personal competence, self-acceptance, and life satisfaction [37]. These characteristics may facilitate stress coping and attenuate stress-induced depression [21]. The lower perceived stress and depression among the adequate resilience group demonstrated in our results might support such a claim. Therefore, the characteristics of resilience can be promoted to prevent IGD and to attenuate perceived stress and depression among the general population.

Two studies have evaluated the buffering effect of resilience on the association between stress and IGD. Wu et al. [36] did not observe significant protective effects of resilience against the effects of stress on IGD. However, Canale et al. [23] identified a moderating role of resilience and demonstrated that higher perceived stress and lower resilience were associated with increased gaming time. The difference in stress measurement methods might have contributed to the inconsistent results. However, the assessment of IGD was performed using questionnaires in the two aforementioned studies. Our study, which used similar measurements to Canale's [23], demonstrated that individuals with IGD had lower resilience and higher perceived stress. Our regression analysis also demonstrated that perceived stress had a higher association with IGD than resilience. Although resilience plays a role in the development of IGD, perceived stress may be another influential factor and should be a target of intervention to prevent IGD.

Individuals with IGD could experience the psychosocial distress results from excessive gaming [35]. However, individuals with IGD usually cope with stress through gaming [15], exhibiting escapist gaming. This might aggravate, not resolve, their psychosocial problems. In the current study, the within-group analysis demonstrated IGD individuals with low reliance had higher, but not significantly, perceived stress than those with adequate resilience. This suggests a limited buffering effect of resilience on stress among individual with IGD relative to that in the general population. This might suggest further intervention aside of promoting resilience should be provided to copy the stress associated with IGD. Therefore, alternative stress coping strategies, such as problem-focus coping, exercise, or mindfulness [38] should be provided to replace escapist gaming for IGD individuals under stress.

Depression is one of the most reported factors associated with IGD [39,40]. With depression controlled, perceived stress and resilience were not significantly associated with IGD. This suggests that depression is the most proximal factor contributing to IGD. According to Baron and Kenny [41], depression may play a mediating role in the association between resilience, perceived stress and IGD. Depression could be the outcome of IGD [26], as IGD leads to psychosocial stress. Without adequate resilience to buffer dysphoric mood and psychosocial stress, individuals of IGD can use gaming as an escape from depression. However, excessive gaming without limitation might lead to further psychosocial problems and result in a vicious cycle. Further, these results also suggest that depression as a mood status has a stronger association with IGD than perceived stress and resilience. This study demonstrated that individuals with IGD had lower resilience and higher depression. Thus, depression could also be the outcome of low resilience under high stress which then contributes to IGD. The causal relationship or bi-direction interaction among resilience, stress, depression, and IGD cannot be confirmed in this cross-sectional study. Nevertheless, comorbid depression should be well assessed and effective intervention—such as antidepressants, cognitive behavior therapy [42], exercise, or promoting resilience—for depression should be provided for individuals with IGD, particularly those with lower resilience or higher perceived stress. Although the depression could be the outcome of IGD [26], gaming could be used to temporarily escape from dysphoric moods for those with limited alternative coping strategies. Thus, depression should be well intervened before aggressive intervention for gaming behavior of individuals with IGD.

4.3. Resilience Characteristic Most Associated with IGD

Discipline was the only resilience characteristic associated with IGD when other items were controlled. Individuals with IGD had lower discipline than controls did. Self-regulation was reported to mediate the association between impulsivity and pathological video gaming among youth [43]. Individuals with lower discipline might have had difficulty in controlling their excessive gaming, leading to a risk of IGD. Conversely, a loss of control in gaming with negative consequences might represent a lifestyle with lower discipline. The causal relationship between discipline and IGD cannot be confirmed with a cross-sectional study. However, our study suggests it is important to promote discipline to prevent risk of IGD among the general population and to prevent the deterioration of daily life functioning among individuals with IGD. Future prospective studies regarding the predictive ability of discipline for IGD or the treatment effect of promoting discipline in IGD may clarify this causal relationship.

5. Limitations

This study had limitations that should be considered when interpreting the findings. First, IGD was evaluated only through a diagnostic interview with participants. Additional information from family members or partners could have increased the validity of the diagnosis. Second, the cross-sectional research design could not confirm causal relationships between resilience, perceived stress or escapist online gaming behaviors and IGD. Lastly, we excluded those take psychotropic medication from this study to prevent its effect on depression and perceived stress. However, it could limit the generation of this study's results to populations with psychotropic medication.

6. Conclusions

Individuals with IGD had lower resilience, higher perceived stress, and higher depression. Participants with low resilience exhibited 3.46 times odds ratio for IGD compared with those with adequate resilience. Further, depression was a more proximal factor to IGD than resilience and mediated the association between resilience and IGD. Interventions to promote coping strategies and treat depression should therefore be provided for individuals with IGD and concurrent high stress or depression. Finally, discipline is the resilience characteristic most associated with IGD. Its implications for IGD interventions deserve further study.

Author Contributions: J.-Y.Y. drafted the manuscript; H.-C.L., W.-P.C., and T.-L.L. acquired and analyzed the data; C.-H.K. designed the study, interpreted the data, and gave the final approval of the version to be published.

References

1. Ferguson, C.J.; Coulson, M.; Barnett, J. A meta-analysis of pathological gaming prevalence and comorbidity with mental health, academic and social problems. *J. Psychiatr. Res.* **2011**, *45*, 1573–1578. [CrossRef] [PubMed]
2. Kuss, D.J.; Griffiths, M.D. Internet and gaming addiction: A systematic literature review of neuroimaging studies. *Brain Sci.* **2012**, *2*, 347–374. [CrossRef] [PubMed]
3. Mentzoni, R.A.; Brunborg, G.S.; Molde, H.; Myrseth, H.; Skouverøe, K.J.M.; Hetland, J.; Pallesen, S. Problematic video game use: Estimated prevalence and associations with mental and physical health. *Cyberpsychol. Behav. Soc. Netw.* **2011**, *14*, 591–596. [CrossRef] [PubMed]
4. Brunborg, G.S.; Mentzoni, R.A.; Frøyland, L.R. Is video gaming, or video game addiction, associated with depression, academic achievement, heavy episodic drinking, or conduct problems? *J. Behav. Addict.* **2014**, *3*, 27–32. [CrossRef] [PubMed]
5. Hellström, C.; Nilsson, K.W.; Leppert, J.; Åslund, C. Effects of adolescent online gaming time and motives on depressive, musculoskeletal, and psychosomatic symptoms. *Upsala J. Med. Sci.* **2015**, *120*, 263–275. [CrossRef]
6. Kim, N.R.; Hwang, S.S.; Choi, J.S.; Kim, D.J.; Demetrovics, Z.; Kiraly, O.; Nagygyorgy, K.; Griffiths, M.D.; Hyun, S.Y.; Choi, S.W. Characteristics and psychiatric symptoms of internet gaming disorder among adults using self-reported DSM-5 criteria. *Psychiatry Investig.* **2016**, *13*, 58–66. [CrossRef] [PubMed]
7. Andreassen, C.S.; Billieux, J.; Griffiths, M.D.; Kuss, D.J.; Demetrovics, Z.; Mazzoni, E.; Pallesen, S. The relationship between addictive use of social media and video games and symptoms of psychiatric disorders: A large-scale cross-sectional study. *Psychol. Addict. Behav.* **2016**, *30*, 252–262. [CrossRef]
8. Kwon, J.H.; Chung, C.S.; Lee, J. The effects of escape from self and interpersonal relationship on the pathological use of Internet games. *Community Ment. Health J.* **2011**, *47*, 113–121. [CrossRef]
9. Park, M.; Kim, Y.J.; Kim, D.J.; Choi, J.S. Differential neurophysiological correlates of information processing in internet gaming disorder and alcohol use disorder measured by event-related potentials. *Sci. Rep.* **2017**, *7*, 9062. [CrossRef]
10. Valentino, R.J.; Lucki, I.; Van Bockstaele, E. Corticotropin-releasing factor in the dorsal raphe nucleus: Linking stress coping and addiction. *Brain Res.* **2010**, *1314*, 29–37. [CrossRef]
11. Zhao, L.Y.; Shi, J.; Zhang, X.L.; Epstein, D.H.; Zhang, X.Y.; Liu, Y.; Kosten, T.R.; Lu, L. Stress enhances retrieval of drug-related memories in abstinent heroin addicts. *Neuropsychopharmacology* **2010**, *35*, 720–726. [CrossRef] [PubMed]

12. Tao, R.; Huang, X.; Wang, J.; Zhang, H.; Zhang, Y.; Li, M. Proposed diagnostic criteria for internet addiction. *Addiction* **2010**, *105*, 556–564. [CrossRef] [PubMed]
13. American Psychiatric Association. *Diagnostic and Statistical Manual of Mental Disorders: DSM-5*, 5th ed.; American Psychiatric Association: Washington, DC, USA, 2013.
14. Martín-Fernández, M.; Matalí, J.L.; García-Sánchez, S.; Pardo, M.; Lleras, M.; Castellano-Tejedor, C. Adolescents with internet gaming disorder (IGD): Profiles and treatment response. *Adicciones* **2016**, *29*, 125–133. [CrossRef] [PubMed]
15. Wu, A.M.; Lai, M.H.; Yu, S.; Lau, J.T.; Lei, M.W. Motives for online gaming questionnaire: Its psychometric properties and correlation with internet gaming disorder symptoms among Chinese people. *J. Behav. Addict.* **2017**, *6*, 11–20. [CrossRef] [PubMed]
16. Király, O.; Tóth, D.; Urbán, R.; Demetrovics, Z.; Maraz, A. Intense video gaming is not essentially problematic. *Psychol. Addict. Behav.* **2017**, *31*, 807–817. [CrossRef] [PubMed]
17. Hagström, D.; Kaldo, V. Escapism among players of MMORPGs—Conceptual clarification, its relation to mental health factors, and development of a new measure. *Cyberpsychol. Behav. Soc. Netw.* **2014**, *17*, 19–25. [CrossRef] [PubMed]
18. Goeders, N.E. The impact of stress on addiction. *European Neuropsychopharmacology* **2003**, *13*, 435–441. [CrossRef] [PubMed]
19. Koob, G.F.; Buck, C.L.; Cohen, A.; Edwards, S.; Park, P.E.; Schlosburg, J.E.; Schmeichel, B.; Vendruscolo, L.F.; Wade, C.L.; Whitfield, T.W.; et al. Addiction as a stress surfeit disorder. *Neuropharmacology* **2014**, *76*, 370–382. [CrossRef]
20. McEwen, B.S. Protective and damaging effects of stress mediators: Central role of the brain. *Dialogues Clin. Neurosci.* **2006**, *8*, 367–381. [CrossRef] [PubMed]
21. Southwick, S.M.; Vythilingam, M.; Charney, D.S. The psychobiology of depression and resilience to stress: Implications for prevention and treatment. *Annu. Rev. Clin. Psychol.* **2005**, *1*, 255–291. [CrossRef]
22. Nam, C.R.; Lee, D.H.; Lee, J.Y.; Choi, A.R.; Chung, S.J.; Kim, D.J.; Bhang, S.Y.; Kwon, J.G.; Kweon, Y.S.; Choi, J.S. The role of resilience in internet addiction among adolescents between sexes: A moderated mediation model. *J. Clin. Med.* **2018**, *7*, 222. [CrossRef] [PubMed]
23. Canale, N.; Marino, C.; Griffiths, M.D.; Scacchi, L.; Monaci, M.G.; Vieno, A. The association between problematic online gaming and perceived stress: The moderating effect of psychological resilience. *J. Behav. Addict.* **2019**, *8*, 1–7. [CrossRef] [PubMed]
24. Wagnild, G. *The Resilience Scale User's Guide for the US English version of the Resilience Scale and the 14-Item Resilience Scale (RS-14)*; Resilience Center: Worden, MT, USA, 2009.
25. Liu, L.; Yao, Y.W.; Li, C.R.; Zhang, J.T.; Xia, C.C.; Lan, J.; Ma, S.S.; Zhou, N.; Fang, X.Y. The Comorbidity between Internet Gaming Disorder and Depression: Interrelationship and Neural Mechanisms. *Front. Psychiatry* **2018**, *9*, 154. [CrossRef] [PubMed]
26. Gentile, D.A.; Choo, H.; Liau, A.; Sim, T.; Li, D.; Fung, D.; Khoo, A. Pathological Video Game Use Among Youths: A Two-Year Longitudinal Study. *Pediatrics* **2011**, *127*, e319–e329. [CrossRef] [PubMed]
27. Strain, J.J. The psychobiology of stress, depression, adjustment disorders and resilience. *World J. Biol. Psychiatry* **2018**, *19*, S14–S20. [CrossRef] [PubMed]
28. Liu, H.; Zhang, C.; Ji, Y.; Yang, L. Biological and psychological perspectives of resilience: Is it possible to improve stress resistance? *Front. Hum. Neurosci.* **2018**, *12*, 326. [CrossRef] [PubMed]
29. Sheehan, D.V.; Lecrubier, Y.; Sheehan, K.H.; Amorim, P.; Janavs, J.; Weiller, E.; Hergueta, T.; Baker, R.; Dunbar, G.C. The mini-international neuropsychiatric interview (M.I.N.I.): The development and validation of a structured diagnostic psychiatric interview for DSM-IV and ICD-10. *J. Clin. Psychiatry* **1998**, *59*, 22–33.
30. Cohen, S.; Kamarck, T.; Mermelstein, R. A global measure of perceived stress. *J. Health Soc. Behav.* **1983**, *24*, 385–396. [CrossRef]
31. Chien, C.P.; Cheng, T.A. Depression in Taiwan: Epidemiological survey utilizing CES-D. *Seishin Shinkeigaku Zasshi* **1985**, *87*, 335–338.
32. Radloff, L.S. The CES-D scale: A self-report depression scale for research in the general population. *Appl. Psychol. Meas.* **1977**, *1*, 385–401. [CrossRef]
33. Busner, J.; Targum, S.D. The clinical global impressions scale: Applying a research tool in clinical practice. *Psychiatry* **2007**, *4*, 28–37. [PubMed]

34. Ruisoto, P.; Contador, I. The role of stress in drug addiction: An integrative review. *Physiol. Behav.* **2019**, *202*, 62–68. [CrossRef] [PubMed]
35. Ko, C.H.; Yen, J.Y.; Chen, S.H.; Wang, P.W.; Chen, C.S.; Yen, C.F. Evaluation of the diagnostic criteria of Internet gaming disorder in the DSM-5 among young adults in Taiwan. *J. Psychiatr. Res.* **2014**, *53*, 103–110. [CrossRef] [PubMed]
36. Wu, A.M.; Chen, J.H.; Tong, K.K.; Yu, S.; Lau, J.T. Prevalence and associated factors of internet gaming disorder among community dwelling adults in Macao, China. *J. Behav. Addict.* **2018**, *7*, 62–69. [CrossRef] [PubMed]
37. Wagnild, G.M.; Young, H.M. Development and psychometric evaluation of the Resilience Scale. *J. Nurs. Meas.* **1993**, *1*, 165–178.
38. Li, W.; Garland, E.L.; Howard, M.O. Therapeutic mechanisms of Mindfulness-Oriented Recovery Enhancement for internet gaming disorder: Reducing craving and addictive behavior by targeting cognitive processes. *J. Addict. Dis.* **2018**, 1–9. [CrossRef]
39. González-Bueso, V.; Santamaría, J.; Fernández, D.; Merino, L.; Montero, E.; Ribas, J. Association between internet gaming disorder or pathological video-game use and comorbid psychopathology: A comprehensive review. *Int. J. Environ. Res. Public Health* **2018**, *15*, 668. [CrossRef]
40. Wang, H.R.; Cho, H.; Kim, D.J. Prevalence and correlates of comorbid depression in a nonclinical online sample with DSM-5 internet gaming disorder. *J. Affect. Disord.* **2018**, *226*, 1–5. [CrossRef]
41. Baron, R.M.; Kenny, D.A. The moderator-mediator variable distinction in social psychological research: Conceptual, strategic, and statistical considerations. *J. Pers. Soc. Psychol.* **1986**, *51*, 1173–1182. [CrossRef]
42. Hickie, I.B. An approach to managing depression in general practice. *Med. J. Aust.* **2000**, *173*, 106–110.
43. Liau, A.K.; Neo, E.C.; Gentile, D.A.; Choo, H.; Sim, T.; Li, D.; Khoo, A. Impulsivity, self-regulation, and pathological video gaming among youth: Testing a mediation model. *Asia Pac. J. Public Health* **2015**, *27*, NP2188–NP2196. [CrossRef] [PubMed]

8

Does Smartphone Addiction Fall on a Continuum of Addictive Behaviors?

Sheila Yu [1,*] and Steve Sussman [1,2]

1 Department of Preventive Medicine, University of Southern California, 2001 N Soto St., Los Angeles, CA 90032, USA; ssussma@usc.edu
2 Department of Psychology, University of Southern California, 3620 South McClintock Ave, Los Angeles, CA 90089, USA
* Correspondence: sheilayu@usc.edu

Abstract: Due to the high accessibility and mobility of smartphones, widespread and pervasive smartphone use has become the social norm, exposing users to various health and other risk factors. There is, however, a debate on whether addiction to smartphone use is a valid behavioral addiction that is distinct from similar conditions, such as Internet and gaming addiction. The goal of this review is to gather and integrate up-to-date research on measures of smartphone addiction (SA) and problematic smartphone use (PSU) to better understand (a) if they are distinct from other addictions that merely use the smartphone as a medium, and (b) how the disorder(s) may fall on a continuum of addictive behaviors that at some point could be considered an addiction. A systematic literature search adapted from the Preferred Reporting Items for Systematic Reviews and Meta-Analyses (PRISMA) method was conducted to find all relevant articles on SA and PSU published between 2017 and 2019. A total of 108 articles were included in the current review. Most studies neither distinguished SA from other technological addictions nor clarified whether SA was an addiction to the actual smartphone device or to the features that the device offers. Most studies also did not directly base their research on a theory to explain the etiologic origins or causal pathways of SA and its associations. Suggestions are made regarding how to address SA as an emerging behavioral addiction.

Keywords: smartphone addiction; problematic smartphone use

---

1. Introduction

After the iPhone entered global markets in 2007, significant technological advancements for smartphones have been made [1]. Smartphones offer a myriad of information sources at the touch of one's fingertips and enhance productivity (e.g., synced calendars, email, alerts and alarms, global positioning system (GPS) maps), as well as provide instant access to entertainment and social networking sites and social media channels (e.g., Facebook, Twitter, Instagram) [1,2]. Due to the high accessibility and mobility of smartphones, widespread and pervasive smartphone use has become the social norm [2], which has resulted in an increase in potential distractions that expose users to various health and other risk factors (e.g., distracted driving or walking, resulting in traffic accidents; physical health detriments, such as neck and shoulder issues, blurred vision, and wrist pain; sleep disturbances; highly sedentary habits; poor academic performance; mental health concerns; financial burdens) [1–5].

One other consequence of excessive smartphone use is the possibility of developing an addiction. The concept of addiction historically has focused on recreational drug use, exhibiting classic characteristics related to repetitive use (i.e., tolerance, withdrawal symptoms [4,5], dependence, social problems [5], and loss of control [4]). Addiction now includes behaviors in addition to substances [1–5], such as gambling disorder and Internet gambling disorder [4], as discussed in the latest fifth edition of the Diagnostic and Statistical Manual of Mental Disorders (DSM–5) [4–6] and in the proposed International Classification of Diseases (ICD)-11 for Mortality and Morbidity Statistics [7]. The recognition of these conditions, however, did not occur immediately, as evidence of neurobiological and psychological mechanisms indicating the addictive nature of these behavioral disorders, and accurate assessment of them, took time [8].

The acknowledgement of PSU [3] has led to a debate on whether the concept of SA is a true addiction and, if it is, if it is distinct from other technological addictions engaged in on the smartphone, such as Internet and gaming addiction. Due to the recency of this phenomenon, there has been a paucity of research on its assessment [4,5]. Assessment of SA should involve reliable instruments (e.g., good internal consistency), and demonstrate adequate content validity as a measure of addiction (attempts at appetitive need fulfillment, preoccupation, loss of control, undesired consequences [9]). In addition, such a measure should capture unique consequences of SA (e.g., use while in social situations that interfere with a flow of conversation or upsets a speaker, use while driving). Limitations of knowledge in this new arena of SA/PSU studies include self-report bias from participants, lack of standardized criteria to measure SA/PSU, and different contexts that need to be considered, which may impose variation in external demands for smartphone use (e.g., sociocultural, professional, social, and academic conflicts) [10].

While there are a variety of limitations, the growing empirical research generally seems to support the concept of SA as a genuine addictive disorder, despite the available data being insufficient in establishing a valid and definitive conceptualization of SA [4]. We propose that SA may fall along a continuum of dysregulated behavior, which is problematic and even incapacitating at some point [8,11]. It is important to explore how authors to date have characterized excessive smartphone misuse and understand how various factors gleaned from current research coalesce to discern a clearer picture of this emerging behavioral addiction.

Research Aims

The goal of this review was to examine the most recent studies of SA/PSU to see the extent to which there appears to be unique features of SA/PSU and how studies assess this behavior, to arrive at an understanding regarding at which point there is likely to be consensus on the condition being an addiction along a spectrum of problematic behaviors.

We also explored proneness to SA/PSU as a function of gender, as some researchers have suggested that SA may be more prevalent among females [12–23]. Other research has suggested that subsets of SA (e.g., social media addiction versus gaming addiction) may differentiate males from females in their smartphone use [12,14,15,24–36].

Additionally, we examined variation as a function of age. Some researchers have suggested that SA may be more prevalent among youth and young adults as compared to older adults and elderly who use smartphones less often than youth [12,13,19,26,30,32,34,35,37–55].

2. Materials and Methods

We conducted a systematic review of the literature on and related to SA/PSU utilizing the Preferred Reporting Items for Systematic Reviews and Meta-Analyses (PRISMA) statement [56] as a general guide. Electronic databases utilized included: MEDLINE/PubMed, ProQuest, GALE, Web of Science, Directory of Open Access Journals, Elsevier's collection, Taylor & Francis Online, Wiley Online Library, SpringerLink, and Sage Journal's collection.

2.1. Inclusion Criteria

We utilized the following search terms: "(smartphone OR "mobile phone") AND (addiction OR "problematic use")", published in peer-reviewed journals between 2017 and 2019. Examining Google Scholar, we noticed a steep influx of SA/PSU articles published beginning 2017 (from 22 appearing in 2007; 41 in 2011; 164 in 2013; and 1020 in 2017). Therefore, we began the search from 2017 since this would best capture the current state of research in the area of SA/PSU research. Of the 170 articles returned from the search, 100 were retained for the current review after screening their titles and abstracts. The references of these articles were also searched, of which eight articles were deemed relevant and were included, allowing us to review 108 articles in total.

2.2. Exclusion Criteria

Articles published in a language other than English, duplicate articles (primary articles were retained), studies that did not substantively extend a parent study (i.e., only adapted established SA/PSU scales to a new language with some validation testing), and irrelevant articles (determined after looking through the abstracts or text; examples of irrelevant studies included those assessing the efficacy of an app serving as an intervention, focusing on the risk factors of SA/PSU rather than SA/PSU itself, and measuring invariance among SA-related scales) were excluded from the review pool (see Figure 1).

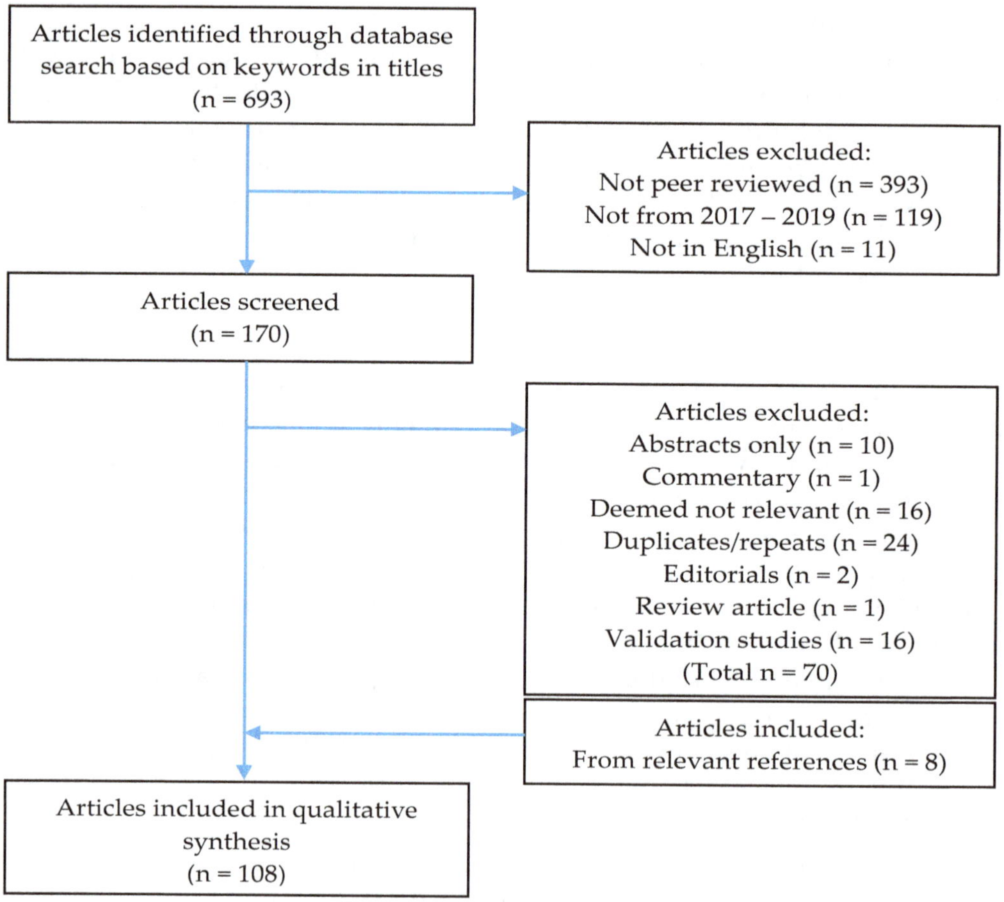

Figure 1. Process of final article selection for the current review.

2.3. Information Synthesis

Since most of the literature on smartphone use were based upon SA and PSU scales, we created a table to compile scales used to measure SA/PSU of smartphones, examining the following (based on Bianchi and Phillips, 2008 [3]): (1) Scale/measurement items, (2) Cronbach's alpha coefficients, and (3) variables and/or factors measured to assess smartphone use. A total of 14 relevant assessments emerged from a review of previous SA/PSU studies (see Table 1).

Table 1. Smartphone addiction/problematic smartphone use assessments in the literature.

Title (Abbreviation): Authors	Year Cat [1]	Items CA [2]	Measures/Factors
Mobile Phone Problem Use Scale (MPPUS): Bianchi and Phillips	2005 PSU	27 0.93	1. Tolerance 2. Escape from other problems 3. Withdrawal 4. Craving 5. Negative life consequences
Mobile Phone Addiction Index (MPAI): Leung	2008 SA	17 0.87	1. Inability to control craving 2. Feeling anxious and lost 3. Withdrawal or escape 4. Productivity loss
Problematic Mobile Phone Use Questionnaire (PMPUQ): Billieux, Van der Linden, and Rochat	2008 PSU	30 0.77	1. Dangerous/prohibited use 2. Dependence 3. Financial problems
Smart Mobile Phone Addiction Scale (MPAS): Hong, Chiu, and Huang	2012 SA	11 0.90	1. Academic problems and effects 2. Time management and problems 3. Substitute satisfaction
Problematic Use of Mobile Phones (PUMP) Scale: Merlo, Stone, and Bibbey	2013 PSU	20 0.94	1. Tolerance 2. Withdrawal 3. Longer time than intended 4. Great deal of time spent 5. Craving 6. Activities given up or reduced 7. Use despite physical/psychological problems 8. Failure to fulfill role obligations 9. Use in physically hazardous situations 10. Use despite social/interpersonal problems
Smartphone Addiction Scale (SAS): Kwon, Lee, Won, Park, Min, Hahn, Gu, Choi, and Kim	2013 SA	48 0.97	1. Daily-life disturbance 2. Positive anticipation 3. Withdrawal 4. Cyberspace-oriented relationship 5. Overuse 6. Tolerance
Short Version for Adolescents (SAS-SV): Kwon, Kim, Cho, Yang	2013 SA	10 0.91	1. Daily-life disturbance 2. Withdrawal 3. Cyberspace-oriented relationship 4. Overuse 5. Tolerance
Smartphone Addiction Scale for College Students (SAS-C): Su, Pan, Liu, Chen, Wang, and Li	2014 SA	22 0.93	1. Withdrawal behavior 2. Salience behavior 3. Social comfort 4. Negative effects 5. Use of application (app) 6. Renewal of app
Smartphone Addiction Management System (SAMS): Lee, Ahn, Choi, and Choi	2014 SA	14 N/A	1. Daily-life disturbance 2. Virtual world orientation 3. Withdrawal 4. Tolerance
Smartphone Addiction Inventory (SPAI): Lin, Chang, Lee, Tseng, Kuo, and Chen	2014 SA	26 0.94	1. Compulsive behavior 2. Functional impairment 3. Withdrawal 4. Tolerance
Korean Smartphone Addiction Proneness Scale (SAPS [3]): Kim, Lee, Lee, Nam, and Chung	2014 SA	29 0.88	1. Disturbance of adaptive functions 2. Withdrawal 3. Tolerance 4. Virtual life orientation
Smartphone Addiction Scale (SPAS): Bian and Leung	2014 SA	19 0.83	1. Disregard of harmful consequences 2. Preoccupation 3. Inability to control craving 4. Productivity loss 5. Feeling anxious and lost
Mobile Phone Problem Use Scale: derivation of a short scale (MPPUS-10): Foerster, Roser, Schoeni, and Röösli	2015 PSU	10 0.85	1. Craving 2. Withdrawal 3. Dependence 4. Loss of control 5. Negative life consequences
Short form of Smartphone Addiction Inventory (SPAI-SF): Lin, Pan, Lin, and Chen	2016 SA	10 0.84	1. Compulsive behavior 2. Functional impairment 3. Withdrawal 4. Tolerance

Notes. [1] Category: Smartphone addiction (SA) or problematic smartphone use (PSU); [2] Cronbach's alpha value; [3] First developed by Korea's National Information Society Agency (2011) "Report on the Development of Korean Smartphone Addiction Proneness Scale for Youth and Adults" (also known as S-Scale) [Korean].

We compared the items across these assessments to see which were common among the scales (see Table 2). Based on Griffiths' (2005) six-component model of addiction, we categorized the measured items based on the components argued to be needed "to be present for a behavior to be operationally defined as addictive": Salience (activity becomes most important, dominating aspect), mood modification (subjective experience of feeling better, whether calming down and/or feeling less destressed), tolerance (more activity needed to feel activity's previous effect), withdrawal (abrupt termination of activity results in unpleasant feeling, psychologically and/or physiologically), conflict (activity causes conflict between addict and others or ones' self-image), and relapse (addictive activity patterns recur) [57].

Table 2. Comparison of major validated scale variables based on Griffiths' component model.

	MPPUS	MPAI	MPAS	SAS	SAS-SV	SPAI	SPAI-SF	SAPS	SPAS	Total
Conflict	√	√	√	√	√	√	√	√	√	9
Withdrawal	√	√	√	√	√	√	√	√	√	9
Tolerance	√	√	√	√	√	√	√	√	√	9
Salience	√	√	√	√	√	√	√	√	√	9
Mood	√	√		√		√		√	√	6
Relapse						√	√	√		3

We also extracted the following information from the studies (see Table 3): (1) First author; (2) year published; (3) whether the study classified smartphone use as an addiction (SA) or problematic smartphone use (PSU); (4) sample size (n); (5) the scale used to assess SA/PSU; (6) if SA/PSU was clearly defined; (7) if studies mentioned the negative attributes and/or risk factors of SA/PSU; (8) if studies distinguished SA/PSU from other technological addictions (e.g., Internet and gaming addiction); (9) if studies differentiated if the addiction is to the actual phone device or to what the phone device offers, such as functions, services, and/or content (e.g., social networking services, apps, etc.); and (10) if studies were structured around a theory or model to explain SA/PSU and how it affects the smartphone user. Under the scale column "adapted", scales refer to scales adapted from SA/PSU assessment scales used in previous studies (e.g., authors compiled x items from scale A and y items from scale B to create their own scale, S) and/or input from field experts.

Table 3. Characteristics of relevant smartphone studies, 2017–2019.

First Author	Year	Cat [1]	Scale	Define [2]	Distinct [3]	D v. F [4]	Theory
Abed	2018	SA	Adapted	No	No	No	n/a
Akodu	2018	SA	SAS-SV	No	No	Yes	n/a
Akturk	2018	SA	SAS-SV	Yes	No	No	n/a
AlAbdulwahab	2017	SA	SAS	No	No	No	n/a
Alavi	2018	SA	MPPUS	No	No	No	Yes [5]
Albursan	2019	SA	Adapted	No	Yes	Yes	n/a
Alhassan	2018	SA	SAS-SV	Yes	No	No	n/a
Alhazmi	2018	SA	SAS-SV	Yes	No	No	n/a
Arefin	2017	SA	Adapted	Yes	Yes	Yes	n/a
Arnavut	2018	SA	SAS-SV	Yes	No	No	n/a
Barnes	2019	SA	Adapted	Yes	Yes	Yes	Yes [6]
Basu	2018	SA	Adapted	Yes	No	No	n/a
Beison	2017	PSU	MPPUS	No	No	No	Yes [7]
Cerit	2018	SA	SAS	Yes	No	No	n/a
Cha	2018	SA	SAPS	Yes	No	No	n/a
Chang	2019	SA	SPAI	Yes	No	No	n/a
Chen	2018	SA	Adapted	No	Yes	Yes	Yes [8]
Chen	2017	SA	Adapted	Yes	No	No	Yes [9]
Chen	2017	SA	SAS-SV	Yes	No	No	n/a
Chiang	2019	SA	SPAI-SF	No	No	No	n/a
Cho	2017	SA	SAPS	Yes	No	No	Yes [10]

Table 3. *Cont.*

First Author	Year	Cat [1]	Scale	Define [2]	Distinct [3]	D v. F [4]	Theory
Cho	2017	SA	AMT [11]	No	No	No	n/a
Choi	2017	SA	SAS	Yes	No	No	n/a
Chou	2019	SA	SPAI-SF	No	No	No	Yes [12]
Chung	2018	SA	SAPS	No	No	No	n/a
Cocoradă	2018	SA	SAS-SV	Yes	No	No	Yes [13]
Contractor	2017	PSU	SAS-SV	Yes	No	No	Yes [14]
De-Sola	2017	SA	MPPUS	Yes	Yes	No	n/a
Ding	2019	PSU	SOCS	No	No	Yes	n/a
Duke	2017	SA	SAS-SV	No	Yes	Yes	n/a
Elhai	2017	PSU	SAS	No	No	No	Yes [15]
Elserty	2018	SA	SAS-SV	Yes	No	No	n/a
Gao	2018	SA	MPAI	Yes	No	No	Yes [16]
Gao	2017	SA	MPAS	No	No	No	n/a
Gezgin	2018	SA	SAS-SV	Yes	No	No	n/a
Gligor	2019	SA	MPDQ [17]	No	No	No	n/a
Gökçearslan	2018	SA	SAS-SV	Yes	No	No	n/a
Habibi	2018	SA	Adapted	Yes	No	No	n/a
Han	2017	SA	MPAI	Yes	Yes	No	Yes [18]
Hao	2019	SA	MPAI	Yes	No	No	n/a
Hawi	2017	SA	SAS-SV	No	No	No	n/a
Heo	2018	SA	SAPS	No	No	No	n/a
Herrero	2019	SA	SPAS	No	No	No	Yes [10]
Herrero	2019	SA	SPAS	Yes	No	No	n/a
Herrero	2019	SA	SPAS	Yes	No	No	n/a
Ihm	2018	SA	Adapted	No	No	No	n/a
Jeong	2019	SA	SAPS	Yes	Yes	No	n/a
Jin	2017	SA	SAS-SV	Yes	No	No	Yes [18,19]
Jo	2018	SA	SAPS	No	No	No	n/a
Khoury	2019	SA	SPAI	No	Yes	No	n/a
Kim	2018	PSU	Adapted	Yes	No	No	Yes [20]
Kim	2017	PSU	Adapted	Yes	No	No	n/a
Kim	2019	SA	SAPS	No	No	No	n/a
Kim	2018	SA	SAPS	Yes	No	No	n/a
Kim	2017	SA	SAPS	No	No	No	Yes [18]
Kim	2017	SA	SAPS	Yes	No	No	Yes [14]
Kim	2017	SA	SAS	No	No	No	n/a
Kim	2018	SA	SAPS	Yes	No	No	Yes [18]
Kita	2018	SA	SAS-SV	Yes	No	No	n/a
Konan	2019	SA	SAS-SV	Yes	No	No	n/a
Konan	2018	SA	SAS-SV	No	No	No	n/a
Kuang-Tsan	2017	SA	MPAS	No	No	No	n/a
Kumcağız	2019	SA	SAS-SV	No	No	No	n/a
Kumcağız	2017	SA	SAS-SV	No	No	No	n/a
Kuss	2018	PSU	PMPUQ	Yes	No	No	Yes [21]
Kwak	2018	SA	Adapted	No	No	No	Yes [22]
Kwan	2017	SA	SAS	Yes	No	Yes	Yes [23,24]
Lan	2018	SA	MPIAS [25]	No	No	No	n/a
Lee	2018	PSU	SAPS	Yes	No	No	Yes [26]
Lee	2017	SA	SAPS	Yes	Yes	No	n/a
Lee	2017	SA	SAPS	No	No	No	n/a
Lee	2017	SA	Adapted	No	No	No	n/a
Lee	2018	SA	Adapted	No	No	No	n/a
Lee	2018	SA	Adapted	No	No	No	n/a
Lee	2018	SA	SAS-SV	No	Yes	No	n/a
Lee	2018	SA	SAS-SV	Yes	Yes	No	Yes [27]
Li	2018	SA	SPAS	No	No	No	Yes [28]
Lian	2018	SA	MPAI	Yes	No	No	Yes [26,29]
Lian	2017	SA	MPAI	Yes	No	No	Yes [26]
Lin	2017	SA	App	Yes	Yes	Yes	n/a
Liu	2018	SA	MPAI	Yes	No	No	Yes [22]

Table 3. *Cont.*

First Author	Year	Cat [1]	Scale	Define [2]	Distinct [3]	D v. F [4]	Theory
Liu	2018	PSU	SAS-SV	Yes	No	Yes	Yes [30]
Liu	2017	SA	MPAI	No	No	No	Yes [31]
Lu	2018	SA	MPAS	No	No	No	n/a
Mahapatra	2018	SA	Adapted	Yes	No	Yes	Yes [32]
Matar B.	2017	SA	SPAI	No	Yes	No	n/a
Megna	2018	SA	SAS-SV	Yes	No	No	n/a
Mei	2018	SA	MPAI	Yes	No	Yes	Yes [33]
Nayak	2018	SA	Adapted	Yes	Yes	No	n/a
Noë	2019	SA	SAS	Yes	Yes	Yes	n/a
Parasuraman	2017	SA	Adapted	No	No	Yes	n/a
Salvi	2018	SA	Adapted	Yes	No	No	n/a
Sekhon	2018	SA	MPPUS	Yes	No	No	n/a
Serin	2019	SA	SAS-SV	Yes	No	No	n/a
Sok	2019	SA	Adapted	No	No	No	n/a
Song	2018	SA	SAS (Lee)	No	No	No	n/a
Sun	2019	SA	SAS (Ku)	Yes	No	No	Yes [34]
Tunc-Aksan	2019	SA	SAS	No	No	Yes	Yes [35]
Wang	2018	SA	SAS-SV	No	No	No	Yes [36,37]
Wang	2017	SA	SAS-SV	No	No	No	Yes [38]
Wolniewicz	2018	PSU	SAS-SV	Yes	Yes	Yes	Yes [15,16]
Xu	2019	PSU	MPAS	Yes	No	No	Yes [22,39]
Yang	2019	SA	MPAI	Yes	No	No	Yes [40]
Yang	2019	PSU	Adapted	Yes	No	No	n/a
Yildiz Durak	2017	SA	SAS	Yes	Yes	No	Yes [41]
Yildiz	2017	SA	SAS-SV	No	No	No	n/a
You	2019	SA	MPAS	No	No	No	Yes [42]
Youn	2018	SA	SAS	No	No	No	n/a

Notes. [1] Category based on study title: Smartphone addiction (SA) or problematic smartphone use (PSU); [2] Define: If SA or PSU was defined; [3] Distinct: If studies distinguished SA from other technological addictions (e.g., Internet, gaming addiction); [4] D v. F: If studies differentiated if the addiction is to the actual phone device or to what the phone device offers, such as functions, services, and/or content (e.g., social networking services, apps, etc.); [5] Psychosocial Theory of Development (Erikson, 1963) and Adolescent Identity Paradigm (Marcia, 1991); [6] Cognitive absorption (Agarwal & Karahanna, 2000); [7] Reward Deficiency Syndrome hypothesis (Blum et al., 1996); [8] Social influence theory (Rashotte, 2007); [9] Four categories of drinking motives (Stewart & Devine, 2000); [10] Big Five personality traits (Norman, 1963); [11] Addiction Measurement Tools of Measuring Smartphone Addiction of Children-Adolescents (Korea Network Information Center); [12] 6-T Internet attitude model (Chou, Wu, & Chen, 2013); [13] Theory of Reasoned Action (Fishbein & Ajzen, 1975); [14] Impulsive pathway perspective (Billieux, 2012); [15] Uses and Gratifications Theory (UGT) (Blumler & Katz, 1974); [16] Compensatory Internet Use Theory (CIUT) (Kardefelt-Winther, 2014); [17] MPDQ: Mobile phone dependence questionnaire; [18] Attachment theory (Bowlby, 1969); [19] Psychoanalytic theory (Kassel et al., 2007); [20] Social enhancement model (Kraut et al., 2002); [21] Biopsychosocial model of addiction (Griffiths, 2005); [22] General strain theory (Agnew, 1992); [23] Theory of parenting style (Baumrind, 1971); [24] First theory of self-regulation (Asgari et al., 2011); [25] MPIAS: Mobile Phone Internet Addiction Scale; [26] Problem behavior theory (PBT) (Jessor, 1977); [27] Power distance belief (Hofstede, 1980); [28] Media system dependency (MSD) theory (Ball-Rokeach & DeFleur, 1976); [29] Social skills deficit theory (Valkenburg & Peter, 2007); [30] Social compensation theory (Zell & Moeller, 2018); [31] Response style theory (Nolen-Hoeksema, 1991); [32] Incentive-Sensitization (Robinson & Berridge, 2003) & Learning Theory (Wallace, 1999); [33] Hierarchy of needs theory (Maslow, 1968); [34] Risky families model (Repetti, 2002); [35] Intrinsic motivation theory (Przybylski, Weinstein, Ryan, & Rigby, 2009); [36] Sensation seeking theory (Zuckerman, 1994); [37] Social support buffering hypothesis (Cohen & Wills, 1985); [38] Cognitive-behavioral model (Davis, 2001); [39] Resilience theory (Fergus & Zimmerman, 2005); [40] Diathesis-stress theories (Monroe & Simons, 1991) and stress-buffering hypothesis (Cohen & Edwards, 1989); [41] Social Cognitive Theory (Bandura, 1986); [42] Sociometer theory of self-esteem (Leary et al., 1995).

To supplement Table 3, we conducted an in-depth analysis on the study samples (see Table 4), specifically (1) the group population, either child/youth (in primary, elementary, middle, or high school), university student (students in college, graduate, and vocational/technical/institute schools were all categorized as university students), or adult; (2) sample size, n; (3) percentage of males in the sample; (4) mean age and age range of participants; (5) participant nationality; (6) sociodemographic characteristics (SDCs) (biometrics, such as body mass index (BMI), height, and weight; number of children; education; income; marital status; region or residence, such as rural or urban; and work/employment status); and (7) reported study biases. SDC data were reported for university students and adults, usually the parents of children.

The point of Table 4 was to determine the generalizability of the studies' results: Can the research findings and conclusions of a particular group of interest be extended to the population at large? If a particular population sample is studied across age and nationality, does that imply that that group is at-risk for SA?

Table 4. Demographic profile of smartphone study samples and reported study biases.

First Author	Pop [1]	n [2]	Males (%)	Age (m (r) [3])	Nationality	SDC [4] (BCEIMRW)	Reported Biases
Abed	Univ	229	35	n/a	Iraqi	MRW	None
Akodu	Univ	77	57	22	Nigerian	B	Sampling
Akturk	Univ	1156	49	n/a	Turkish	CEI	Sampling
AlAbdulwahab	Univ	78	50	21	Saudi	B	None
Alavi	Univ	500	21	28 (18–31+)	Iranian	EM	Sampling
Albursan	Univ	2008	45	22 (17–28)	Arab		Sampling
Alhassan	Adult	935	34	32 (18–55+)	Saudi	EIR	Multiple
Alhazmi	Univ	181	48	24	Saudi	BM	Sampling
Arefin	Univ	247	54	(18–27)	Bangladeshi		Sampling
Arnavut	Adult	714	58	(18–30+)	Turkish		Sampling
Barnes	Univ	140	31	(18–35+)	American	E	Multiple
Basu	Univ	388	60	20	Indian	R	Sampling
Beison	Univ	100	25	20 (18–23)	American [5]	EI	None
Cerit	Univ	214	20	20 (18–26)	Turkish		Recall
Cha	MS	1824	51	16	Korean	IW	Multiple
Chang	ES/Adult	5089	52/31	n/a/43	Taiwanese	EIM	Multiple
Chen	Univ	2000	49	21 (17–23)	Taiwanese		Multiple
Chen	Univ	384	54	n/a	Chinese		Multiple
Chen	Univ	1441	48	20 (17–26)	Chinese	R	Multiple
Chiang	ES/MS	2155	52	n/a	Taiwanese	EIM	Multiple
Cho	Adult	400	52	(20–40+)	Korean	EW	Multiple
Cho	PS/Adult	303	7/51	(20–40+)/(0–6)	Korean	EIW	Sampling
Choi	HS	1020	52	n/a	Korean	R	Sampling
Chou	HS/Adult	1444	43/n/a	n/a/n/a	Taiwanese	EI	Recall
Chung	MS/HS	1796	46	15 (13–18)	Korean		Sampling
Cocoradă	HS/Univ	717	35	20	Romanian		Multiple
Contractor	Adult	346	42	34	American [5]	IMW	Multiple
De-Sola	Adult	1126	48	33 (16–65)	Spanish	ER	Multiple
Ding	Univ	849	56	n/a	Chinese		Multiple
Duke	Adult	262	36	32	German		Recall
Elhai	Adult	308	54	33	American [5]	EIMW	Multiple
Elserty	Univ	420	32	20	Egyptian	B	None
Gao	Univ	1105	29	21 (16–25)	Chinese	I	Multiple
Gao	Univ	722	48	20 (15–24)	Chinese	CIR	Multiple
Gezgin	HS	161	58	16	Turkish		Multiple
Gligor	Univ	150	44	27	Romanian	R	Multiple
Gökçearslan	Univ	885	41	n/a	Turkish	I	None
Habibi	HS	271	n/a	17	Indonesian		None
Han	Univ	543	41	20 (17–22)	Chinese		Sampling
Hao	Univ	847	51	20 (18–24)	Chinese	CR	Sampling
Hawi	Univ	381	59	21 (17–27)	Lebanese		Multiple
Heo	HS	790	23	n/a	Korean		None
Herrero	All	526	52	(15–55+)	Spanish	ER	None
Herrero	All	241	55	(15–55+)	Spanish	ER	Sampling
Herrero	All	416	52	(15–55+)	Spanish	ER	Selection
Ihm	Youth	2000	50	12	Korean		Recall
Jeong	HS	768	58	n/a	Korean	IM	Multiple
Jin	Univ	297	55	20 (17–24)	Chinese	I	Sampling
Jo	All	7003	45	(14–39)	Korean	R	Recall
Khoury	Univ	100	48	(18–25)	Brazilian [5]	IM	Response
Kim	Adult	615	51	30 (19–40)	American [5]		Recall
Kim	All	930	52	26 (13–40)	American [5]	M	Recall
Kim	MS/HS	4512	45	15	Korean	IM	Multiple
Kim	Youth	3380	51	(10–19)	Korean	EIMRW	Information
Kim	Univ	200	37	22 (19–28)	Korean		Sampling
Kim	Univ	608	30	23	Korean	I	Multiple
Kim	HS	1479	48	n/a	Korean	B	Sampling
Kim	Univ	313	42	22 (17–29)	Korean		Sampling
Kita	YA	221	65	19 (17–22)	Israeli		Sampling

Table 4. *Cont.*

First Author	Pop [1]	n [2]	Males (%)	Age (m (r) [3])	Nationality	SDC [4] (BCEIMRW)	Reported Biases
Konan	Univ	496	25	n/a	Turkish		None
Konan	Univ	330	36	(20–24)	Turkish		None
Kuang-Tsan	Univ	332	65	(18–22)	Taiwanese		Sampling
Kumcağız	HS	352	44	16 (14–19)	Turkish	E W	Multiple
Kumcağız	Adult	428	37	40 (21–65)	Turkish	CEIM W	Sampling
Kuss	All	273	26	28 (16–65)	Various		None
Kwak	MS	1170	42	n/a	Korean	I	Sampling
Kwan	Univ	211	35	22	Hong Kong		None
Lan	Univ	1044	48	21	Chinese		Information
Lee	Youth	231	40	16 (13–18)	Korean		Sampling
Lee	MS	370	49	13	Korean		Multiple
Lee	MS/HS	3000	53	n/a	Korean		Sampling
Lee	MS/HS	1125	51	n/a	Korean	EI R	Multiple
Lee	Univ	125	49	n/a	Korean		None
Lee	Univ	324	9	n/a	Korean		Multiple
Lee	MS	490	100	14	Korean	E	Multiple
Lee	Adult	778	63/58 [6]	35/25 [6]	Various	EI	Information
Li	Adult	527	46	27 (18–35)	Chinese	EIM W	Sampling
Lian	Univ	716	54	20 (18–24)	Chinese	R	Sampling
Lian	Univ	682	58	19 (18–24)	Chinese		Recall
Lin	Univ	79	72	22	Taiwanese		Sampling
Liu	HS	899	46	17 (14–19)	Chinese		Sampling
Liu	Univ	465	31	19 (16–24)	Chinese		Sampling
Liu	HS	1196	53	17 (14–20)	Chinese		Multiple
Lu	MS	1311	54	15	Various		Sampling
Mahapatra	HS/Univ	330	58	(15–20)	Indian		Multiple
Matar B.	Univ	688	53	21	Lebanese	W	Recall
Megna	Adult	52	46	27 (18–35)	Italian		None
Mei	Univ	1034	47	20	Chinese	C I R	Multiple
Nayak	Univ	429	35	20 (16–29)	Indian		None
Noë	Adult	64	53	25 (19–46)	British	E W	Sampling
Parasuraman	Adult	409	42	23 (18–55)	Malaysian	E W	Sampling
Salvi	Univ	100	59	21 (18–25)	Indian		None
Sekhon	Univ	80	50	(20–24)	Indian		Sampling
Serin	Univ	287	14	n/a	Turkish	CEIM	Multiple
Sok	Univ	139	16	n/a	Korean		Sampling
Song	PS/Adult	328	n/a/0	(3–5)/n/a	Korean	E W	Multiple
Sun	HS	1041	56	12 (11–15)	Chinese		Multiple
Tunc-Aksan	HS	296	54	n/a	Turkish	E	None
Wang	MS	655	55	17 (15–19)	Chinese		Multiple
Wang	MS	768	44	17 (15–19)	Chinese	E W	Multiple
Wolniewicz	Univ	296	43	20	American [5]	E W	Multiple
Xu	MS	316	47	14 (12–16)	Chinese		Sampling
Yang	HS	1258	53	17 (14–20)	Chinese		Sampling
Yang	Univ	218	58	18 (16–19+)	Taiwanese		Multiple
Yildiz Durak	MS/HS	612	52	13 (10–18)	Turkish	CEI R	Multiple
Yildiz	HS	262	50	17 (14–19)	Turkish		Sampling
You	Univ	653	50	20 (17–25)	Chinese	EI	Sampling
Youn	Youth	158	53	15 (12–19)	Korean	EI	Multiple

Notes. [1] Pop: Population general group (PS: Primary school; ES: Elementary school; MS: Middle school; HS: High school; Univ: University, college, or institute of technology students; YA: Young adult); [2] Sample size n; [3] m (r): mean age (range, if available); [4] SDC: Common sociodemographic characteristics besides gender, age, and ethnicity (B = biometrics: height, weight, BMI; C = number of children; E = education; I = income; M = marital status; R = regional/residence: urban or rural; W: work/employment status); [5] Reports racial status (e.g., African-American/Black, American Indian, Asian, Native Hawaiian/other Pacific Islander, White) and ethnicity (e.g., Hispanic/Latino, Not Hispanic/Latino); [6] Of 778 total, 431 US and 347 Chinese participants: male % and mean age of US and Chinese, respectively.

To supplement Table 4 on the characteristics of the studies' samples (refer to Table 5), we examined the quality of the data collection process by noting if samples were selected as a convenience sample or randomly selected and if a sample size calculation was calculated before participant recruitment. We also categorized the data collected as consequences pertaining to: Academics (grades, academic performance), physiological (headache, eye/neck/hand pain), psychological (experiencing depression, loneliness, cravings), social (peer relationships), or usage; and whether it was objective or subjective (such as an objective clinical diagnosis of depression or a subjective self-report of experiencing depression).

Additionally, we assessed the operationalization of theory by noting if the SA/PSU scale used in the study met Griffiths' criteria for behavioral addictions: Conflict, mood modification, relapse, salience, tolerance, and withdrawal. The 2004 Surgeon General's report, *The Health Consequences of Smoking*, developed a framework for interpreting evidence, specifying a four-level hierarchy for interpreting evidence: (a) Evidence is sufficient to infer a causal relationship (multiple scientifically supported evidence), (b) evidence is suggestive but not sufficient to infer a causal relationship (scientifically supported evidence), (c) evidence is inadequate to infer the presence or absence of a causal relationship (evidence that is not scientifically supported and/or is sparse, of poor quality, or conflicting), or (d) evidence is suggestive of no causal relationship (no evidence) [58]. We also noted if the assumption of addiction, referencing back to the title assumption of whether the authors viewed excessive smartphone use as SA or PSU, influenced the study results.

Table 5. The quality of samples, level of evidence, and theoretical framework of the studies.

First Author	Sel [1]	SSS [2]	Evidence [3]	Obj [4]	Int [5]	Griffiths [6]	Inf [7]
Abed	R	No	PhPs	S	I	n/a	Yes
Akodu	C	No	Ph	O	Sg	C STW	Yes
Akturk	C	Yes	S	S	Sg	C STW	Yes
AlAbdulwahab	C	Yes	Ph	S	I	CM STW	Yes
Alavi	C	Yes	Ps	O	I	CM STW	Yes
Albursan	R	No	Ps	S	I	n/a	Yes
Alhassan	R	No	Ps	S	I	C STW	Yes
Alhazmi	R	Yes	Ph	S	I	C STW	Yes
Arefin	C	No	A	O	Sg	CM STW	Yes
Arnavut	R	No	U	S	I	C STW	Yes
Barnes	C	No	Ps	S	I	C STW	Yes
Basu	R	Yes	U	S	I	CM STW	Yes
Beison	n/a	No	S	S	Sg	CM STW	Yes
Cerit	R	Yes	Ph	S	I	CM STW	Yes
Cha	R	No	PhPsU	S	I	CMRSTW	Yes
Chang	R	No	SU	S	I	CMRSTW	Yes
Chen	C	No	PsS	S	I	n/a	PSU [8]
Chen	C	No	Ps	S	I	CMRSTW	Yes
Chen	R	No	PhPs	S	I	C STW	Yes
Chiang	R	No	Ps	S	I	C TW	Yes
Cho	R	No	Ps	S	I	CMRSTW	Yes
Cho	R	No	Ps	S	I	n/a	Yes
Choi	n/a	No	U	S	I	C TW	Yes
Chou	R	No	U	S	I	C TW	Yes
Chung	R	No	Ph	S	I	CMRSTW	Yes
Cocoradă	C	No	PsU	S	I	C STW	Yes
Contractor	C	No	Ps	S	I	C STW	Yes
De-Sola	C	No	Ps	S	I	CM STW	Yes
Ding	R	No	PsU	S	I	CMRST	Yes
Duke	C	No	U	S	I	C STW	Yes
Elhai	C	No	PsU	S	I	CM STW	Yes
Elserty	C	No	PhU	S	I	C STW	Yes
Gao	C	No	Ps	S	I	CM STW	Yes
Gao	C	No	Ps	S	I	C RSTW	Yes
Gezgin	C	No	PsU	S	I	C STW	Yes
Gligor	n/a	No	Ps	S	I	CM STW	Yes
Gökçearslan	C	No	PsS	S	I	C STW	Yes
Habibi	n/a	No	Ps	S	I	C STW	Yes
Han	R	No	Ps	S	I	CM STW	Yes
Hao	R	No	PsU	S	I	CM STW	Yes
Hawi	R	No	Ps	S	I	C STW	Yes
Heo	C	Yes	Ps	S	I	CMRSTW	Yes
Herrero	R	No	PsSU	S	I	CM STW	Yes
Herrero	R	No	Ps	S	I	CM STW	Yes
Herrero	R	No	Ps	S	I	CM STW	Yes
Ihm	R	No	S	S	I	CMRSTW	Yes
Jeong	n/a	No	PsS	S	I	CMRSTW	Yes
Jin	C	No	Ps	PsS	I	C STW	Yes
Jo	n/a	No	Ps	S	I	CMRSTW	Yes
Khoury	R	No	Ph	O	Sg	CMRSTW	Yes

Table 5. *Cont.*

First Author	Sel [1]	SSS [2]	Evidence [3]	Obj [4]	Int [5]	Griffiths [6]	Inf [7]
Kim	R	No	Ps	S	I	C STW	Yes
Kim	R	No	Ps	S	I	C STW	Yes
Kim	R	No	Ps	S	I	CMRSTW	Yes
Kim	R	No	S	S	I	CMRSTW	Yes
Kim	n/a	Yes	Ps	S	I	CMRSTW	Yes
Kim	C	No	Ph	S	Sg	CMRSTW	Yes
Kim	n/a	No	Ph	S	I	CM STW	Yes
Kim	C	No	Ps	S	I	CMRSTW	Yes
Kita	C	No	S	O	Sg	C STW	Yes
Konan	R	No	PsS	S	I	C STW	Yes
Konan	C	No	Ps	S	I	C STW	Yes
Kuang-Tsan	C	No	S	S	Sg	C RSTW	Yes
Kumcağız	C	No	S	S	I	CM STW	Yes
Kumcağız	C	No	S	S	I	C STW	Yes
Kuss	C	No	Ps	S	I	C RSTW	Yes
Kwak	C	No	PsS	S	Sg	CMRSTW	Yes
Kwan	C	No	PsS	S	I	CM STW	Yes
Lan	R	No	Ps	S	Sg	n/a	Yes
Lee	C	Yes	PsS	S	Sg	CMRSTW	Yes
Lee	C	No	Ps	O	Sg	CMRSTW	PSU [8]
Lee	n/a	No	S	S	Sg	CMRSTW	Yes
Lee	R	No	Ph	S	I	C STW	Yes
Lee	R	No	S	O	Sg	CMRSTW	Yes
Lee	C	No	S	S	I	CM STW	Yes
Lee	n/a	No	Ps	S	I	C STW	Yes
Lee	n/a	No	Ps	S	I	C STW	Yes
Li	C	No	S	S	I	CM STW	Yes
Lian	C	No	S	S	I	CM STW	Yes
Lian	C	No	S	S	I	CM STW	Yes
Lin	n/a	No	U	O	Sg	n/a	Yes
Liu	R	No	Ps	S	I	CM STW	Yes
Liu	C	No	PsS	S	I	C STW	Yes
Liu	C	No	PhPs	S	I	CM STW	Yes
Lu	C	No	S	S	I	C RSTW	Yes
Mahapatra	C	No	APsS	S	I	C STW	Yes
Matar B.	R	No	PsU	S	I	CMRSTW	Yes
Megna	C	No	Ph	O	Sg	C STW	Yes
Mei	C	Yes	Ps	S	I	CM STW	Yes
Nayak	R	No	AU	S	I	C STW	Yes
Noë	C	No	U	O	Sg	CM STW	Yes
Parasuraman	C	No	U	S	I	n/a	Yes
Salvi	n/a	No	Ph	O	Sg	n/a	Yes
Sekhon	n/a	No	Ps	S	I	CM STW	Yes
Serin	C	No	Ps	S	I	C STW	Yes
Sok	C	Yes	PsSU	S	I	n/a	Yes
Song	C	No	S	S	I	CMRSTW	Yes
Sun	n/a	No	PsS	S	I	n/a	Yes
Tunc-Aksan	R	No	APsS	S	I	CM STW	Yes
Wang	n/a	No	PsS	S	I	C STW	Yes
Wang	n/a	No	PsS	S	I	C STW	Yes
Wolniewicz	C	No	PsU	S	I	C STW	Yes
Xu	n/a	No	APs	S	I	C RSTW	Yes
Yang	R	No	Ps	S	I	CM STW	Yes
Yang	C	No	PhPsU	S	I	C S W	Yes
Yildiz Durak	C	No	Ps	S	I	CM STW	Yes
Yildiz	C	No	Ps	S	I	CSTW	Yes
You	C	No	Ps	S	I	C RSTW	Yes
Youn	C	No	PsS	S	I	CM STW	Yes

Notes. [1] Sel: Selection of sample: C = convenience sample, R = randomly selected; [2] SSS: Sufficiency of sample size: Yes or No; [3] Evidence: Type of data presented: A = academic, Ph = physiological, Ps = psychological, S = social, U = usage; [4] Obj: Objectivity: O = objective, S = subjective; [5] IE: Interpretation of the level of evidence: Sf = sufficient, Sg = suggestive but not sufficient, I = inadequate, NR = suggestive of no causal relationship; [6] Griffiths: C = conflict, M = mood modification, R = relapse, S = salience, T = tolerance, W = withdrawal; [7] Inf: Assumption of addiction influencing study results: Yes or No; [8] Was titled an SA study but conclusions use PSU terminology.

3. Results

3.1. The Scales Used to Assess SA/PSU and Their Internal Consistency

The majority of the studies in the current review (96 out of 108) fell under the SA category (89%). Excluding one study that did not use a scale, there were nine major scales used among the studies, in order of frequency: Smartphone Addiction Scale Short Version (SAS-SV) (26%), Smartphone Addiction Proneness Scale (SAPS) (13%), Smartphone Addiction Scale (SAS) (9%), Mobile Phone Addiction Index (MPAI) (8%), Mobile Phone Addiction Scale (MPAS) (5%), Mobile Phone Problem Use Scale (MPPUS) (4%), Smartphone Addiction Scale (SPAS) (4%), Smartphone Addiction Inventory (SPAI) (3%), and SPAI Short Form (SPAI-SF) (2%). Overall, most studies either used SAS or SAS-SV (35%) or some adapted form of an SA/PSU-assessment scale based on scales from previous studies and/or input from field experts (26%). Excluding the adapted scale studies, 8 of the 12 PSU studies (67%) used SA scales to assess problematic use instead of a PSU scale, and 3 of the 95 SA studies (3%) used PSU scales to assess SA instead of SA scales (refer to Table 3).

In terms of meeting Griffiths' criteria for behavioral addictions, all of the major scales met conflict, withdrawal, tolerance, and salience. Six of the nine met mood modification and only three met relapse (refer to Table 2). Excluding nine studies in which specific adapted scale items were unavailable, one study that did not use a scale, and 79 that used one of the nine major scales, the remaining 19 studies used an adapted SA/PSU scale that met at least half of Griffiths' criteria for behavioral addictions (mean of 4.79, SD of 0.92): One study (5% of 19) met three criteria, seven (37%) met four, six (32%) met five, and five (26%) met all six.

All scales demonstrated validity: All scales provided a Cronbach's alpha (CA) value as a measure of internal consistency, and performed factor structure analyses, ensuring that factor fit properly explains correlations among outcomes [59,60]. Other evaluations of validity also included testing the concurrent validity of the scale with other established scales. The CA of the nine major scales ranged from 0.83 to 0.97, with a mean of 0.90 and standard deviation (SD) of 0.05 (refer to Table 1).

3.2. How Studies Defined SA/PSU

In total, 87 of the 108 studies (81%) attempted a working definition of SA/PSU, of which 56 explicitly stated the definition in the paper (64%), while the rest simply characterized SA/PSU by its negative risk factors or listed associated traits. Nearly all of the studies (96%) mentioned the negative risk factors associated with SA/PSU, including physical (insomnia, pain in neck and wrists, eye soreness, etc.) and physiological concerns (depression, anxiety, loneliness, etc.). SA has been defined as a maladaptive dependency on and/or obsessive-compulsive use of the smartphone device [18], a state of being immersed in uncontrollable smartphone usage [41], and the inability to properly regulate smartphone usage to the point of experiencing adverse consequences in one's daily life (Billieux, 2012) [21]. Interestingly, PSU has been similarly defined as "an excessive or uncontrolled use of smartphone" (also Billieux, 2012) [61]. It is interesting to note that the same reference has been used to define both SA and PSU, highlighting the interchangeability of the two terms.

Overall, 64 out of 108 studies (59%) mentioned other technological addictions, such as Internet and gaming addiction, in their paper. Of the 64 studies, only 13 (20%) explicitly argued that SA is separate and distinct from Internet addiction (2 out of 4 PSU studies; 11 out of 47 SA studies). In total, 20 studies out of 108 (19%) (4 out of 13 PSU studies; 16 out of 95 SA studies) mentioned whether SA is an addiction to the actual smartphone device or to the functions/services/content that the smartphone offers users, such as social networking services and various apps that are usually not found on other devices (refer to Table 3).

3.3. Theories Adopted Across These Studies

More than half of the studies (63%) did not explicitly base their study upon a specific established theory (refer to Table 3). Nine of 12 (75%) PSU studies used a theory (five of nine, 42%) or a concept, model, or hypothesis (four of nine, 33%) to guide their research; while 31 of 96 SA studies (29%) used a theory (23 of 96, 24%) or a concept or model (eight of 96, 8%) to guide their study (refer to Table 3).

The following four theories in the current review stood out as guiding points on understanding SA and how its pathways may work. First, social influence theory (Kelman,1974) helps to illustrate how socially influential factors predict a user's intended and actual behavior in virtual settings, which is affected by three social processes: "Compliance (normative influence from others' expectations), internalization (congruence of one's goals with others' goals), and identification (conception of one's self in terms of the group's defining features)" [39]. This theory could help to explain SA among impressionable youths, who are more prone to peer pressure to what their peers may deem cool, which could include engaging in addictive behaviors on the smartphone (e.g., games, social media, streaming videos on Twitch), as well as among adults whose lifestyles are affected by today's heavily connected environment, which makes smartphone use a social norm.

The second theory, the theory of reasoned action (Fishbein & Ajzen, 1975), explains that a person's actual behavior is determined by their intention to behave in a certain way, being influenced both by their own attitudes and the social context. The attitudes towards the smartphone (positive, negative, fear of missing out, and task switching) were considered key predictors of addiction [62]. This perspective focuses on the intrapersonal reasons a person may fall into SA, with positive attitudes potentially bringing about positive reinforcement to keep engaging in the cycle of excessive smartphone use. Other theories helping to illustrate user adoption and acceptance of information technologies include diffusion of innovations (Rogers, 1962), the theory of planned behavior (Ajzen, 1985), and the technology acceptance model (TAM) (Davis, 1989) [25].

However, the previous theories are limited in explaining how attitudes, perceptions, and beliefs are shaped around information technologies. To address this conceptual shortfall, cognitive absorption (CA) (Agarwal & Karahanna, 2000) was proposed as a motivating factor of usage behavior through "cognitive complexity beliefs". CA was defined as "a state of deep involvement with software ... where highly engaging and engrossing experiences result in users' 'deep attention' and complete immersion and engagement with an activity" [25]. The multidimensional construct of CA has five dimensions: Temporal dissociation, focused immersion, heightened enjoyment, control, and curiosity, which follow closely with Griffiths' biopsychosocial model of addiction.

Another relevant theory, the uses and gratifications theory (UGT), "helps understand background characteristics and individual differences motivating people to choose using *particular* types of mass media. UGT can explain how people with certain types of psychological and/or demographic characteristics may be drawn to increasingly use specific types of smartphone features" to achieve gratification [63]. Why are some people more prone to using Instagram and obsessing over how many "likes" they have accrued on their posts? What is it about some people having to constantly check their Twitter to see if their "tweets" are trending or how many "retweets" they have received? This theory could play a role in defining and characterizing social media addiction as a subset of SA.

3.4. Group-Specific Variation in SA

Of the total 108 studies, 84 (78%) focused on adolescents or emerging adults (ranging from elementary, middle, and high school students (32 of 84 studies, 38%) to college/university students (50 of 84, 59%) (the remaining two studies looked at both high school and university students)) and mentioned that smartphone use was highly prevalent among this youth/young adult group as compared to a more elderly group. Fourteen studies (13% of 108) focused on adults, and 10 studies included both child and adult participants, usually family members (10% of 108) (refer to Table 4).

Nineteen studies (18%) reported that gender was a significant predictor of SA, specifically that being female was significantly associated with higher tendencies toward SA or smartphone dependency or that SA/dependency/risk for SA was more prevalent in females than in males. Sixteen studies (15%) suggested that females may be more likely to be addicted to social media while males may be more likely to be addicted to gaming. However, no consistent findings regarding the subtypes of SA by gender were uncovered.

3.5. Generalizability of Study Results and Biases

Across all studies (refer to Table 4), the average percent of male participants was 46% (SD = 13). Twenty-four countries were represented in this review, with 90 studies (83%) categorized as a South, Southeast, or East Asian country (in order of frequency: South Korea, China, Turkey, Taiwan, India, Saudi Arabia, Lebanon, Bangladesh, Hong Kong, Indonesia, Iran, Iraq, and Malaysia).

All studies reported gender and age, and seven reported ethnicity (six studies with American adult participants and one with Brazilian adult participants). We also considered other common sociodemographic characteristics (SDCs) measures, including biometrics (e.g., height, weight, and BMI); number of children; education, income, marital, and work/employment status; and region (northern, southern, western, or eastern) or residence (urban or rural). Fifty of the 108 studies (46%) did not measure any SDCs, 27 (25%) looked at 1 SDC, 18 (17%) looked at 2, 9 (8%) looked at 3, and 4 (4%) looked at 4 SDCs.

About a third of the studies (35%) reported sampling bias (from convenience sampling), which did not allow for generalization of the findings outside of the study group population. For example, the results from studies focusing on university students may not apply to the general public. Recall bias of participants' self-reports on actual smartphone use and/or dependence, information bias, social desirability bias, response bias, and selection bias were also noted. Thirty-nine of the studies (36%) also reported multiple biases while 17 (16%) did not report any biases.

Only two studies used longitudinal data [64,65], and none of the others conducted follow-up assessments on the cross-sectional analyses of smartphone use and behavior. That is, limitations included: The use of cross-sectional data, which limits the ability to draw causal inferences, especially when determining the direction of association between SA/PSU and risk factors of interest; small sample size; not being able to determine whether study characteristics preceded SA/PSU development or were the outcome of smartphone use; use of less-than-optimal instruments tending to be subjective rather than objective; incentive-influenced survey answers; and attrition. The studies that did not report biases or limitations may have overlooked noting the potential ones mentioned above.

Nearly all of the authors recommended one or more of the following: Conducting future studies to further investigate the relationship between SA/PSU and related health risks, thoroughly identifying positive and negative outcomes, conducting longitudinally designed research studies with broader sample profiles; creating public health educational programs to inform the public of the physical and psychological risks associated with SA/PSU, and developing proper evidence-based strategies and interventions to address SA/PSU.

3.6. Quality of Samples and Level of Evidence

Examining data collection methods (refer to Table 5), about a half of the studies (49%) reported using convenience sampling, about a third (34%) reported random sampling, and the rest (17%) did not clearly report a sampling method. Most of the studies (90%) did not calculate an appropriate sample size before recruiting participants. In terms of sample sizes (with a range of 52–7003), 17 studies (16%) had 200 participants or less, 41 (38%) fell in the 201–500 range, 24 (22%) in the 501–1000 range, and 26 (24%) had more than 1001 participants.

In terms of associations with SA/PSU, 1 study focused on academic data, 11 (10%) presented physiological data (e.g., craniovertebral angle, skin conductance), 40 (37%) psychological data (e.g., depression, anxiety), 16 (15%) social data (e.g., social connectedness, alexithymia), 8 (7%) smartphone usage data (e.g., duration, types of functions used), and 28 (26%) reported a mix of those categories.

Most of the studies were subjective reports (90%). Ten of the 11 objective reports (one academic, four physiological, one psychological, two social, and two smartphone usage) were deemed suggestive (but not sufficient or indicative) of a causal association with SA/PSU. The remaining objective report (psychological) was deemed insufficient because the link between SA and national identity was not clear to us. Seven of the 97 subjective reports (six social, one psychological) were deemed suggestive (but not sufficient or indicative) because unlike other psychological reports (within which subjective reports can be verified with objective testing, or physiological measures), certain social aspects (e.g., loneliness, family history of alcohol addiction, need for social assurance, life satisfaction, parental neglect, friends' support, and peer relationships) are hard to measure with objective testing and so subjective data is helpful and could be relatively valid and reliable in those cases.

4. Discussion

4.1. Smartphone Addiction on a Continuum of Addictive Behaviors

4.1.1. Is Smartphone Addiction Really an Entity of Its Own?

With smartphone use engrained as the social norm today, and the pervasive use ever increasing despite an awareness of the health risks and adverse consequences, now the question is if excessive smartphone use is truly an addiction (SA) or just problematic smartphone use (PSU). This review highlights that SA articles already assume that SA is an addiction and frame the research as such, while PSU articles explore reasons why PSU falls short of meeting the necessary criteria to be considered a true addiction. The growing literature on excessive smartphone use has conceptualized the disorder as an addictive behavior. Specifically, advocates of PSU argue that the ethiopathological pathways and processes have not yet been identified in SA research, suggesting that SA interventions are simply targeting the symptoms rather than the underlying causes [66]. We agree that research on SA etiology is necessary in order for the disorder to be properly and accurately diagnosed. Although that will take a considerable amount of time and effort to accrue, hopefully our future capabilities to capture sound psychosocial as well as neurobiological evidence will be established. There has also been criticism that the only support to date of SA being an addiction is limited to "exploratory studies relying on self-report data which is collected via convenience sampl[ing]" [4]. Although the majority of recent reports have been subjective, there have been attempts to collect objective data that are promising, especially if those studies are planning on following up on the data in the future. It seems more studies are also trying to carry out randomized studies with larger sample sizes in order to expand on the empirical data available in the field of SA research.

The current review found that all of the assessment scales measuring SA/PSU met at least half of Griffiths' criteria, which need to be met in order for a disorder to be considered an addiction, according to Griffiths. However, PSU advocates counter that conforming excessive smartphone use within addiction models, such as Griffiths', could oversimplify the disorder and result in clinical irrelevance [66]. Specifically, attempts at conceptualizing tolerance with respect to SA may be insufficient, as inferring tolerance based on the increasing use of the smartphone could vary by several factors, such as age (e.g., teens pressured by peers to participate in social media use), subscription status (subscriptions to apps are paid in full or need to be paid monthly), relationship status (single versus in a relationship), occupation status (student, works desk job), and significant life events (starting or ending a romantic relationship) [4]. Although it could indeed oversimply the condition, Griffiths' model has been widely used as a biopsychosocial framework to operationalize addictive components, and so it is a good starting point to conceptualize the level of addiction to the smartphone. Also, once again, in order to truly verify conceptualizations like tolerance, there is a need for neurobiological evidence (e.g., "alteration/sensitization in specific cerebral circuitries" [4]) to confirm tolerance levels increasing in a smartphone user.

We considered using the "Surgeon General's criteria" (the "Hill criteria") for causality, noting the: (1) Consistency, (2) strength, (3) specificity, (4) temporal relationship, and (5) coherence of the association between SA/PSU and the variables of interest. However, we chose not to include consistency, as none of the studies conducted follow-up studies in different populations under different circumstances, or specificity, which researchers have criticized to be useless or misleading [67]. However, the vast majority of the studies only met the coherence criteria. Additionally, since all but two studies were longitudinal, temporality could not be assessed. Future studies could consider addressing the consistency, strength, and temporal relationship of the association by conducting longitudinal and follow-up studies, with adequate sample sizes ensuring power in the analyses.

4.1.2. Assuming SA Is an Addiction, Is It an Addiction to the Device or on the Device?

What used to be a novelty-type activity about a decade ago has now become more of a normative behavior [68]; excessive smartphone use is one of the more recent forms of human–machine interaction, raising public health alarms. However, the current review notes that despite the growing body of research, many studies still do not clearly define SA. In fact, in some of the literature, SA and PSU are still interchangeable terms. To add to the ambiguity, only about one in five articles make the distinction that SA is an addiction specifically to the mobile features provided by the smartphone (texting; various social media apps, such as Twitter and Instagram) that desktops and even laptops cannot match in terms of ease of portability and handheld capabilities. The vast majority of recent articles did not make a clear distinction of SA from related addictions, such as Internet or gaming addiction, suggesting that researchers may assume that SA is actually a subset of technological addictions. Those articles focused more on the mediating role of associated variables (e.g., emotional intelligence and coping style [48]) on SA and/or the moderating role of variables on the relation between risk factors of SA and SA (e.g., whether perceived social support and depression would moderate the relationship between sensation seeking and adolescent SA [49]) rather than differentiating SA from other technological addictions or specifying that SA is an addiction distinct from other addictions (e.g., gaming, gambling, shopping, socializing, sex) based on what the smartphone offers users.

We believe that the only difference between smartphone and Internet addiction (IA) is that SA is essentially IA presented through a highly portable device. IA is a potential addiction restricted to a stationary type of device. In contrast, excessive smartphone use is more prevalent due to its ease of access and portability, and the smartphone itself has become the most common device of choice for people today to access the Internet. Currently, the smartphone is the medium of problematic overuse of apps, games, and social networking site interactions. In the future, perhaps a new behavioral addiction will be virtual reality addiction through use of high-tech contact lens—the ever-changing and improving technological advancements will make possibilities (and potential problems) endless. However, for today, we argue that SA is an emerging addiction to the smartphone content specifically through the smartphone device.

4.1.3. Generalizability of Results and At-Risk Populations

The emergence of SA as an addiction is highlighted by the fact that people from various countries are affected by SA, which is not localized to just one continent but worldwide. Although several factors (e.g., not all sociodemographic characteristics of samples being measured, biases, cross-sectional limitations of inferencing causality, insufficient sample sizes, inability to determine directionality of SA and its risk factors, attrition) did not allow for generalization of the findings outside of the study group population, the results still suggested that children and young adults are more affected by SA than other age groups and that men and women are affected by SA in different ways.

In terms of SA affecting youth, one study reported that those at risk of developing SA displayed more severe levels of behavioral and emotional problems, lower self-esteem, and poorer quality of communication with their parents compared with those at normal risk [45]. In terms of gender differences, one study observed that girls who frequently use their smartphones may have a greater tendency to use social networking apps (e.g., Facebook) to upload pictures/share their lives online and therefore have a higher degree of smartphone attachment as compared to boys. Girls have also been reported to form and maintain social relationships and be engaged emotionally through constant app connection while boys mostly use smartphones to communicate through texts [36]. However, not all people at risk fall neatly into those observed categories. Implications of these differences require further research among similar group populations (e.g., youths, females versus males, students) around the world to better understand age, gender, and cultural variations in SA that may exist, which could help guide future tailored interventions.

4.2. Limitations

For this review, we narrowed our article pool by searching for only "smartphone"/"mobile phone" and "addiction"/"problematic use" terms. We did not actively search for "android", "iPhone", "cell phone", "cellular device", "compulsive use", "phubbing", "snubbing", and "nomophobia", which could have potentially made us miss articles relevant to this review. However, we were able to locate a few relevant articles after reviewing the reference sections of selected articles. Much more research is needed that investigates differences as a function of demographic variables, such as gender, age, or ethnicity. Another limitation is that our interpretations of categorizing certain variables into their respective groupings may not match others' opinions. For example, while we may propose that a certain subjective report is suggestive of a causal relationship with SA/PSU, another researcher may disagree and say that it is insufficient evidence. Another example would be missing a guiding theory used in articles, making Table 3 incomplete.

5. Conclusions

Most studies to date seem to assume that SA is a valid behavioral addiction, many forming their assumptions based on Griffiths' component model of addiction, and framing their study based on that assumption. The interchangeable use of the terms SA and PSU, inconsistent methodological approaches used to study SA (e.g., varied use of SA/PSU scales among research), lack of standardized diagnostic criteria, and unclear distinctions of SA from other related addictions make it difficult to make a conclusive statement on the status of SA, which could be considered "an ill-defined and heterogeneous construct" [67]. With no unifying theory on SA, all theories mentioned in the current research highlight the complexity of SA: One theory cannot simply explain SA, but rather several theories and models possibly need to be integrated to better explain its distinct addictive traits in this new technologically advanced era. Much more research is needed to confirm the uniqueness of SA, which encompasses the addictive activities engaged in on the smartphone, which includes apps that are not available on other devices. It is most plausible, based on the current studies, to infer that SA falls on a continuum of additive behaviors, from mild PSU to more extreme addictive behavior, where the consequences need to be addressed, prevented, and potentially treated before the adverse health effects debilitate the smartphone user.

Author Contributions: Conceptualization, methodology, analysis, writing—original draft preparation, S.Y.; writing—Review and editing, supervision, S.S. All authors have read and agreed to the published version of the manuscript.

Acknowledgments: We would like to thank Dmitri Rozgonjuk and Regina van den Eijnden for their support on this paper.

References

1. Elhai, J.D.; Dvorak, R.D.; Levine, J.C.; Hall, B.J. Problematic smartphone use: A conceptual overview and systematic review of relations with anxiety and depression psychopathology. *J. Affect. Disord.* **2017**, *207*, 251–259. [CrossRef] [PubMed]
2. Sapacz, M.; Rockman, G.; Clark, J. Are we addicted to our cell phones? *Comput. Hum. Behav.* **2016**, *57*, 153–159. [CrossRef]

3. Bianchi, A.; Phillips, J.G. Psychological predictors of problem mobile phone use. *Cyberpsychol. Behav.* **2005**, *8*, 39–51. [CrossRef] [PubMed]
4. Billieux, J.; Maurage, P.; Lopez-Fernandez, O.; Kuss, D.J.; Griffiths, M.D. Can Disordered Mobile Phone Use Be Considered a Behavioral Addiction? An Update on Current Evidence and a Comprehensive Model for Future Research. *Curr. Addict. Rep.* **2015**, *2*, 156–162. [CrossRef]
5. Choi, S.W.; Kim, D.J.; Choi, J.S.; Ahn, H.; Choi, E.J.; Song, W.Y.; Kim, S.; Youn, H. Comparison of risk and protective factors associated with smartphone addiction and Internet addiction. *J. Behav. Addict.* **2015**, *4*, 308–314. [CrossRef]
6. American Psychiatric Association. *Diagnostic and Statistical Manual of Mental Disorders*, 5th ed.; American Psychiatric Association: Arlington, VA, USA, 2013.
7. ICD-11 for Mortality and Morbidity Statistics. Available online: https://icd.who.int/browse11/l-m/en (accessed on 1 October 2019).
8. Sussman, S. *Substance and Behavioral Addictions: Concepts, Causes, and Cures*, 1st ed.; Cambridge University Press: Cambridge, UK, 2017.
9. Sussman, S.; Sussman, A.N. Considering the Definition of Addiction. *Int. J. Environ. Res. Public Health* **2011**, *8*, 4025–4038. [CrossRef]
10. Panova, T.; Carbonell, X. Is smartphone addiction really an addiction? *J. Behav. Addict.* **2018**, *7*, 252–259. [CrossRef]
11. Sussman, S.; Rozgonjuk, D.; van den Eijnden, R.J.J.M. Substance and behavioral addictions may share a similar underlying process of dysregulation. *Addiction* **2017**, *112*, 1717–1718. [CrossRef]
12. Alhassan, A.A.; Alqadhib, E.M.; Taha, N.W.; Alahmari, R.A.; Salam, M.; Almutairi, A.F. The relationship between addiction to smartphone usage and depression among adults: A cross sectional study. *BMC Psychiatry* **2018**, *18*, 148. [CrossRef]
13. Chen, C.; Zhang, K.; Gong, X.; Zhao, S.; Lee, M.; Liang, L. Examining the effects of motives and gender differences on smartphone addiction. *Comput. Hum. Behav.* **2017**, *75*, 891–902. [CrossRef]
14. Chun, J.S. Conceptualizing effective interventions for smartphone addiction among Korean female adolescents. *Child. Youth Serv. Rev.* **2018**, *84*, 35–39. [CrossRef]
15. Elserty, N.S.; Helmy, N.A.; Mounir, K.M. Smartphone addiction and its relation to musculoskeletal pain in Egyptian physical therapy students. *Eur. J. Physiother.* **2018**, 1–9. [CrossRef]
16. Hao, Z.; Jin, L.; Li, Y.; Akram, H.; Saeed, M.F.; Ma, J.; Ma, H.; Huang, J. Alexithymia and mobile phone addiction in Chinese undergraduate students: The roles of mobile phone use patterns. *Comput. Hum. Behav.* **2019**, *97*, 51–59. [CrossRef]
17. Jeong, Y.J.; Suh, B.; Gweon, G. Is smartphone addiction different from Internet addiction? comparison of addiction-risk factors among adolescents. *Behav. Inf. Technol.* **2019**, 1–16. [CrossRef]
18. Jin, Y.; Sun, C.; An, J.; Li, J. Attachment Styles and Smartphone Addiction in Chinese College Students: The Mediating Roles of Dysfunctional Attitudes and Self-Esteem. *Int. J. Ment. Health Addict.* **2017**, *15*, 1122–1134. [CrossRef]
19. Jo, H.; Na, E.; Kim, D.J. The relationship between smartphone addiction predisposition and impulsivity among Korean smartphone users. *Addict. Res. Theory* **2017**, *26*, 1–8. [CrossRef]
20. Konan, N.; Çelik, O.T. The Mediator Role of Interaction Anxiety in the Relationship between Social Support Perception and Smartphone Addiction. *J. Educ. Future* **2019**, *15*, 63–75.
21. Kwan, H.; Leung, M. The Structural Model in Parenting Style, Attachment Style, Self-regulation and Self-esteem for Smartphone Addiction. *J. Psychol. Behav. Sci.* **2017**, *3*, 85–103. [CrossRef]
22. Sekhon, A. Gender differences in mobile phone addiction and its association with stress among medical students. *Indian J. Health Wellbeing* **2018**, *9*, 232–234.
23. Yang, Z.; Asbury, K.; Griffiths, M.D. An Exploration of Problematic Smartphone Use among Chinese University Students: Associations with Academic Anxiety, Academic Procrastination, Self-Regulation and Subjective Wellbeing. *Int. J. Ment. Health Addict.* **2019**, *17*, 596–614. [CrossRef]
24. Arnavut, A.; Nuri, C.; Direktör, C. Examination of the relationship between phone usage and smartphone addiction based on certain variables. *An. Psicol.* **2018**, *34*, 446–450. [CrossRef]
25. Barnes, S.; Pressey, A.; Scornavacca, E. Mobile Ubiquity: Understanding the Impact of Cognitive Absorption on Smartphone Addiction. *Comput. Hum. Behav.* **2018**, *90*, 246–258. [CrossRef]

26. Chen, B.; Liu, F.; Ding, S.; Ying, X.; Wang, L.; Wen, Y. Gender differences in factors associated with smartphone addiction: A cross-sectional study among medical college students. *BMC Psychiatry* **2017**, *17*, 1–9. [CrossRef] [PubMed]
27. Chiang, J.T.; Chang, F.C.; Lee, K.W.; Hsu, S.Y. Transitions in smartphone addiction proneness among children: The effect of gender and use patterns. *PLoS ONE* **2019**, *14*, 1–12. [CrossRef]
28. Chung, J.E.; Choi, S.A.; Kim, K.T.; Yee, J.; Kim, J.H.; Seong, J.W.; Seong, J.M.; Kim, J.Y.; Lee, K.E.; Gwak, H.S. Smartphone addiction risk and daytime sleepiness in Korean adolescents: Smartphone addiction and sleep problems. *J. Paediatr. Child Health* **2018**, *54*, 800–806. [CrossRef]
29. Duke, E.; Montag, C. Smartphone addiction, daily interruptions and self-reported productivity. *Addict. Behav. Rep.* **2017**, *19*, 90–95. [CrossRef]
30. Kim, S.G.; Park, J.; Kim, H.T.; Pan, Z.; Lee, Y.; McIntyre, R.S. The relationship between smartphone addiction and symptoms of depression, anxiety, and attention-deficit/hyperactivity in South Korean adolescents. *Ann. Gen. Psychiatry* **2019**, *9*, 1–8. [CrossRef]
31. Kuang-Tsan, C.; Fu-Yuan, H. Study on Relationship Among University Students' Life Stress, Smart Mobile Phone Addiction, and Life Satisfaction. *J. Adult Dev.* **2017**, *24*, 109–118. [CrossRef]
32. Kuss, D.J.; Kanjo, E.; Crook-Rumsey, M.; Kibowski, F.; Wang, G.Y.; Sumich, A. Problematic Mobile Phone Use and Addiction Across Generations: The Roles of Psychopathological Symptoms and Smartphone Use. *J. Technol. Behav. Sci.* **2018**, *3*, 141–149. [CrossRef]
33. Lee, H.; Kim, J.W.; Choi, T.Y. Risk Factors for Smartphone Addiction in Korean Adolescents: Smartphone Use Patterns. *J. Korean Med. Sci.* **2017**, *32*, 1674–1679. [CrossRef]
34. Lee, C.; Lee, S.J. Prevalence and predictors of smartphone addiction proneness among Korean adolescents. *Child. Youth Serv. Rev.* **2017**, *77*, 10–17. [CrossRef]
35. Nayak, J.K. Relationship among smartphone usage, addiction, academic performance and the moderating role of gender: A study of higher education students in India. *Comput. Educ.* **2018**, *123*, 164–173. [CrossRef]
36. Yang, S.Y.; Lin, C.Y.; Huang, Y.C.; Chang, J.H. Gender differences in the association of smartphone use with the vitality and mental health of adolescent students. *J. Am. Coll. Health* **2018**, *66*, 693–701. [CrossRef] [PubMed]
37. Abed, S.N.; Abd, R.K.; Salim, I.D.; Jamal, N.A.R. Health problems of Mobile Phone Addiction for sample of students and their health awareness at institute technical of kut. *J. Pharm. Sci. Res.* **2018**, *10*, 412–415.
38. Alavi, S.S.; Ghanizadeh, M.; Mohammadi, M.R.; Kalhory, S.M.; Jannatifard, F.; Sepahbodi, G. The Survey personal and national identity between individual with cell phone addiction disorder and normal smartphone users. *Iran. J. Psychiatry* **2018**, *13*, 15–21.
39. Chen, C.Y. Smartphone addiction: Psychological and social factors predict the use and abuse of a social mobile application. *Inf. Commun. Soc.* **2018**, 1–14. [CrossRef]
40. Kim, J.H. Smartphone-mediated communication vs. face-to-face interaction: Two routes to social support and problematic use of smartphone. *Comput. Hum. Behav.* **2017**, *67*, 282–291. [CrossRef]
41. Kim, H.J.; Min, J.Y.; Min, K.B.; Lee, T.J.; Yoo, S. Relationship among family environment, self-control, friendship quality, and adolescents' smartphone addiction in South Korea: Findings from nationwide data. *PLoS ONE* **2018**, *13*, 1–13. [CrossRef]
42. Kim, Y.; Lee, N.; Lim, Y. Gender differences in the association of smartphone addiction with food group consumption among Korean adolescents. *Public Health* **2017**, *145*, 132–135. [CrossRef]
43. Kumcagiz, H. Quality of Life as a Predictor of Smartphone Addiction Risk Among Adolescents. *Technol. Knowl. Learn.* **2019**, *24*, 117–127. [CrossRef]
44. Lee, J.E.; Jang, S.I.; Ju, Y.J.; Kim, W.; Lee, H.J.; Park, E.C. Relationship between Mobile Phone Addiction and the Incidence of Poor and Short Sleep among Korean Adolescents: A Longitudinal Study of the Korean Children & Youth Panel Survey. *J. Korean Med. Sci.* **2017**, *32*, 1166–1172. [CrossRef] [PubMed]
45. Lee, J.; Sung, M.J.; Song, S.H.; Lee, Y.M.; Lee, J.J.; Cho, S.M.; Park, M.K.; Shin, Y.M. Psychological Factors Associated with Smartphone Addiction in South Korean Adolescents. *J. Early Adolesc.* **2018**, *38*, 288–302. [CrossRef]
46. Mahapatra, S. Smartphone addiction and associated consequences: Role of loneliness and self-regulation. *Behav. Inf. Technol* **2019**, *38*, 833–844. [CrossRef]

47. Sok, S.R.; Seong, M.H.; Ryu, M.H. Differences of Self-Control, Daily Life Stress, and Communication Skills between Smartphone Addiction Risk Group and General Group in Korean Nursing Students. *Psychiatr. Q* **2019**, *90*, 1–9. [CrossRef] [PubMed]
48. Sun, J.; Liu, Q.; Yu, S. Child neglect, psychological abuse and smartphone addictionamong Chinese adolescents: The roles of emotional intelligence and coping style. *Comput. Hum. Behav.* **2019**, *90*, 74–83. [CrossRef]
49. Wang, P.; Lei, L.; Wang, X.; Nie, J.; Chu, X.; Jin, S. The exacerbating role of perceived social support and the "buffering" role of depression in the relation between sensation seeking and adolescent smartphone addiction. *Personal. Indivd Differ.* **2018**, *130*, 129–134. [CrossRef]
50. Wang, P.; Zhao, M.; Wang, X.; Xie, X.; Wang, Y.; Lei, L. Peer relationship and adolescent smartphone addiction: The mediating role of self-esteem and the moderating role of the need to belong. *J. Behav. Addict.* **2017**, *6*, 708–717. [CrossRef]
51. Xu, T.T.; Wang, H.Z.; Fonseca, W.; Zimmerman, M.A.; Rost, D.H.; Gaskin, J.; Wang, J.L. The relationship between academic stress and adolescents' problematic smartphone usage. *Addict. Res. Theory* **2019**, *27*, 162–169. [CrossRef]
52. Yang, X.; Zhou, Z.; Liu, Q.; Fan, C. Mobile Phone Addiction and Adolescents' Anxiety and Depression: The Moderating Role of Mindfulness. *J. Child Fam. Stud.* **2019**, *28*, 822–830. [CrossRef]
53. Yildiz Durak, H. Investigation of nomophobia and smartphone addiction predictors among adolescents in Turkey: Demographic variables and academic performance. *Soc. Sci. J.* **2018**, in press. [CrossRef]
54. Yıldız, M. Emotion regulation strategies as predictors of internet addiction and smartphone addiction in adolescents. *J Educ. Sci. Psychol.* **2017**, *7*, 66–78.
55. Youn, H.; Lee, S.I.; Lee, S.H.; Kim, J.Y.; Kim, J.H.; Park, E.J.; Park, J.S.; Bhang, S.Y.; Lee, M.S.; Lee, Y.J.; et al. Exploring the Differences between Adolescents' and Parents' Ratings on Adolescents' Smartphone Addiction. *J. Korean Med. Sci.* **2018**, *33*, 1–11. [CrossRef] [PubMed]
56. Moher, D.; Liberati, A.; Tetzlaff, J.; Altman, D.G.; PRISMA Group. Preferred reporting items for systematic reviews and meta-analyses: The PRISMA statement. *PLoS Med.* **2009**, *6*, 1–6. [CrossRef]
57. Griffiths, M. A 'components' model of addiction within a biopsychosocial framework. *J. Subst. Use* **2005**, *10*, 191–197. [CrossRef]
58. Office of the Surgeon General (US); Office on Smoking and Health (US). *The Health Consequences of Smoking: A Report of the Surgeon General*; Centers for Disease Control and Prevention (US): Atlanta, GA, USA, 2004.
59. Kwon, M.; Lee, J.Y.; Won, W.Y.; Park, J.W.; Min, J.A.; Hahn, C.; Gu, X.Y.; Choi, J.H.; Kim, D.J. Development and Validation of a Smartphone Addiction Scale (SAS). *PLoS ONE* **2013**, *8*, 1–7. [CrossRef] [PubMed]
60. Lin, Y.H.; Chang, L.R.; Lee, Y.H.; Tseng, H.W.; Kuo, T.B.; Chen, S.H. Development and validation of the Smartphone Addiction Inventory (SPAI). *PLoS ONE* **2014**, *9*, 1–5. [CrossRef] [PubMed]
61. Kim, J.H. Psychological issues and problematic use of smartphone: ADHD's moderating role in the associations among loneliness, need for social assurance, need for immediate connection, and problematic use of smartphone. *Comput. Hum. Behav.* **2018**, *80*, 390–398. [CrossRef]
62. Cocoradă, E.; Maican, C.I.; Cazan, A.M.; Maican, M.A. Assessing the smartphone addiction risk and its associations with personality traits among adolescents. *Child. Youth Serv. Rev.* **2018**, *93*, 345–354. [CrossRef]
63. Elhai, J.D.; Levine, J.C.; Dvorak, R.D.; Hall, B.J. Non-social features of smartphone use are most related to depression, anxiety and problematic smartphone use. *Comput. Hum. Behav.* **2017**, *69*, 75–82. [CrossRef]
64. Herrero, J.; Torres, A.; Vivas, P.; Urueña, A. Smartphone Addiction and Social Support: A Three-year Longitudinal Study. *Psychosoc. Interv.* **2019**, *28*, 111–118. [CrossRef]
65. Herrero, J.; Urueña, A.; Torres, A.; Hidalgo, A. Socially Connected but Still Isolated: Smartphone Addiction Decreases Social Support Over Time. *Soc. Sci. Comput. Rev.* **2017**, *37*, 73–88. [CrossRef]
66. Billieux, J.; Philippot, P.; Schmid, C.; Maurage, P.; De Mol, J.; Van der Linden, M. Is Dysfunctional Use of the Mobile Phone a Behavioural Addiction? Confronting Symptom-Based Versus Process-Based Approaches. *Clin. Psychol. Psychother.* **2015**, *22*, 460–468. [CrossRef] [PubMed]
67. Rothman, K.J.; Greenland, S. *Hill's Criteria for Causality. Encyclopedia of Biostatistics, 2nd ed*; John Wiley & Sons, Ltd.: Hoboken, NJ, USA, 2005. [CrossRef]
68. Pinna, F.; Dell'Osso, B.; Di Nicola, M.; Janiri, L.; Altamura, A.C.; Carpiniello, B.; Hollander, E. Behavioural addictions and the transition from DSM-IV-TR to DSM-5. *J. Psychopathol.* **2015**, *21*, 380–389.

9

A Marketing Approach to a Psychological Problem: Problematic Smartphone Use on Adolescents

Adnan Veysel Ertemel [1,*] and Ela Ari [2]

1 Istanbul Commerce University, Faculty of Business Administration, International Trade Department, 34445 Istanbul, Turkey

2 Istanbul Medipol University, Faculty of Humanities and Social Sciences, Psychology Department, 34810 Istanbul, Turkey; eari@medipol.edu.tr

* Correspondence: avertemel@ticaret.edu.tr

Abstract: *Background:* Smartphones have become an indispensable part of the daily lives of adolescents in the 21st century, which is characterized by a highly digitized modern world. Besides their many advantages, smartphones might pave the way to compulsive usage and addictive experiences. To remedy this problem, this study proposes an authentic approach which integrates consumer behavior theories and techniques such as unhook and gamification. An education program has been designed based on these approaches to decrease the problematic smartphone use. *Method:* The participants of the education program consisted of 305 students (48.2% girls and 51.8% boys) with a mean age of 14.57 (SD = 0.74). The Demographic Form and Smartphone Addiction Scale for Adolescents (SASA) were conducted before the education program and three weeks after the education. *Results:* The results of the paired sample *t*-test analysis before and after the education program revealed that the SASA total scores decreased significantly ($p < 0.01$). There are significant differences in terms of gender, mothers' education and class levels. *Conclusion:* This research emphasizes the role of an interdisciplinary approach to the addiction problem. The content used in the education program includes strategies that originally aimed at increasing consumption. The effectiveness of the program can be enhanced further in the future along with self-regulatory additions.

Keywords: problematic smartphone use; adolescence; marketing; unhook; gamification

---

1. Introduction

With more than 3.1 [1] billion worldwide users as of 2019, which is expected to reach 3.8 billion by 2021 [2], smartphones have permanently changed our daily routines. They have become the de facto means for communication, socialization and access to information; and hence become inseparable in our lives [3]. When separated, individuals may encounter the following incidents: physiological withdrawal-like symptoms [4], increased anxiety [5] and even phantom vibration syndrome which can be described as the sensation that one's smartphone is vibrating even though there is no notification coming [6], a syndrome experienced by the majority of users [7].

Not surprisingly, problematic smartphone use, which can be categorized as a form of technological addiction [8], has become a major global concern across societies [3]. Technology addiction may be characterized as a non-chemical behavioral addiction involving human-computer interaction [9]. On the other hand, problematic smartphone use, which is also interchangeably called as smartphone addiction or smartphone use disorder [10], can be defined as the overuse of smartphones in a manner that is difficult to control and has harmful effects on the other areas of life [11].

As smartphones are devices that can be carried anywhere and are available anytime, problematic smartphone use causes various serious potential problems. Among those problems pointed in the literature are their negative effect in interpersonal relations, [12], personal health [13] well-being [14,15], including decreased academic performance and decreased physical activity [16] as well as depression symptoms [17]. Validating this phenomenon, American Psychiatric Association addressed this behavior in Diagnostic and Statistical Manual of Mental Disorders-5 (DSM-5) by introducing the non-substance addiction as a psychiatric diagnosis, although there are still controversies on the topic [18].

Contemporary research on behavioral psychology points out that addictions arise out of problematic habit-driven behavior, which is a natural outcome of ineffective self-regulation and self-control [19]. As such, this repetitive habitual behavior increases the risk of personal and social problems [20]. Frequent interruptions were found to result in loss of productivity [21] and higher tendency of attention deficit hyperactivity disorder [22]. Even the mere existence of a smartphone on a table when studying was found to result in reduced cognitive capacity and up to a 10% decrease in IQ [23,24]. Studies show that it takes 23 min on average for a fully concentrated individual to come back to the previous state after being interrupted with a notification message [25]. Worsening the case, the probability that the individual will self-interrupt increases by 8%.

As devices are being carried around all the time, Oulasvirta et al. [26] distinguish smartphone usage behavior as a series of 'short duration, isolated, reward-based' (SIRB) sessions as opposed to other technological devices like tablets and laptops. In this sense, informational rewards reinforce the checking behavior ultimately, performing it out of habit. As smartphones give access to a broad variety of sources for seeking information, socializing and entertainment, the overall reward value of "checking" habits increases as well.

Until recent times, severe criticisms of technology platforms due to their addictive-by-design experiences have gone unnoticed. However, the last couple of years witness a change in this case. As a result of the increasing awareness of these addictive-by-design techniques and the lobbying activities, technology platforms have started to adopt a more responsible code of conduct. As an example, Instagram and some other social media platforms changed their infinite scroll feature so that the users can scroll back up to two days. Again, as of 2019, Instagram started to hide the number of 'likes' to a post to avoid a meaningless competition of having more likes.

Problematic smartphone use can be attributed to many factors. In the last decade, however, it is argued that digital platforms' architected, finely tuned experiences that are designed to be addictive to deliberately make consumers spend prolonged periods of time on screens result in more problematic smartphone use [27–31]. Therefore, as opposed to looking from a mere psychological perspective, the need to adopt a multidisciplinary approach to prevent problematic smartphone use is brought into consideration.

Looking from a marketing perspective, we propose that using the same techniques that increase consumption—but in reverse manner—can effectively work in preventing problematic smartphone use. In the remainder of the paper, the defining characteristics of the modern digital marketing environment are discussed first. Afterwards, the mechanics of deliberately designed habit-forming experiences are explored. Finally, a consciousness-based preventive educational program on adolescents is proposed. The results of the study conducted among 305 students in 14 schools located in Istanbul, Turkey are also analyzed and discussed.

Adolescents were chosen as the target group since their acquaintance with smartphones is relatively new as opposed to their older counterparts, which implies that their smartphone behavior is not ossified yet. A study conducted late in 2019 in Turkey revealed that the most problematic smartphone use is seen in young adolescents and this problematic behavior rate decreases as the age of the users increases [32]. Another study conducted in Turkey published that 90.7% of the youngest age group (16–24). Internet use is listed as the heaviest compared to all other age groups. This group partially includes adolescents (10–19 years) which implies that this age group is the most susceptible to problematic smartphone use [33].

A recent global mobile consumer survey conducted in 28 countries across six continents revealed that Turkish consumers rank the highest in hourly checking of social networks and also highest in playing mobile games. Turkish consumers also ranked highest (26%) indicating physical health problems related with heavy smartphone usage [32]. These figures justify that adolescents are more prone to the risks associated with problematic smartphone use when compared to adults. Nevertheless, adolescents are more open to guidance for change. Undertaking such a study in Turkey is especially important since Turkey is classified as one of the countries with the highest risk potential of problematic smartphone use. Recent figures highlight that the percentage of Turkish users using WhatsApp heavily is 94% and Instagram with 80% is way higher than that of the European Union averages which is reported as 55% and 35%, respectively [32]. These rates place Turkey either to the first or the second place all over the world and above the averages of European countries.

In recent years, digital health related smartphone apps specifically designed to help individuals achieve positive behavior change started to emerge. These apps frequently use persuasive technology itself as a tool to reduce unhealthy, problematic smartphone use. The techniques used incorporate gamification, self-monitoring and goal setting [34].

However, to our knowledge, there is no structured education program that uses gamification, hook and the like techniques, in reverse manner, to decrease problematic smartphone use among adolescents.

1.1. New Marketing Strategies Appealing to the Unconscious

The highly competitive modern marketing environment of the 21st century imposes unique challenges. Whether online or offline, the abundance of marketing messages coming from a variety of sources has caused consumers to have difficulty in devoting their time and attention to those messages. With the advent of the Internet of things (IoT) and big data, consumers currently witness an even higher level of digitalization, which takes the aforementioned phenomenon to a different level.

In such a world, digital ecosystems are characterized by attention economy [35] in which marketers offer their services in exchange for the consumers' attention. Monetization occurs indirectly through advertisers. Facebook, Instagram, YouTube, Twitter are typical examples which do not charge consumers but monetize their attention in this attention economy.

Since appealing to the conscious mind in the attention economy becomes increasingly difficult marketers have started to resort to alternative strategies that appeal rather to the unconscious. As such, digital platforms, particularly in the last decade, are in an arms race to grab and keep the consumers' attention using sophisticated techniques in today's always on and connected world.

The flow theory, which has the aim of achieving the flow state, an emotional state embracing perceptual distortion and enjoyment [36] is one such strategy. Built on flow theory, new marketing strategies like gamification and user experience design which are collectively named as illusional marketing strategies [37,38] provide shortcuts to consumers by enabling them to take action without effortful thinking. The following sections provide further details on the marketing strategies, namely gamification and hook strategy, which make up the main focus of this paper, and are developed to design addictive experiences by appealing to the unconscious.

1.1.1. Gamification

Gamification can be described as the use of game design features in non-game contexts [39]. Through a gamified process, game elements and mechanics like achievements, progress bars, badges, leader boards, levels and points are employed to engage users [40]. In the context of marketing, gamification refers to a new marketing strategy that aims at changing the consumers' behavior in predetermined ways to foster engagement and ultimately to buy products [41,42]. In order to attain this goal, designation of an engaging experience plays a key role. Previous studies show that gamified and engaging experiences may result in brand recall and buying behavior [43].

Marketing scholars classify gamification as a different kind of persuasive marketing [44], which raises more ethical concerns than other persuasive marketing strategies like product packaging, personalized digital marketing, etc. Some other scholars define gamification as a form of stealth marketing which refers to configuring a product in such a way that people are not aware that the marketer is trying to persuade them to buy it [45]. These concerns arise out of the degree and type of engagement between the brand and consumers due to the highly engaging gamified experience. Deep sense of participatory engagement in gamification can also be compared to co-creation marketing [46,47] in which consumers' co-produce products by actively engaging in the design process [48]. However, gamification can have subversive results.

1.1.2. Hook Strategy

Hook is a recent marketing strategy similar to gamification, based on behaviorist thinking related to marketing software products. It has its roots in Persuasive Technology Lab in Stanford University, founded by BJ Fogg, back in 1998. This relatively new field has been named 'captology', which is an acronym for 'computers as persuasive technologies'. The ultimate goal in captology is to provide meaningful input into how software products can be designed to change consumer beliefs and behaviors [49].

Habitual behavior is central to such strategies. Habit-driven, automatic behaviors occupy the majority of the daily life and are performed with little, or no conscious thinking at all. Previous studies show that following a trigger-action-reward loop, a desirable habit can be imposed on an individual [50–52].

Impressed with Fogg's work, Eyal [53] developed the Hook model, which is grounded on the reinforcement theory in forming habitual behavior, which goes back to reinforcement experiments [54]. The Hook model advises a four-step loop to make the desired behavior a habitual one. The first step is the trigger, which refers to an external or internal stimulus that tells the user what to do next and how to behave next. The second step, action, refers to the actions of the user based on the information provided by the stimulus. The third stage, namely reward, refers to the acquisition of a variable reward as a consequence of the actions mentioned above. The last step, investment, means having the users make a deliberate effort to invest in the platform as in the form of time, effort, social capital investment to increase the likelihood of the repetitive behavior.

The Hook model can be illustrated through a typical Instagram usage habit. The process starts with a notification message, which is an external trigger. The model aims at starting with an external trigger and gradually making it an internal one. Internal triggers are states of mind and emotions. For the behavior to be habitual, the emotion should be somewhat vague and negative like loneliness, boredom, uncertainty, etc. Vague emotions allow the desired behavior to become a habit by avoiding reaching the consciousness level while negative emotions cause the individual to take action more easily [28].

Action refers to the behavior of entering the Instagram application. The key in the action step is to make the desired behavior as effortless as possible. This is because the level of effort required in the behavior directly affects the habitual nature of the behavior [53]. In this context, instead of requiring the user to enter a password, smartphones now enable a mindless sort of authentication by fingerprint or retina scans. This allows consumers to take the action step literally in an effortless manner. Auto-activation of the smartphone camera by a single swipe and the similar features serve the same goal.

The next step is the variable reward. It is what the notification is all about. For example, the user might have uploaded a photo album that consists of many photos. The variable reward is the discovery of which photo got the most likes, how many likes are received in total, who have commented and what they said about the posts and so on. The fact that the reward is variable allows the unconscious to be stimulated by surprise, causing dopamine release in the brain and regarding the perception of the reward as reinforcing [55]. Immediate variable rewards work perfectly well when the brain is in the unconscious mode [55] by gradually associating the reward with the trigger.

Additionally, it has been documented that this state of mind causes an individual's long run self to have no control over his or her decisions [56], which in turn causes a compulsive and addictive behavioral pattern.

The last step, investment to the platform, refers to invest in a small effort on the platform in such a way that calls for the repetition of the behavior over time, and finally makes it impossible to break off from the cycle. In Instagram application, this investment is the number of followers and the photo archive accumulated so far. The more investment is made in the platform, the more addictive it becomes. The system aims to replace the external trigger with the internal trigger in the long term. In Instagram application, the internal trigger is the desire not to miss the opportunity to capture a photo of the moment. An individual's Spotify list, for example, is perceived as valuable since he/she has spent a considerable amount of effort creating that list.

The addictive nature of various digital platforms was confirmed in various studies [31,57]. Some authors who investigated the gamification strategy also warn that the application of variable rewards may create gambling-like addictive experiences, which may lead to consumers being unable to exercise their free will [58]. The flow state is a state of mind characterized with enjoyment and perceptual distortion in time and space contributing to the addictive behavior [36]. The Hook model could be classified as a more sophisticated form of gamification since it targets the unconscious, applying gamification elements such as variable rewards and is designed to be addictive in nature. In this study, both hook and gamification strategies will be included in the education program considering their potential to create new habitual behavior [30].

Finally, this study first sought to explore the demographic factors influence on the adolescents' problematic smartphone use, namely gender, age, grades and parental education [59–62]. Afterwards, the main focus of the study is to find out how does a marketing based education program reduces the problematic smartphone use of adolescents. Further, and last of all, the study investigates how the smartphone problematic use changed after the education according to the above stated demographic factors as gender, age, and grades except parents' education. For all these research aims, the following hypotheses are formulated under three main categories, which are before the education program, about the education program and after the education program. Thus, the following hypotheses guided the present study.

Before the education program;

Hypothesis 1 (H1). *The problematic smartphone use differs according to demographic factors.*

Hypothesis 1 (H1a). *The problematic smartphone use differs on the basis of gender.*

Hypothesis 1 (H1b). *Age and problematic smartphone use are related.*

Hypothesis 1 (H1c). *The problematic smartphone use differs on the basis of the adolescents' grades.*

Hypothesis 1 (H1d). *The problematic smartphone use of adolescents differs on the basis of their parents' education level.*

About the education program;

Hypothesis 2 (H2). *The adolescents' problematic smartphone use will decrease after receiving a marketing based education program including gamification and unhook strategies.*

After the education program,

Hypothesis 3 (H3). *The problematic smartphone use differs according to demographic factors after the education program.*

Hypothesis 3 (H3a). *The problematic smartphone use decrease differs on the basis of gender after the education.*

Hypothesis 3 (H3b). *Age and the problematic smartphone use after the education are related.*

Hypothesis 3 (H3c). *The problematic smartphone use differs on the basis of the adolescents' grades after the education.*

2. Method

2.1. Participants

The sample consisted of 337 students from 14 different schools. Out of 337 participants, 32 were excluded since they were outliers or had missing data. In total, 144 girls (47.2%) and 161 boys (52.8%) participated in the study. Their mean age was 14.57 (SD = 0.74).

2.2. Procedure

2.2.1. Before the Education Program

The researchers have promoted the free education program to decrease problematic smartphone use on the social media platforms of the associated university. After that, the university corporate communications and public relations department e-mailed about the education program to school counselors of various schools residing in Istanbul. Following this, the education program was scheduled with the school counselors who requested it. Afterwards, school counselors have chosen the class sections randomly. Then, the school counselors sent to their families two weeks before the parental permission form including an information sheet about the research and a certificate of consent about the adolescent's participation to the education program and research.

On the day of the education after the education, those students who volunteer to participate signed an assent form. If the adolescents did not sign the assent form they were not included in the study. Thus, only 337 out of 1055 students signed the assent form. Then, the researcher explained the procedures to the participants to complete the surveys. The participants were allowed to ask questions if they encountered problems while completing the questionnaires, and the research assistants helped them to resolve their problems.

2.2.2. Description of the Education Program

The intervention included a PowerPoint presentation accompanied by several striking videos that highlight the non-neutral characteristic of technology. The adolescents were also given flyers that highlight the key points as reminders of the education and a check-list of to-do items to be performed throughout the three-week observation period.

The whole program was delivered in one day using two breaks. The education program consisted of eight modules. Each module of the program roughly lasted about 15 min. The first module consisted of creating awareness about the problematic use of smartphones. The educator presented famous technology figures' examples and introduced statistics about the problematic smartphone use.

The module included evidence based striking facts and insights on how Silicon Valley-based technology platforms create addictive experiences. For example, Twitter, Instagram and Facebook platforms create a "craving" effect on users by making them wait (on variable time) to get their liking feedback.

Once the participants were oriented and motivated to be a conscious smartphone user, then the next module was implemented, which showed how to measure and keep track of the participants' screen time. The educator explained in detail the hook strategy that marketers employ to engage users.

The next module was about presenting the participants how to unhook from their smartphones. Snapchat's Snap Streaks feature could be regarded as a deceptive example to hook strategy. This feature shows the number of consecutive days someone has messaged to his or her respective friend as a badge. Adolescents see it as an indication of how strong their relationships are with their acquaintances and hence they do not want to break the streak. During the education program, some participants reflected by stating that when they were to be offline for a certain period of time (during a holiday with their family, etc.) they gave their user credentials to one of their close friends and asked them to send dummy messages to their stated friends so as not to break their snap streaks.

In order to practice unhook strategies, the participants were first asked to identify the applications that made them feel unhappy. These applications were removed with the guidance of the educator. Additionally, in this module, the participants were persuaded to hide the social media applications that hooked them inside a folder. The home screen was cleared up and the time consuming applications were saved in another folder.

During the third module, participants learned how to turn off all the notifications. Also the educator instructed to mute the group messages and to remove the last seen or read information from the account menu under the privacy settings. Once all the sources of distractions were removed, the fourth module was initiated.

It was in the fourth module that a digital diet program was introduced. The fifth module integrated mindfulness applications as well as attention focusing techniques to control unconscious use. The sixth module included strategies to increase the quality of the participants' social relationships. The adverse effects of being available all the time and its damaging impact on personal productivity were explained along with supportive research findings. Afterwards, steps that could be taken to prevent the problem were introduced. On WhatsApp, for example, the adolescents were advised to avoid immediate reply to not-so-urgent incoming messages and to put a deliberate delay so that the other party's anticipation for an immediate reply was lowered. Then, the educator taught the participants to build the communication rules and facilitate the quality of social communication without phone. Recent studies showed that 72% of adolescents (as opposed to 48% of adults) feel an urge to respond to an incoming call or a message immediately [63]. This phenomenon can be attributed to the wrong interpersonal communication etiquette as well as low self-control and peer pressure. Therefore, the education module also incorporated the proper etiquette for communication that relieves the individual from feeling the urge to respond to everything immediately.

All through the seventh module a gamification strategy was used to engage the adolescents with the use of #iamincontrol hashtag use. This module of the education was about adolescents' controlling their lives. The participants learned how to protect an area they identified as a phone-free zone. The educator taught when, where and how to leave their phone in their daily routines.

The participants were also offered many activities they could plan together with their loved ones. Along the modules, the participants were asked to do homework and were supported with manuals, digital diet planners, activities list and handy calendars. Once all the content was delivered, the researcher scheduled a follow-up meeting three weeks after with the same school.

2.2.3. After the Education Program

Three weeks later, the scales and checklist were collected from the participants with the help of the school counselors. The participants who conducted the demographic questionnaires and the smartphone addiction scale before the education were distributed an id number so that it matched the collected surveys after the program. The researchers prepared an evaluation form to test the effectiveness of each task in the education program. Then, the participants were asked to rate about the effectiveness of each step in the program. Finally, they rated these steps according to their own usage benefits.

2.3. *Measures*

Demographic Form: The form includes gender, age, parents' education, parents' occupation, social media use of the family and the adolescent, purpose of use for the smartphone and the time they started using it and how much time they spent on it on a daily basis.

The Smartphone Addiction Scale for Adolescents

The Smartphone Addiction Scale for Adolescents (SASA) measures smartphone addiction. SASA was developed by Kwon et al. [60]. The Turkish validation study conducted by Demirci et al. (2014) consisted of 6 point Likert scales ranging from 1 (Definitely No) to 6 (Definitely Yes), 36-items and 7 factors as disturbing daily life and tolerance, withdrawal symptoms, positive anticipation, overuse, social network dependency, physical symptoms and cyberspace-oriented relationships [61].

The correlations between the subscales ranged from 0.22 to 0.51 The highest total scales values indicated a higher risk for problematic smartphone addiction. The Cronbach's α's of the seven factors were found respectively as 0.85, 0.81, 0.74, 0.62, 0.59, 0.64, 0.34 and 0.89 for the total scale in this study, which are very close to the validated scale. The Pearson correlations coefficients varied between the SASA factors and total varied between 0.18 and 0.75, indicating statistically significant positive relations (all p's < 0.01). Since it is a reliable and valid tool of measurement, SASA was conducted to assess the change in the smartphone usage before and after the education program.

2.4. *Statistical Analysis*

The data analysis was conducted using SPSS 21 for Windows. Descriptive statistics were calculated to investigate the demographic data. In order to test first and third set of hypotheses, the demographics of the participants were compared by independent sample *t*-tests analysis of variance tests. Pearson moment correlation analysis was run to evaluate the relationships between continuous demographics (e.g., age) and the factors of SASA. In order to test Hypothesis 2 which aims to evaluate of the effectiveness of education, paired sample *t*-test was used to compare before and after SASA scores.

2.4.1. Demographic Results

Three hundred and five participants were included in this study. 144 (47.2%) were female, and 161 (52.8%) were male. Only 44 (14.4%) of the participants indicated that they had cyber friendship, which they had met online and then later got to know in person. Table 1 listed gender, grades, electronics they possess, purpose of use, applications they have and parents' education.

2.4.2. Difference Tests Results before the Education

Smartphone use variable was the reported use of smartphone time as minutes per day (X_{use} = 139.84, SD = 83.68). The daily use of smartphones was declared to be less than 180 minutes for 75%, between 180 to 300 min for 21.5% and more than 300 min for 3.5% of the sample.

The first set of hypotheses explored the problematic smartphone use difference in terms of gender (H1a), age (H1b), adolescents' grades (H1c) and parents' education (H1d). In order to test gender differences, an independent sample *t*-test was conducted. As a result, there were no significant difference between boys (X_{boys} = 81.06) and girls (X_{girls} = 84.99) in terms of total SASA before the education ($p > 0.05$).

Then, to test the age and SASA relation (H1b), a Pearson moment correlation analysis was conducted. The findings revealed no significant relationship between age and SASA scores (r = 0.01, $p > 0.05$).

In order to test the problematic smartphone use difference on the basis of the adolescents' grades (H1c) an analysis of variance test showed that SASA scores before the education do differ significantly according to the students' grade levels. A Tukey post hoc test indicated that the SASA scores increased significantly at 10th grade (X_{Pep} = 16.19 X_{9th} = 17.26 X_{10th} = 19.33 X_{11th} 17.06 $F_{(305)} = 3.59$, $p < 0.05$ d = 0.3).

Table 1. Demographics of the Participants.

N = 305	Frequency	Percentage
Gender		
Female	144	47.2
Male	161	51.8
Grades		
Prep (14 yrs)	44	14.4
9th Grade (15 yrs)	210	68.9
10th Grade (16 yrs)	31	10.2
11th Grade (17 yrs)	20	6.6
The distribution of electronics they do possess		
Smartphone	305	100
Computer	187	61.3
Pad	82	26.9
Console	57	18.7
Smartphone purpose of use		
Education/Research	275	90.2
Entertainment/Game	239	78.4
Free Time	207	67.9
Social Media	238	78.0
Communication	217	71.1
Shopping	124	40.7
Applications participants have		
WhatsApp	302	99.0
Instagram	247	81.0
Facebook	75	24.6
TicToc	10	3.3
Snapchat	102	33.4
Twitter	58	19.0
Pinterest	67	22.0
YouTube	222	72.8
Twitch	43	14.1
Mother's Education		
Middle School	125	41.0
High School	78	25.6
College	102	33.4
Father's Education		
Middle School	89	29.2
High School	91	29.8
College	125	41.0

In order to measure the problematic smartphone difference on the basis of the parents' education (H1d) an analysis of variance test indicated that the adolescents' SASA scores vary according to their mothers' education level. A Tukey post hoc test showed that there was a significant difference between high school graduates and college graduates' mothers in terms of their children's SASA scores ($X_{MiddleSchool} = 17.39$ $X_{HighSchool} = 18.13$ $X_{College} = 16.52$; $F_{(305)} = 3.62$, $p < 0.05$). Another analysis of variance test revealed that fathers' education also differed in terms of their children's SASA scores. A Tukey post hoc test showed that there was a significant difference between high school graduates and college graduates fathers' in terms of their children's SASA scores ($X_{MiddleSchool} = 16.95$ $X_{HighSchool} = 18.22$ $X_{College} = 16.89$; $F_{(305)} = 3.21$, $p < 0.05$ d = 0.3).

2.4.3. Difference Tests Results after the Education

In order to test the second hypothesis, which evaluated the influence of the education program, a paired sample *t*-test analysis before and after the education program was conducted. As shown in Table 2, the results revealed a significant decrease in disturbing daily life and tolerance ($X_{pretest} = 2.93$ $X_{posttest} = 2.68$), withdrawal symptoms ($X_{pretest} = 2.09$ $X_{posttest} = 1.97$), positive anticipation ($X_{pretest} =$

3.18 $X_{posttest} = 2.84$), overuse ($X_{pretest} = 2.61$ $X_{posttest} = 2.44$), physical symptoms ($X_{pretest} = 2.67$ $X_{posttest} = 2.51$) dimensions and in the total SASA scale ($X_{pretest} = 17.30$ $X_{posttest} = 16.19$). Cyberspace oriented relationships and social network dependence factors did not change significantly after the education program (p 's > 0.05). Thus, the effectiveness of the education program has been proven for total and five factors except cyberspace oriented relationships and social network dependence factors as can be seen in Table 2.

Table 2. Paired sample t test results before and after the education program.

Factors	Mean Difference	St. Dev	t	p
1. Disturbing daily life and tolerance	0.25	0.81	5.29	<0.01 **
2. Withdrawal symptoms	0.12	0.75	2.56	<0.01 **
3. Positive anticipation	0.34	0.88	6.73	<0.01 **
4. Cyberspace oriented relationships	0.03	0.74	0.75	0.45
5. Overuse	0.17	0.89	3.32	<0.01 **
6. Social network dependence	0.06	1.05	1.06	0.29
7. Physical symptoms	0.15	0.89	2.97	<0.01 **
Total SASA	1.11	3.45	5.61	<0.01 **

Notes: ** deemed significant at the 0.01 level.

In order to test the third set of hypotheses that explore the difference of the problematic smartphone use in terms of gender (H3a), age (H3b) and adolescents' grades (H3c). Firstly, an independent sample t-test was conducted to compare boys' and girls' SASA scores after the education program (H3a). The results revealed that male adolescents' total SASA dropped significantly more than those of the girls with a medium effect size ($X_{female} = 17.17$ $X_{male} = 15.31$; $t_{(305)} = 3.63$, $p < 0.01$ d = 0.42). Additionally, the SASA scores of the participants after the education have been subtracted from the SASA scores before the education. Boys' change is significantly higher than that of girls' change ($X_{girls} = -0.58$ $X_{boys} = -1.58$; $t_{(305)} = 2.55$, $p < 0.01$ d = 0.30).

Following this, to test the age and SASA relation after the education program (H3b), a Pearson moment correlation analysis was conducted. The findings revealed no significant relationship between age and SASA scores after the education program ($r = -0.01$, $p > 0.05$).

After the completion of the education, an analysis of variance test indicated that SASA scores varied significantly according to the adolescent's grades. A Tukey post hoc test showed that only the SASA scores of preparation grade and 10th graders were significantly different ($X_{Pep} = 14.56$ $X_{9th} = 16.36$ $X_{10th} = 17.33$ $X_{11th} = 16.23$; $F_{(305)} = 2.66$, $p < 0.05$ d = 0.02).

2.5. Feedback Results about the Program

The percentage of the participants who practice no-tolerance rule to phubbing friends, those who prefer to look to their smartphone screens instead of themselves in a physical conversation were 62% and 56% of them have found this method to be somewhat or absolutely useful. The corresponding percentages for turning-off all notifications (except from real people) were 55% and 58%, putting all WhatsApp group messages to silent mode were 68% and 65% and turning off the last seen time and read receipt of WhatsApp messages were 58% and 56% respectively.

Initially, many adolescents had reported that they had hard time trying them. After experiencing these methods, however, many of them reflected that they feel more in control of technology and can now focus more easily on their tasks.

3. Discussion

This study first aims to investigate the role of demographic factors, namely gender, age, grades and parents' education level of adolescents in assessing their tendency for smartphone addiction before the education. The first hypothesis related to demographics' differentiation in terms of problematic smartphone use is examined separately for gender, age, grades and parental education. The problematic smartphone use did not differ on the basis of gender nor has been associated with age. Only the problematic smartphone use differs for grades and parental education. The second hypothesis, which constitutes the main objective of this study, is about inquiring the effectiveness of a novel education program for reducing problematic smartphone use in adolescents. In order to achieve this, a marketing based education program has been developed and then later measured the effect before and three weeks after the program. The change in problematic smartphone use showed a significant decrease. Moreover, the last hypothesis is related to the demographic factors, specifically gender, age and grades. These demographics are critical in order to understand which ones differed after the education for future references. Gender and grades differed in terms of decreases in problematic smartphone addiction.

Concerning the first hypothesis, the current study revealed that there is no statistically significant difference between girls and boys in terms of their SASA scores before the education. Thus, the first hypothesis of this study is rejected confirming the previous studies [59,60]. There are many studies that indicated female addiction is higher than males [64–66]. These studies attribute females' higher tendency for mobile addiction to females' being more likely to engage in interpersonal communication and social relationships via their mobile phone [67,68]. Moreover, Demirci et al.'s (2014) study conducted in Turkey indicated higher SASA scores for female participants. The fact that the difference between boys and girls is not significant in this present study can be explained first by age factor. The participants of this study consisted of adolescents while Demirci et al.'s (2014) study consisted of college students. Second, not only the age group might have brought out the discrepancy between these studies but also the six years' difference (2014–2020) might have changed the rates. Indeed, gender gap is predicted to decrease over the years with the advances in technology spreads, which also explains the current gender similarity in terms of addiction [69]. The total SASA scores of the adolescents in this study (girls were 84.99 and boys were 81.06) are higher but the gender difference has closed compared to previous findings [60] as (females were 78.7 and males were 72.2). As a matter of fact, this finding confirm that the gender gap is closing and problematic smartphone use has gradually become more prevalent among adolescents in recent years [32].

This study could not find a statistically significant relationship between age and problematic smartphone use. As Demirci et al. (2014) study [60] also found non-significant negative relationship between age and smartphone addiction, the results are in line with the previous study. Some studies, particularly in the Internet addiction domain, find such negative but significant relation between adolescents' age and addiction level stating that this risky behavior is temporary in the adolescence period. This phenomenon is said to wear off with increased familiarity with the technology [70,71].

The problematic smartphone use differed significantly on the basis of the adolescents' grades. Beginning around age 10 adolescent risk taking, reward sensitivity behaviors start increasing, then peak between 13 and 16, and then decline [72–74]. The problematic smartphone use according to grades is in line with the risk preference trend. The earlier grades' SASA scores are lower than the later ones, then there is a peak at 10th graders and then it drops again.

The higher the maternal and paternal education level the lower were the SASA scores except for college graduates. The college graduate parents are mostly white collar workers who might spend less time and control over the adolescents which might have caused more problematic smartphone use. Thus, this finding of the present study partially confirms the previous studies in the literature [66,67]. In the light of these findings, we can conclude that, both parents' education and attention, which ultimately contributes to a more beneficial attitude towards adolescents [66].

The main aim this study is to reduce the problematic smartphone use after a marketing based education program. The education program started with explaining the negative consequences of problematic smartphone use in terms of its harm on cognitive capacity, academic performance and social relationships. Afterwards, the internal mechanics of addictive design elements of digital products are explained in detail. The program followed by going through the steps in the hook model aimed at exercising the opposite behavior in each step to prevent unconscious, compulsive smartphone usage and ensure conscious and healthy usage behavior. The education program was coupled with a follow-up meeting three weeks after the education. The education module aimed at building awareness on the specifics of addictive mechanisms that ultimately hook users.

Concerning the second hypothesis, the results are very promising since the comparison of SASA scores before and after the education program has proven significant decrease in problematic smartphone use. The disturbing daily life and tolerance, withdrawal symptoms, positive anticipation, overuse, physical symptoms dimensions and the total SASA scores decreased significantly after the education program. The cyberspace-oriented relationships and social network dependence factors did not change significantly after the education program. When the cyberspace-oriented relationship factors' questions items are checked closely, there is a distinction between cyber friends and friends. Only a small percent of the participants did make cyber friendship (14.1%). This fact might be due to the more conservative nature of families in Turkey [75] in which adolescents are still protected closely. Finally, the social network dependence factor did not change significantly after the education. The two items that measured social dependence did include social applications as Facebook and Twitter. The participants' reports indicated that the rate of use for Facebook (24.6%) and Twitter (18.5%) is considerably low. Since most of the participants do not use these applications, these questions might have misdirected them.

Concerning the third hypothesis, the boys' SASA scores decreased more compared to those of the girls. The addiction literature provides evidence of that women had 2.7 more risk at smartphone addiction than men [76]. When women try to be abstinent, they show greater anxiety and stress compared to men [77,78]. First, it might be less stressful to reduce the problematic smartphone use for boys than girls. Furthermore, girls tend to strengthen their friendships, which keeps them on the smartphones and receive more emotional support, while boys aim to use smartphones to extend their weak social relations [79]. The education program's emphasis on how to build social relationship without the use of smartphones might have reduced boys' problematic smartphone use more than the girls. Girls define smartphones as central component of their personal existence [80] which could bring more resistance to reduce their smartphone use.

It was found that there is no significant relationship with adolescents' age and smartphone addiction levels after the education program. There are in the literature longitudinal and cross sectional studies where the expected behavior and age were not correlated after the intervention either [81,82]. A meta-analysis about the intervention programs applied to subjects under 18 years of age revealed that age did not have an influence on the success of the programs [83]. However, the later study mentioned about the possibility of cognitive developmental level, which might be related to grades.

The problematic smartphone use differed significantly on the basis of the adolescents' grades after the education. As a matter of fact, this finding pattern is very similar to the case before education. This illustrates that adolescents at earlier grades are still more open to guidance for healthier and more proper communication suggestions. This can be also explained by the fact that the education could be more influential when the habitual behavior of using a smartphone has recently started.

The results also reveal that, with a 97.2% usage rate, smartphone use is much more prevalent than the use of any other technology products. The results also show that among the responding adolescents, 57.6% check their social media from their smartphone more than 10 times a day. WhatsApp was found to be the most frequently installed mobile app; almost all the responding adolescents (98.2%) use it. Instagram (80.5%) was found to be the second mostly used app among the adolescents.

Overall, the results of the study suggest that educational guidance for healthy usage of technology is missing or not adequate in the visited schools. Unfortunately, the current educational system fails to provide even the basic communication etiquette to adolescents. That is, adolescents do not know and are eager to learn the proper way to communicate with their peers (importance of face to face communication etc.). This is especially valid for younger adults as opposed to their older counterparts.

Limitations and Implications for Future Research

Due to the peculiar characteristics of this special age group, namely adolescents, self-reported inventories like the one in this study have self-assessment bias risk. The results may also differ in terms of participants' self-involvement level, sincerity, beliefs etc. In addition, this study has been conducted in a relatively more conservative culture, which might have driven participants to give desirable answers.

All in all, the program is distinguished in that an improvement is achieved using a structured program. However, in the future, longer and more thorough educational programs could be designed to achieve more lasting effect. In addition, such an educational program could have much more impact if coupled with a digital health app usage that tracks individual behavior.

4. Conclusions

Technology platforms have been creating increasingly more addictive experiences that result in spending prolonged periods of time on screens, which ultimately leads to more profitability in the attention economy. Some of these addictive features include the lack of stop sign facilitated by infinite scroll feature, the hooking technique that relies mainly on the unconscious and employs mechanisms like variable rewards.

Problematic smartphone use increasingly becomes more of a concern globally especially among adolescents. In this study, a marketing approach was adopted in an education program. Consumer-engaging methodologies are used to increase awareness on specifics of hooking strategies and to disengage adolescents from their phones. The results are significant in that an apparent improvement in problematic smartphone use is accomplished with a short and structured education program. Although there are some mindfulness-based intervention studies that have proven to reduce smartphone use [84], to our knowledge, this is the first study in which a marketing-focused education program has been developed to approach smartphone addiction. The program also offered practical, ready-to-use tips to restrain oneself from unconscious, compulsive smartphone use.

This study makes significant contributions to the existing literature in several aspects. Firstly, looking from a marketing perspective, it uses the strategies employed to increase compulsive, unconscious smartphone usage, but in reverse direction to prevent excessive and hence problematic smartphone use. In addition, an educational program was introduced with a special emphasis placed on the conscious usage of smartphones.

Living without digital technologies has become almost impossible. This is particularly true as global pandemics (i.e., Covid-19 virus a.k.a. Corona virus) and the like developments are poised to change our daily habits radically. However, the key question in our relationship with technology is about which party will be in control. Unconscious, compulsive smartphone usage lets technology control users. It will be only by educating the society with the proper way of smartphone use that we can turn the situation the other way around.

The conducted study was scheduled as a one-time education. However, if these eight modules could be spread across the eight-week period with more supportive homework and with more detailed monitoring, the benefits could be improved. Future studies could integrate cognitive behavioral approaches and more gamified activities in order to hook adolescents back to their own future.

Author Contributions: Conceptualization, project administration, organization of the schools, as well as education content and delivery were prepared by A.V.E. Methodology, scale and demographics selections, data preparation and analysis were done by E.A. Writing, reviewing and editing were distributed equally between the two authors. All authors have read and agreed to the published version of the manuscript.

Acknowledgments: We would like to acknowledge Istanbul Commerce University for funding to our project and Oya Özkardeş for her guidance. Special thanks to project fellows Dilara Güler and Zehra Özalp for their technical support in data analysis, Ahu Dereli Dursun and İpek Sarıgöz for her rigorous work in editing process.

References

1. We Are Social. Global Report. 2019. Available online: https://wearesocial.com/global-digital-report-2019 (accessed on 10 September 2019).
2. Ericsson, A.B. *Mobility Report 2015*; Ericsson: Stockholm, Sweden, 2017.
3. Cheever, N.A.; Rosen, L.D.; Carrier, L.M.; Chavez, A. Out of sight is not out of mind: The impact of restricting wireless mobile device use on anxiety levels among low, moderate and high users. *Comput. Hum. Behav.* **2014**, *37*, 290–297. [CrossRef]
4. Clayton, R.B.; Leshner, G.; Almond, A. The extended iSelf: The impact of iPhone separation on cognition, emotion, and physiology. *J. Comput. Mediat. Commun.* **2015**, *20*, 119–135. [CrossRef]
5. Wise, R.A.; Koob, G.F. The development and maintenance of drug addiction. *Neuropsychopharmacology* **2014**, *39*, 254. [CrossRef] [PubMed]
6. Kruger, D.J.; Djerf, J.M. High ringxiety: Attachment anxiety predicts experiences of phantom cell phone ringing. *Cyberpsychol. Behav. Soc. Netw.* **2016**, *19*, 56–59. [CrossRef]
7. Drouin, M.; Kaiser, D.H.; Miller, D.A. Phantom vibrations among undergraduates: Prevalence and associated psychological characteristics. *Comput. Hum. Behav.* **2012**, *28*, 1490–1496. [CrossRef]
8. Lin, Y.H.; Chang, L.R.; Lee, Y.H.; Tseng, H.W.; Kuo, T.B.; Chen, S.H. Development and validation of the Smartphone Addiction Inventory (SPAI). *PLoS ONE* **2014**, *9*, e98312. [CrossRef]
9. Griffiths, M.D. Behavioural addiction and substance addiction should be defined by their similarities not their dissimilarities. *Addiction* **2017**, *112*, 1718–1720. [CrossRef]
10. Griffiths, M. Gambling on the Internet: A brief note. *J. Gambl. Stud.* **1996**, *12*, 4–471. [CrossRef]
11. Park, N.; Lee, H. Social implications of smartphone use: Korean college students' smartphone use and psychological well being. *Cyberpsychol. Psychol. Behav. Soc. Netw.* **2012**, *15*, 491–497. [CrossRef]
12. Augner, C.; Hacker, G.W. Associations between problematic mobile phone use and psychological parameters in young adults. *Int. J. Public Health* **2012**, *57*, 437–441. [CrossRef]
13. Chóliz, M. Mobile-phone addiction in adolescence: The test of mobile phone dependence (TMD). *Prog. Health Sci.* **2012**, *2*, 33–44.
14. Leung, L. Linking psychological attributes to addiction and improper use of the mobile phone among adolescents in Hong Kong. *J. Child. Media* **2008**, *2*, 93–113. [CrossRef]
15. Samaha, M.; Hawi, N.S. Relationships among smartphone addiction, stress, academic performance, and satisfaction with life. *Comput. Hum. Behav.* **2016**, *57*, 321–325. [CrossRef]
16. Thomee, S.; Harenstam, A.; Hagberg, M. Mobile phone use and stress, sleep disturbances, and symptoms of depression among young adults a prospective cohort study. *BMC Public Health* **2011**, *11*, 66. [CrossRef] [PubMed]
17. David, P.; Kim, J.H.; Brickman, J.S.; Ran, W.; Curtis, C.M. Mobile phone distraction while studying. *New Media Soc.* **2015**, *17*, 1661–1679. [CrossRef]
18. American Psychiatric Association. *Diagnostic and Statistical Manual of Mental Disorders*, 5th ed.; American Psychiatric Association: Washington, DC, USA, 1994.
19. LaRose, R.; Lin, C.A.; Eastin, M.S. Unregulated Internet usage: Addiction, habit, or deficient self-regulation. *Media Psychol.* **2003**, *5*, 225–253. [CrossRef]
20. Marlatt, G.A.; Baer, J.S.; Donovan, D.M.; Kivlahan, D.R. Addictive behaviors: Etiology and treatment. *Annu. Rev. Psychol.* **1988**, *39*, 223–252. [CrossRef]
21. Duke, É.; Montag, C. Smartphone addiction, daily interruptions and self-reported productivity. *Addict. Behav. Rep.* **2017**, *6*, 90–95. [CrossRef]
22. Lachmann, B.; Sindermann, C.; Sariyska, R.Y.; Luo, R.; Melchers, M.C.; Becker, B.; Montag, C. The role of empathy and life satisfaction in internet and smartphone use disorder. *Front. Psychol.* **2018**, *9*, 398. [CrossRef]
23. Ward, A.F.; Duke, K.; Gneezy, A.; Bos, M.W. Brain drain: The mere presence of one's own smartphone reduces available cognitive capacity. *J. Assoc. Consum. Res.* **2017**, *2*, 140–154. [CrossRef]
24. Krznaric, R. *Carpe Diem: Reclaiming Seize the Day in a Distracted World*, 1st ed.; Penguin: London, UK, 2017.
25. Mark, G.; Gudith, D.; Klocke, U. The Cost of Interrupted Work: More Speed and Stress. In Proceedings of the SIGCHI Conference on Human Factors in Computing Systems 2008, Florence, Italy, 5–10 April 2008; pp. 107–110.

26. Oulasvirta, A.; Rattenbury, T.; Ma, L.; Raita, E. Habits make smartphone use more pervasive. *Pers. Ubiquitous Comput.* **2012**, *16*, 105–114. [CrossRef]
27. Ertemel, A.V.; Aydın, G. Technology addiction in the digital economy and suggested solutions. *Addicta Turk. J. Addict.* **2018**, *5*, 665–690.
28. Alter, A. *Irresistible: The Rise of Addictive Technology and the Business of Keeping Us Hooked*, 1st ed.; Penguin: London, UK, 2017.
29. Harris, T. How a Handful of Tech Companies Control Billions of Minds Every Day. 2017. Available online: https://www.ted.com/talks/tristan_harris_the_manipulative_tricks_tech_companies_use_to_capture_your_attention (accessed on 10 December 2019).
30. Chou, T.J.; Ting, C.C. The role of flow experience in cyber-game addiction. *Cyberpsychol. Behav.* **2003**, *6*, 663–675. [CrossRef] [PubMed]
31. Alrobai, A.; Phalp, K.; Ali, R. Digital Addiction: A Requirements Engineering Perspective. In *International Working Conference on Requirements Engineering: Foundation for Soft-Ware Quality*; Springer: Berlin/Heidelberg, Germany, 2014; pp. 112–118.
32. Deloitte Global Mobile User Survey. Available online: https://www2.deloitte.com/tr/tr/pages/technology-media-and-telecommunications/articles/TR-GMCS-2019.html (accessed on 12 December 2019).
33. TurkStat. *Annual Report on Information and Communication Technology (ICT) Usage in Households and by Individuals*; Turkish Statistical Institute: Ankara, Turkey, 2018.
34. Bychkov, D.; Young, S.D. Facing Up to Nomophobia: A Systematic Review of Mobile Phone Apps that Reduce Smartphone Usage. In *Big Data in Engineering Applications*; Springer: Singapore, 2018; pp. 161–171.
35. Davenport, T.H.; Beck, J.C. *The Attention Economy: Understanding the New Currency of Business*; Harvard Business Press: Harvard, MA, USA, 2001.
36. Csikszentmihalyi, M.; Csikszentmihalyi, I.S. *Optimal Experience: Psychological Studies of Flow in Consciousness*; Cambridge University Press: Cambridge, UK, 1992.
37. Ertemel, A.V. *Dijital çağda Illüzyonel Pazarlama*, 1st ed.; Abaküs Kitap: İstanbul, Turkey, 2016.
38. Ertemel, A.V. The Importance of Unconscious Mind for Consumer Engagement in the Digital Age: A Model Proposal. In Proceedings of the 23th National Marketing Conference, Trabzon, Turkey, 9 September 2017.
39. Deterding, S.; Dixon, D.; Khaled, R.; Nacke, L. From Game Design Elements to Gamefulness: Defining Gamification. In Proceedings of the 15th International Academic Mindtrek Conference: Envisioning Future Media Environments, Tampere, Finland, 28–20 September 2011.
40. Xu, F.; Weber, J.; Buhalis, D. The Gamification of Tourism. In *Information and Communication Technologies in Tourism*; Xiang, Z., Tussyadiah, I., Eds.; Springer: Wien, Austria, 2014.
41. Rafttopoulos, M. Toward gamification transparency: A conceptual framework for the development of responsible gamified enterprise systems. *J. Gaming Virtual Worlds* **2014**, *6*, 159–178. [CrossRef]
42. Shahri, A.; Hosseini, M.; Phalp, K.; Taylor, J.; Ali, R. Toward a Code of Ethics for Gamification at Enterprise. In *The Practice of Enterprise Modeling*; Frank, V., Loucoploulos, P., Pastor, O., Petrounias, I., Eds.; Springer: Berlin, Germany, 2014; pp. 235–245.
43. Vashisht, D.; Sreejesh, S. Impact of Game Speed and Persuasion Knowledge on Brand Recall and Brand Attitude. In Proceedings of the Twelfth AIMS International Conference on Management, Kerala, India, 2–5 January 2015; pp. 231–234.
44. Thorpe, A.S.; Roper, S. The ethics of gamification in a marketing context. *J. Bus. Ethics* **2019**, *155*, 597–609. [CrossRef]
45. Kaikati, A.M.; Kaikati, J.G. Stealth marketing: How to reach consumers surreptitiously. *Calif. Manag. Rev.* **2004**, *46*, 6–23. [CrossRef]
46. Gamble, J.; Gilmore, A. A new era of consumer marketing An application of co-creational marketing in the music industry. *Eur. J. Mark.* **2013**, *47*, 1859–1888. [CrossRef]
47. Etgar, M. A descriptive model of the consumer co-production process. *J. Acad. Mark. Sci.* **2008**, *36*, 97–108. [CrossRef]
48. Black, I.; Veloutsou, C. Working consumers: Co-creation of brand identity, consumer identity and brand community identity. *J. Bus. Res.* **2017**, *70*, 416–429. [CrossRef]
49. Fogg, B.J. *Persuasive Technology: Using Computers to Change What We Think and Do*; Morgan Kaufmann: Boston, MA, USA, 2003.

50. Duhigg, C. *The Power of Habit: Why We Do What We Do in Life and Business*, 1st ed.; Random House Trade Paperbacks: New York, NY, USA, 2012.
51. Judah, G.; Gardner, B.; Aunger, R. Forming a flossing habit: An exploratory study of the psychological determinants of habit formation. *Br. J. Health Psychol.* **2013**, *18*, 338–353. [CrossRef]
52. Lally, P.; Van Jaarsveld, C.H.; Potts, H.W.; Wardle, J. How are habits formed: Modelling habit formation in the real world. *Eur. J. Soc. Psychol.* **2010**, *40*, 998–1009. [CrossRef]
53. Eyal, N. *Hooked: How to Build Habit-Forming Products*, 1st ed.; Portfolio Books: London, UK, 2014.
54. Ferster, C.B.; Skinner, B.F. *Schedules of Reinforcement*, 1st ed.; Appleton-CenturyCrofts: New York, NY, USA, 1957.
55. Metcalfe, J.; Mischel, W. A hot/cool-system analysis of delay of gratification: Dynamics of willpower. *Psychol. Rev.* **1999**, *106*, 3–19. [CrossRef] [PubMed]
56. Bernheim, B.D.; Rangel, A. Behavioral public economics: Welfare and policy analysis with non-standard decision-makers. *Natl. Bur. Econ. Res.* **2005**, 11518. [CrossRef]
57. Cover, R. Digital addiction: The cultural production of online and video game junkies. *Media Int. Aust. Inc. Cult. Policy* **2004**, *113*, 110–123. [CrossRef]
58. Marczewski, A. The ethics of gamification. XRDS: Crossroads. *ACM Mag. Stud.* **2017**, *24*, 56–59.
59. Kwon, M.; Lee, J.Y.; Won, W.Y.; Park, J.W.; Min, J.A.; Hahn, C.; Kim, D.J. Development and validation of a smartphone addiction scale (SAS). *PLoS ONE* **2013**, *8*, e56936. [CrossRef]
60. Demirci, K.; Orhan, H.; Demirdas, A.; Akpinar, A.; Sert, H. Validity and reliability of the Turkish Version of the Smartphone Addiction Scale in a younger population. *Bull. Clin. Psychopharmacol.* **2014**, *24*, 226–234. [CrossRef]
61. Fırat, S.; Gül, H.; Sertçelik, M.; Gül, A.; Gürel, Y.; Kılıç, B. The relationship between problematic smartphone use and psychiatric symptoms among adolescents who applied to psychiatry clinics. *Psychiatry Res.* **2018**, *270*, 97–103. [CrossRef]
62. Rosen, L.; Carrier, L.M.; Miller, A.; Rokkum, J.; Ruiz, A. Sleeping with technology: Cognitive, affective, and technology usage predictors of sleep problems among college students. *Sleep Health J. Natl. Sleep Found* **2016**, *2*, 49–56. [CrossRef]
63. Commonsense. Available online: https://www.commonsensemedia.org/technology-addiction-concern-controversy-and-finding-balanceinfographic (accessed on 10 October 2019).
64. Frangos, C.C.; Fragkos, K.C.; Kiohos, A. Internet addiction among Greek university students: Demographic associations with the phenomenon, using the Greek version of Young's Internet Addiction Test. *Int. J. Econ. Sci. Appl. Res.* **2010**, *3*, 49–74.
65. Weiser, E.B. Gender Differences in Internet Use Patterns and Internet Application Preferences: A Two-Sample Comparison. *Cyberpsychol. Behav.* **2000**, *3*, 167–178. [CrossRef]
66. Billieux, J.; Van Der Linden, M.; Rochat, L. The role of impulsivity in actual and problematic use of the mobile phone. *Appl. Cogn. Psychol.* **2008**, *22*, 1195. [CrossRef]
67. Hong, F.Y.; Chiu, S.I.; Lin, H.Y. The development and current states of private college student mobile phone addiction scale. *Chung Cheng Educ. Stud.* **2012**, *11*, 87–116.
68. Chiu, S.I.; Hong, F.Y.; Chiu, S.L. An Analysis on the Correlation and Gender Difference between College Students' Internet Addiction as well as Mobile Phone Addiction in Taiwan. *ISRN Addict.* **2013**. [CrossRef]
69. Sherman, R.C.; End, C.; Kraan, E.; Cole, A.; Campbell, J.; Birchmeier, Z.; Klausner, J. The Internet gender gap among college students: Forgotten but not gone. *Cyberpsychol. Behav.* **2000**, *3*, 885–894. [CrossRef]
70. Shek, D.T.; Yu, L. Adolescent internet addiction in Hong Kong: Prevalence, change, and correlates. *J. Pediatric Adolesc. Gynecol.* **2016**, *29*, S22–S30. [CrossRef]
71. Widyanto, L.; McMurran, M. The psychometric properties of the internet addiction test. *Cyberpsychol. Behav.* **2004**, *7*, 443. [CrossRef]
72. Steinberg, L. A social neuroscience perspective on adolescent risk-taking. *Dev. Rev.* **2008**, *28*, 78–106. [CrossRef]
73. Steinberg, L. A dual systems model of adolescent risk-taking. *Dev. Psychobiol.* **2010**, *52*, 216. [CrossRef]
74. Steinberg, L.; Albert, D.; Cauffman, E. Age differences in sensation seeking and impulsivity as indexed by behavior and self-report: Evidence for a dual systems model. *Dev. Psychobiol.* **2008**, *44*, 1764. [CrossRef]
75. Engin, C.; Pals, H. Patriarchal attitudes in Turkey 1990–2011: The influence of religion and political conservatism. *Soc. Politics Int. Stud. Gend. State Soc.* **2018**, *25*, 383–409. [CrossRef]

76. Lee, H.; Kim, J.W.; Choi, T.Y. Risk factors for smartphone addiction in Korean adolescents: Smartphone use patterns. *J. Korean Med. Sci.* **2017**, *32*, 1674–1679. [CrossRef] [PubMed]
77. Hogle, J.M.; Curtin, J.J. Sex differences in negative affective response during nicotine withdrawal. *Psychophysiology* **2006**, *43*, 344–356. [CrossRef] [PubMed]
78. Becker, J.B.; McClellan, M.L.; Reed, B.G. Sex differences, gender and addiction. *J. Neurosci. Res.* **2017**, *95*, 136–147. [CrossRef] [PubMed]
79. Park, N. Gender difference in social networking on smartphones: A case study of Korean college student smartphone users. *Int. Telecommun. Policy Rev.* **2014**, *21*, 1–18.
80. Geser, H. Are Girls (Even) More Addicted? Some Gender Patterns of Cell Phone Usage. In *Sociology in Switzerland: Sociology of the Mobile Phone*; Online Publications: Zuerich, Switzerland, 2006.
81. Reinehr, T.; Temmesfeld, M.; Kersting, M.; De Sousa, G.; Toschke, A.M. Four-year follow-up of children and adolescents participating in an obesity intervention program. *Int. J. Obes.* **2007**, *31*, 1074–1077. [CrossRef]
82. Shochet, I.M.; Dadds, M.R.; Holland, D.; Whitefield, K.; Harnett, P.H.; Osgarby, S.M. The efficacy of a universal school-based program to prevent adolescent depression. *J. Clin. Child Psychol.* **2001**, *30*, 303–315. [CrossRef]
83. Durlak, J.A.; Wells, A.M. Primary prevention mental health programs for children and adolescents: A meta-analytic review. *Am. J. Commun. Psychol.* **2001**, *25*, 115–152. [CrossRef]
84. Li, L.; Niu, Z.M.; Mei, S.L. The mindfulness cognitive behavioral group therapy of medical student'smartphone addiction in group counseling course. *China High. Med. Educ.* **2017**, *5*, 37–38.

10

Confirmatory Factor Analysis of the Malay Version of the Smartphone Addiction Scale among Medical Students in Malaysia

Siti Rubiaehtul Hassim [1], Wan Nor Arifin [1,*], Yee Cheng Kueh [1] and Nor Azwany Yaacob [2]

1 Biostatistics and Research Methodology Unit, School of Medical Sciences, Universiti Sains Malaysia, Kubang Kerian 16150, Malaysia; bisyarah_istikharah@yahoo.com (S.R.H.); yckueh@usm.my (Y.C.K.)
2 Department of Community Medicine, School of Medical Sciences, Universiti Sains Malaysia, Kubang Kerian 16150, Malaysia; azwany@usm.my
* Correspondence: wnarifin@usm.my

Abstract: Background: At present, the validity and reliability evidence of the Malay version of the Smartphone Addiction Scale (SAS-M) is only available by exploratory factor analysis (EFA). The aim of this study is to validate and determine the psychometric properties of the SAS-M by confirmatory factor analysis (CFA). Methods: A cross-sectional study was conducted among 323 medical students in Universiti Sains Malaysia. The students were given questionnaire forms consisting of socio-demographic information, the SAS-M and the Malay version of the Internet Addiction Test (MVIAT). The CFA was conducted using robust maximum likelihood estimator. The internal consistency reliability was determined by Raykov's rho coefficient. The concurrent validity was assessed by the Pearson's correlations between the factor scores of the SAS-M and the MVIAT. Results: The analysis showed the five-factor model of the SAS-M has an acceptable model fit after the inclusion of 12 correlated errors (SRMR = 0.067, RMSEA 0.059 (90% CI: 0.054, 0.065), CFI = 0.895, TLI = 0.882). The factor loadings ranged from 0.320 to 0.875. The internal consistency reliability was good (Raykov's rho = 0.713 to 0.858) and it showed good concurrent validity with the MVIAT. Conclusions: The CFA showed that the SAS-M is a valid and reliable self-administered questionnaire to measure the level of smartphone addiction among medical students.

Keywords: confirmatory factor analysis; Malay version; medical student; smartphone addiction; validation study

---

1. Introduction

Nowadays, a smartphone is an essential and popular communication tool that makes our daily life more convenient. As compared to a phone with basic features, a smartphone packs more computing capability and connectivity [1]. A smartphone performs many of the functions of a computer and comes with an operating system that allows it to run mobile applications [2,3]. The hardware capability, connectivity and inclusion of operating systems allow a smartphone to have a wide range of software, Internet and multimedia (music, video, camera and gaming) functionality, alongside main phone functions such as voice calls and text messaging [3]. All these functions come in the form of a pocket-sized device and its popularity is inevitable [4]. Widespread and pervasive smartphone use has become the social norm because of the high accessibility and mobility of the device [5].

In Malaysia, the smartphone penetration rate stands at a staggering 97.9% based on the latest report by the Department of Statistics, Malaysia in 2019 [6]. The smartphone has become the most common device to access the Internet based on the survey by the Malaysian Communications and Multimedia Commission (MCMC) in 2018, which reported 93.1% of Internet users used smartphones to go online [7]. Based on another survey by MCMC in 2017, other common uses of smartphones are text and voice messaging (98.5%), voice calls (93.8%), social media (88.1%), entertainment (83.7%), map/navigation (73.6%), email (60.0%) and video calls (53.2%) [8]. Judging from these nationwide surveys, the findings clearly show that the smartphone permeates the life of all Malaysians.

There is an increasing concern about the negative effects that come from its overuse, and these may interfere with our daily life [4]. De-Sola Gutiérrez et al. [9] define smartphone addiction as an excessive attention and uncontrolled dedication to one's smartphone. It is a behavior that manifests tolerance, withdrawal symptoms and dependence, along with social problems [10]. Studies on the effects of smartphone use on students have revealed many negative sides of smartphone addiction [11]. Smartphone addiction is associated with low academic performance [12,13], poor attention during learning sessions [12,14], poor psychological health [15,16], poor social interaction [17–19] and low life satisfaction [13].

Studies have also attributed problematic smartphone use with the social media use of smartphones [12,20].

A number of local studies have also supported the negative effects of smartphone use among students in Malaysia. In a study among undergraduate students, Ithnain, Ghazali and Jaafar [21] concluded that smartphone addiction is associated with depression and anxiety. In another study among medical students, Hadi et al. [22] found the association of smartphone addiction with poor psychological health. A recent study reported that 60.7% of undergraduate students had problematic smartphone use, and this was found to be associated with anxiety, depression, stress and a deterioration in academic performance [23]. An earlier study also supported the relationship between problematic phone use with lower academic performance [24].

Given the importance of assessing smartphone-related problems, so far nine major scales have been used in studies, which are the Smartphone Addiction Scale (SAS), Smartphone Addiction Scale Short Version (SAS-SV), Smartphone Addiction Proneness Scale (SAPS), Mobile Phone Addiction Index (MPAI), Mobile Phone Addiction Scale (MPAS), Mobile Phone Problem Use Scale (MPPUS), Smartphone Addiction Scale (SPAS), Smartphone Addiction Inventory (SPAI), and SPAI Short Form (SPAI-SF) [5]. Of these scales, most studies used either the SAS-SV or SAS [5]. Kwon et al. [10] developed the SAS which consists of 33 items and six factors. It was the first questionnaire for the measurement and diagnosis of smartphone addiction, and they showed that the SAS has good validity and reliability [10]. Alternatively, the authors of the SAS also developed the short version of the questionnaire (SAS-SV) which clusters 10 items under one factor [25]. The SAS-SV is intended for easy administration among adolescents, while the SAS is mainly for use among adults [10,25]. The SAS-SV showed comparably good validity and reliability to the longer version of the questionnaire [25]. The SAS-SV has been translated and validated in several languages; Arabic [26], Chinese [27], French [28], German [4], Italian [29], Portuguese [30], Spanish [28] and Turkish [31]. The SAS has been translated and validated in Arabic [26], Japanese [32], Romanian [33] and Thai [34]. In order to facilitate further research on smartphone addiction in Malaysia, Ching et al. [35] translated the SAS into the Malay language (SAS-M) and they showed that the SAS-M is valid and reliable for use among students. The SAS-M has been used in a number of research projects [21,23] in Malaysia to study the effects of smartphone use on students.

However, in both of the SAS-M validation studies [10,35], the researchers used exploratory factor analysis (EFA) to analyze the internal factor structure of the SAS. As compared to EFA, confirmatory factor analysis (CFA) provides stronger evidence to support the validity of the factor structure of a measure [36]. Although CFA provides a better option of analysis, both studies [10,365 were exploratory in nature, which justified the use of EFA. CFA requires specialized software, for example Mplus [37] and *lavaan* R package in R software environment [38,39], while EFA can be easily conducted in many kinds of statistical software. This could have hindered the use of CFA in previous SAS validation studies (with exception of [32,33]). Thus, this study aimed to validate and determine the psychometric properties of the SAS-M by CFA to provide stronger validity and reliability evidence to the earlier EFA study [35].

2. Materials and Methods

2.1. Study Setting and Participants

A cross-sectional study was conducted among Year 1 to Year 5 undergraduate medical students from School of Medical Sciences, Universiti Sains Malaysia (USM), Kubang Kerian, Kelantan, Malaysia. The data collection was done between October 2016 and December 2016. The sample size was determined for the CFA, which required at least 300 respondents for a scale with seven or less factors with item communality of <0.45 [40]. After taking into consideration a 20% drop-out rate, the target sample size was 375 respondents.

The students were selected by stratified random sampling based on the list obtained from the academic office, with the group size per year of study as the stratification variable. The selected students were then invited to participate in the study. The nature of the study and the confidentiality of their responses was explained. Those who consented to participate in the study signed informed consent forms and were given questionnaire forms to be completed. Each questionnaire form consists of socio-demographic information (age, gender, race and family income), purpose of using smartphones, the SAS-M and the MVIAT. The students returned the completed questionnaire forms to the researchers on the same day.

2.2. Instruments

2.2.1. The Malay Version of the Smartphone Addiction Scale (SAS-M)

The English version of the SAS questionnaire [10,35] is a self-administered, 6-point Likert type scale consisting of 33 items that belong to six factors, which are: 1. Cyberspace oriented relationship (7 items): S20–S26; 2. Daily Life Disturbance (5 items): S1–S5; 3. Tolerance (3 items): S31–S33; 4. Overuse (4 items): S27–S30; 5. Positive Anticipation (8 items): S6–S13; and 6. Withdrawal (6 items): S14–S19. Each item has a response scale from 1 (strongly disagree) to 6 (strongly agree). Higher scores indicate a higher degree of smartphone addition [10,35]. The SAS showed good internal consistency reliability (Cronbach's alpha = 0.967 (total), 0.825 to 0.913 (subscales)) and concurrent validity ($r = 0.32$ to 0.61) [10].

The Malay version of the SAS (SAS-M) was validated among medical students in Malaysia [35]. It showed good internal consistency reliability (Cronbach's alpha = 0.940 (total), 0.837 to 0.877 (subscales)), test-retest reliability (intraclass correlation (ICC) = 0.85) and concurrent validity ($r = 0.645$) with the Malay version of the Internet Addiction Test (MVIAT). Based on EFA, the number of extracted factors from SAS-M matched the original SAS [35]. As detailed in the study [35], a new factor "Primacy" replaced the "Tolerance" factor from the original SAS, and there were a number of changes to the placement of items under each factor.

In contrast to the original SAS, the SAS-M questionnaire [35] consists of 33 items that belong to six factors, which are: 1. Cyberspace oriented relationship (7 items): S19–S24, S26; 2. Daily Life Disturbance (6 items): S1–S5, S33; 3. Primacy (5 items): S10-S14; 4. Overuse (7 items): S25, S27–S32; 5. Positive Anticipation (4 items): S6–S9; and 6. Withdrawal (4 items): S15–S18.

2.2.2. The Malay Version of the Internet Addiction Test (MVIAT)

The Internet Addiction Test (IAT) is the most commonly used questionnaire to diagnose internet addiction [35]. The questionnaire is a self-administered, 5-point Likert type scale consisting of 20 items, and each item has a response scale from 1 (never) to 5 (always), reflecting the frequency of the symptoms [41]. Higher scores indicate higher degree of pathological use of the internet [41]. The Malay version of the IAT (MVIAT) was validated among a group of medical students in Malaysia; it showed good internal consistency reliability (Cronbach's alpha = 0.91) and parallel reliability with the IAT (intraclass correlation coefficient (ICC) = 0.88, $p < 0.001$) [41]. The MVIAT [41] showed five extracted factors, which are: 1. Lack of control (8 items): T1, T2, T10, T11, T12, T14, T16, T17; 2. Neglect of Duty (7 items): T3, T6, T8, T9, T18, T19, T20; 3. Problematic Use (2 items): T4, T15; 4. Social relationship disruption (2 items): T5, T13; and 5. Email Primacy (1 item): T7.

2.3. Statistical Analysis

The data analysis was performed in R software environment [39]. The CFA was performed using *lavaan* and *semTools* R packages [38,42]. Robust maximum likelihood estimator was used because the data were not normally distributed [36]. The model fit assessment was based on the following fit indices (robust) with their respective cut-off values [36]: χ^2 ($p > 0.05$), comparative fit index (CFI) and Tucker-Lewis fit index (TLI) ≥ 0.95 (good) or ≥ 0.90 (acceptable), root mean square error of approximation (RMSEA) ≤ 0.08, and standardized root mean square residual (SRMR) ≤ 0.08. Model-to-model comparison was based on Akaike information criterion (AIC) and Bayesian information criterion [36]. The model with the lowest values of AIC and BIC was chosen as the best fitting model for the CFA. Items with factor loadings of >0.3 were considered acceptable [40]. Multicollinearity between the factors was identified when factor-to-factor correlation was $r > 0.85$ [36]. The internal consistency reliability was determined by Raykov's rho coefficient [43]. Raykov's rho values of ≥0.7 were considered to reflect good reliability [40].

The concurrent validity was assessed by Pearson's correlation coefficient (r) for the correlations between factor scores of the SAS-M and MVIAT. The strength of correlation was interpreted according to Colton [44]: no or little correlation (0.00–0.25), fair correlation (0.26–0.50), moderate correlation (0.51–0.75), and perfect correlation (0.76–1.00).

2.4. Ethical Consideration

The approval for this research was obtained from the Human Research Ethics Committee of Universiti Sains Malaysia (JEPeM Code: USM/JEPeM/16030107). The confidentiality of the data was maintained and only the researchers had access to the data. The permission to conduct the study among the medical students in USM was obtained from the academic office. The permission to use the SAS-M and the MVIAT was obtained from the original authors.

3. Results

A total of 323 medical students agreed to participate in the study. The socio-demographic characteristics of the respondents are displayed in Table 1. The mean (SD) age of the students was 21.39 (1.71) years. The majority of them were female (64.4%), of Malay race (53.6%) and those coming from families with a monthly income of more than RM5000 (38.7%).

The CFA of the six-factor model of SAS-M (Model 1) showed that the model did not fit the data. After the inclusion of 12 correlated errors to the model, the CFA showed an acceptable model fit (Model 2). The factors were not multicollinear because all r values were less than 0.85, which indicated good discrimination between the factors. The model fit details, factor-to-factor correlation and correlated errors are presented in Table 2.

The factor loadings for all items exceeded the cut-off value of 0.3 (0.320 to 0.875). The reliability for each factor was good (Raykov's rho = 0.713 to 0.858). The factor loadings and Raykov's rho values by factor are displayed in Table 3.

The strength and direction of the correlation between the factor scores of the SAS-M and MVIAT are shown in Table 4. The result shows significant correlations between the related SAS-M and MVIAT factors in the range of 0.258 to 0.511, which indicated concurrent validity of the SAS-M.

Table 1. Socio-demographic characteristics of the medical students (N = 323).

Variable		*N* (%)
Age (Mean [SD])		21.39 (1.71)
Year of Study	Year 1	62 (19.2)
	Year 2	59 (18.3)
	Year 3	63 (19.5)
	Year 4	61 (18.9)
	Year 5	78 (24.1)
Gender	Male	115 (35.6)
	Female	208 (64.4)
Race	Malay	173 (53.6)
	Chinese	77 (23.8)
	India	64 (19.8)
	Others	9 (2.8)
Monthly family income (Ringgit Malaysia; RM)	<RM1000	33 (10.2)
	RM1000–1999	49 (15.2)
	RM2000–2999	39 (12.1)
	RM3000–3999	48 (14.9)
	RM4000–4999	28 (8.7)
	>RM5000	125 (38.7)

Table 2. Model fit indices and correlated errors of the CFA.

Models	χ^2 (df), p	SRMR	RMSEA (90% CI)	CFI	TLI	AIC	BIC
Model 1	1213.1 (480), < 0.001	0.075	0.074 (0.069, 0.079)	0.834	0.817	31,194.3	31,623.5
Model 2 *	931.3 (468), < 0.001	0.067	0.059 (0.054, 0.065)	0.895	0.882	30,895.2	31,369.7

* Correlated errors in Model 2: S3↔S4 (r = 0.410, $p \leq 0.001$), S14↔S15 (r = 0.481, $p \leq 0.001$), S31↔S32 (r = 0.378, $p \leq 0.001$), S33↔S31 (r = 0.336, $p \leq 0.001$), S21↔S23 (r = 0.371, $p \leq 0.001$), S10↔S13 (r = 0.292, $p \leq 0.001$), S23↔S26 (r = 0.353, $p \leq 0.001$), S21↔S26 (r = 0.259, p = 0.001), S20↔S21 (r = 0.218, p = 0.002), S1↔S2 (r = 0.274, p = 0.002), S14↔S17 (r = 0.220, p = 0.001), S22↔S30 (r = 0.282, p = 0.001). Correlation between factors in Model 2: S1↔S2 (r = 0.538, $p \leq 0.001$), S1↔S3(r = 0.762, $p \leq 0.001$), S1↔S4(r = 0.635, $p \leq 0.001$), S1↔S5 (r = 0.422, $p \leq 0.001$), S1↔S6 (r = 0.844, $p \leq 0.001$), S2↔S3 (r = 0.483, $p \leq 0.001$), S2↔S4 (r = 0.694, $p \leq 0.001$), S2↔S5 (r = 0.292, p = 0.004), S2↔S6 (r = 0.623, $p \leq 0.001$), S3↔S4 (r = 0.587, $p \leq 0.001$), S3↔S5 (r = 0.676, $p \leq 0.001$), S3↔S6 (r = 0.808, $p \leq 0.001$), S4↔S5 (r = 0.388, $p \leq 0.001$), S4↔S6 (r = 0.697, $p \leq 0.001$), S5↔S6 (r = 0.513, $p \leq 0.001$). Abbreviations: F = factor; S = SAS item; CFA = confirmatory factor analysis; SRMR = standardized root mean square residual; RMSEA = root mean square error of approximation; CFI = comparative fit index; TLI = Tucker-Lewis fit index; AIC = Akaike information criterion; BIC: Bayesian information criterion.

Table 3. The factor loadings and Raykov's rho values by factor.

Factor	Question No.	Factor Loading	Raykov's Rho
F1. Cyberspace oriented relationship	S19	0.592	0.756
	S20	0.621	
	S21	0.546	
	S22	0.791	
	S23	0.651	
	S24	0.531	
	S26	0.562	
F2. Daily life disturbance	S1	0.592	0.713
	S2	0.637	
	S3	0.543	
	S4	0.485	
	S5	0.654	
	S33	0.582	

Table 3. *Cont.*

Factor	Question No.	Factor Loading	Raykov's Rho
F3. Primacy	S10 S11 S12 S13 S14	0.667 0.783 0.792 0.809 0.735	0.858
F4. Overuse	S25 S27 S28 S29 S30 S31 S32	0.483 0.320 0.585 0.699 0.836 0.786 0.586	0.798
F5. Positive anticipation	S6 S7 S8 S9	0.752 0.875 0.677 0.668	0.831
F6. Withdrawal	S15 S16 S17 S18	0.767 0.743 0.699 0.604	0.800

Table 4. Pearson's correlation coefficients (p-values) between the Malay Version of the Smartphone Addiction Scale (SAS-M) and Malay version of the Internet Addiction Test (MVIAT) factor scores.

	SAS-M					
MVIAT	***Cyberspace oriented Relationship***	***Daily Life Disturbance***	***Primacy***	***Overuse***	***Positive Anticipation***	***Withdrawal***
Lack Of control	0.331 (<0.001)	0.437 (<0.001)	0.338 (<0.001)	0.511 (<0.001)	0.211 (<0.001)	0.466 (<0.001)
Neglect of duty	0.455 (<0.001)	0.454 (<0.001)	0.320 (<0.001)	0.422 (<0.001)	0.116 (0.220)	0.463 (<0.001)
Problematic use	0.400 (<0.001)	0.367 (<0.001)	0.291 (<0.001)	0.310 (<0.001)	0.101 (0.270)	0.393 (<0.001)
Socialrelationship	0.402 (<0.001)	0.383 (<0.001)	0.258 (<0.001)	0.214 (<0.001)	0.051 (0.360)	0.426 (<0.001)
Email primacy	0.243 (<0.001)	0.130 (0.130)	0.097 (0.270)	0.107 (0.270)	0.099 (0.270)	0.158 (0.030)

4. Discussion

EFA was used to analyze the internal structure of the original SAS [10] and the Malay version of the SAS [35]. As CFA can provide a stronger evidence in support of the validity of the factor structure [36], this study provided the psychometric properties and model fit assessment of the SAS-M by CFA.

The results of this study showed that the six-factor model of the SAS-M has an acceptable model fit after the inclusion of 12 correlated errors. These correlated errors can be justified on the basis of method effect that reflects additional item covariation, for example between similarly worded items [36]. In the context of the SAS and the SAS-M, the correlation is possible because all items contained the "smartphone" word, and most items contain the "feeling" word. One notable example in this study is between S20 and S21; both item statements start with "Feeling" (SAS) or "Berasa" (SAS-M).

To the authors' knowledge, this is the first study that reports the CFA of the SAS-M. For the CFA of the SAS, there are a very limited number of studies that used the CFA method [32,33]. The five-factor model is supported mainly by SRMR and RMSEA values that were clearly below the cut-off value of 0.08, while the support from CFI and TLI values were just close enough to the cut-off value of more than 0.90. In contrast, the CFA of the Romanian version of the SAS supported bi-factor model [13], and similar to this study the RMSEA and SRMR values were below 0.08 (0.064 and 0.054 respectively), while the CFI and TLI values were below 0.90 (0.870 and 0.848 respectively). For the Japanese version, they could not confirm the factor structure by CFA and resorted to using EFA which extracted four factors instead of six from the original SAS [32]. In this study, the approach to the CFA was to maintain the six-factor structure found in the earlier EFA [35], to keep all 33 items and to avoid overfitting the model. For these reasons, although it was possible to add more correlated errors to obtain higher CFI and TLI values, the modification to the model was stopped when these values were very close to the cut-off value of 0.90 to qualify as an acceptable model fit. In addition, similar to Vintila et al. [33], the decision to accept the model fit was also based on two other fit indices, which were RMSEA and SRMR. In both studies, the RMSEA and SRMR values were below 0.08 which indicated good model fit.

The factor loadings in each of the factors of the SAS-M showed all items were acceptable in view of the recommended cut-off value of 0.3 [40]. The factor loadings in this study ranged from 0.320 to 0.875. The result is comparable to the factor loadings obtained from the EFA of the SAS-M [35], which ranged from 0.415 to 0.897. The internal consistency reliability for each factor was also good, which ranged from 0.713 to 0.858 (by Raykov's rho). However, these values were lower than the EFA, which ranged from 0.837 to 0.877 (by Cronbach's alpha) [35]. This can be attributed to the Raykov's rho formula, which also takes into account the correlated error covariances in the calculation of the reliability [43].

In this study, most of the factor scores of the SAS-M were correlated to the MVIAT factor scores at fair-to-moderate strength. Similar to the earlier SAS-M validation study [35], there was negligible correlation between the "Positive anticipation" factor score with all MVIAT factor scores. In contrast to the earlier study which examined the correlation between SAS-M factor scores with the total score of the MVIAT [35], this study examined the correlation with each MVIAT factor score. The correlation was low between all factor scores of the SAS-M and "Email primacy" factor score of the MVIAT, and between the "Overuse" factor score of the SAS-M and "Social relationship disruption" factor score of the MVIAT. The poor correlation between the SAS-M and "Email primacy" of the MVIAT could be because email was not the main cause of smartphone addiction. Previous studies indicated that the addiction is better attributed to the social media use of smartphone [12,20]. The poor relationship between "Overuse" of the SAS-M and "Social relationship disruption" of the MVIAT in this study was unexpected because this finding contradicts previous studies which associate problematic smartphone use with poor social interaction [17–19]. This could be a population-specific finding (medical students), which warrants a further investigation in future studies.

There are two important limitations of this study that must be highlighted. First, the sample that was used for this study came from a single medical school in Malaysia, which might not represent all medical students in Malaysia. This limitation also affects the earlier study by Ching et al. [35], which also consists of a sample from a single medical school. Thus, it is recommended to cross-validate the SAS-M among medical students from other universities in Malaysia. Second, similar to the study by Ching et al. [35], all participants were medical students. The homogeneity of the sample makes it difficult to generalize the findings to students from other field of studies. In contrast, the validation of the original SAS was done among adult participants from companies and universities [10]. Thus, the validity of the SAS-M could be limited to a medical student population. To address this limitation, it is recommended to cross-validate the questionnaire in other heterogeneous samples in future studies. Despite these limitations, it was decided that in this study medical students would be selected as the sample to reflect closely the population in the EFA study by Ching et al. [35]. By restricting the sample to medical students, this will allow a direct comparison between the factor structure extracted by EFA and the one confirmed by CFA in the selected population.

5. Conclusions

This study provided the validity evidence and psychometric properties of the SAS-M by CFA. The results showed that the SAS-M is a valid and reliable self-administered questionnaire to measure the level of smartphone addiction among medical students. The generalizability of this validity evidence can be further supported by conducting confirmatory studies among medical students in other universities in Malaysia. In addition, the use of SAS-M in other populations requires further research in the form of cross-validation studies to explore and confirm its psychometric properties in these populations.

Author Contributions: Conceptualization, S.R.H. and N.A.Y.; methodology, S.R.H.; W.N.A.; Y.C.K. and N.A.Y.; software, S.R.H. and W.N.A.; validation, W.N.A.; Y.C.K. and N.A.Y.; formal analysis, S.R.H.; W.N.A.; investigation, S.R.H. and N.A.Y.; resources, W.N.A. and Y.C.K.; data curation, S.R.H. and W.N.A.; writing—original draft preparation, S.R.H; writing—review and editing, W.N.A.; supervision, W.N.A.; Y.C.K. and N.A.Y.; project administration, S.R.H. All authors have read and agreed to the published version of the manuscript.

Acknowledgments: We are grateful to the medical students in School of Medical Sciences, Universiti Sains Malaysia for their participation in this study. We also thank the academic office of the medical school for allowing use to conduct the study.

References

1. Rashvand, H.F.; Hsiao, K.F. Smartphone intelligent applications: A brief review. *Multimed. Syst.* **2015**, *21*, 103–119. [CrossRef]
2. "Smartphone", Oxford Advanced Learner's Dictionary. Available online: https://www.oxfordlearnersdictionaries.com (accessed on 28 February 2020).
3. Wikipedia Contributors. "Smartphone", Wikipedia, the Free Encyclopedia. Available online: https://en.wikipedia.org/w/index.php?title=Smartphone (accessed on 28 February 2020).
4. Duke, E.; Montag, C. Smartphone addiction, daily interruptions and self-reported productivity. *Addict. Behav. Rep.* **2017**, *6*, 90–95. [CrossRef] [PubMed]
5. Yu, S.; Sussman, S. Does Smartphone Addiction Fall on a Continuum of Addictive Behaviors? *Int. J. Environ. Res. Public Health* **2020**, *17*, 422. [CrossRef] [PubMed]
6. Department of Statistics Malaysia. *Press Release: ICT Use and Access by Individuals and Households Survey Report, Malaysia, 2018*; Department of Statistics Malaysia: Putrajaya, Malaysia, 2019.
7. Malaysian Communications and Multimedia Commission. *Internet Users Survey 2018*; Malaysian Communications and Multimedia Commission: Cyberjaya, Selangor, Malaysia, 2018.
8. Malaysian Communications and Multimedia Commission. *Hand Phone Users Survey 2017*; Malaysian Communications and Multimedia Commission: Cyberjaya, Selangor, Malaysia, 2017.
9. De-Sola Gutiérrez, J.; Rodríguez de Fonseca, F.; Rubio, G. Cell-phone addiction: A review. *Front. Psychiatry* **2016**, *7*, 175. [CrossRef] [PubMed]
10. Kwon, M.; Lee, J.Y.; Won, W.Y.; Park, J.W.; Min, J.A.; Hahn, C.; Gu, X.; Choi, J.H.; Kim, D.J. Development and validation of a smartphone addiction scale (SAS). *PLoS ONE* **2013**, *8*, e56936. [CrossRef]
11. Singh, M.K.K.; Samah, N.A. Impact of Smartphone: A Review on Positive and Negative Effects on Students. *Asian Soc. Sci.* **2018**, *14*, 83–89. [CrossRef]
12. Rozgonjuk, D.; Saal, K.; Täht, K. Problematic smartphone use, deep and surface approaches to learning, and social media use in lectures. *Int. J. Environ. Res. Public Health* **2018**, *15*, 92. [CrossRef]
13. Samaha, M.; Hawi, N.S. Relationships among smartphone addiction, stress, academic performance, and satisfaction with life. *Comput. Hum. Behav.* **2016**, *57*, 321–325. [CrossRef]
14. Froese, A.D.; Carpenter, C.N.; Inman, D.A.; Schooley, J.R.; Barnes, R.B.; Brecht, P.W.; Chacon, J.D. Effects of classroom cell phone use on expected and actual learning. *Coll. Stud. J.* **2012**, *46*, 323–332.
15. Hwang, K.H.; Yoo, Y.S.; Cho, O.H. Smartphone overuse and upper extremity pain, anxiety, depression, and interpersonal relationships among college students. *J. Korea Contents Assoc.* **2012**, *12*, 365–375. [CrossRef]

16. Lee, Y.K.; Chang, C.T.; Lin, Y.; Cheng, Z.H. The dark side of smartphone usage: Psychological traits, compulsive behavior and technostress. *Comput. Human Behav.* **2014**, *31*, 373–383. [CrossRef]
17. Misra, S.; Cheng, L.; Genevie, J.; Yuan, M. The iPhone effect: The quality of in-person social interactions in the presence of mobile devices. *Environ. Behav.* **2014**, *48*, 275–298. [CrossRef]
18. Przybylski, A.K.; Weinstein, N. Can you connect with me now? How the presence of mobile communication technology influences face-to-face conversation quality. *J. Soc. Pers. Relatsh.* **2013**, *30*, 237–246. [CrossRef]
19. Kuss, D.J.; Griffiths, M.D. Online social networking and addiction—A review of the psychological literature. *Int. J. Environ. Res. Public Health* **2011**, *8*, 3528–3552. [CrossRef]
20. Carbonell, X.; Chamarro, A.; Oberst, U.; Rodrigo, B.; Prades, M. Problematic use of the internet and smartphones in university students: 2006–2017. *Int. J. Environ. Res. Public Health* **2018**, *15*, 475. [CrossRef]
21. Ithnain, N.; Ghazali, S.E.; Jaafar, N. Relationship between smartphone addiction with anxiety and depression among undergraduate students in Malaysia. *Int. J. Health Sci. Res.* **2018**, *8*, 163–171.
22. Hadi, A.A.; Nawawi, H.M.M.; Shamsuri, N.; Rahim, N.N.; Pasi, H. Smartphone Addiction and Its Relationship with Psychological Health among Clinical Years Medical Students of International Islamic University Malaysia (IIUM), Kuantan. *IIUM Med. J. Malays.* **2019**, *18*, 10.
23. Nasser, N.S.; Loh, J.L.; Rashid, A.A.; Sharifat, H.; Ahmad, U.; Ibrahim, B.; Mustafa, S.; Hoo, F.K.; Ching, S.M.; Suppiah, S. *A Cross-Sectional Survey on Smartphone Usage Pattern, the Level of Mobile Phone Dependence and Psychosocial Effects among Undergraduate Students in a Malaysian University*; MedRxiv Preprint; Cold Spring Harbor Laboratory Press: New York, NY, USA, 2020. [CrossRef]
24. Ng, S.F.; Hassan, N.S.I.C.; Nor, N.H.M.; Malek, N.A.A. The Relationship between Smartphone Use and Academic Performance: A Case of Students in a Malaysian Tertiary Institution. *Malays. Online J. Educ. Technol.* **2017**, *5*, 58–70.
25. Kwon, M.; Kim, D.J.; Cho, H.; Yang, S. The smartphone addiction scale: Development and validation of a short version for adolescents. *PLoS ONE* **2013**, *8*, e83558. [CrossRef]
26. Sfendla, A.; Laita, M.; Nejjar, B.; Souirti, Z.; Touhami, A.A.O.; Senhaji, M. Reliability of the Arabic smartphone addiction scale and smartphone addiction scale-short version in two different moroccan samples. *CyberPsychol. Behav. Soc. Netw.* **2018**, *21*, 325–332. [CrossRef]
27. Luk, T.T.; Wang, M.P.; Shen, C.; Wan, A.; Chau, P.H.; Oliffe, J.; Viswanath, K.; Chan, S.S.C.; Lam, T.H. Short version of the Smartphone Addiction Scale in Chinese adults: Psychometric properties, sociodemographic, and health behavioral correlates. *J. Behav. Addict.* **2018**, *7*, 1157–1165. [CrossRef] [PubMed]
28. Lopez-Fernandez, O. Short version of the Smartphone Addiction Scale adapted to Spanish and French: Towards a cross-cultural research in problematic mobile phone use. *Addict. Behav.* **2017**, *64*, 275–280. [CrossRef]
29. De Pasquale, C.; Sciacca, F.; Hichy, Z. Italian validation of smartphone addiction scale short version for adolescents and young adults (SAS-SV). *Psychology* **2017**, *8*, 1513–1518. [CrossRef]
30. Andrade, A.L.M.; Kim, D.J.; Caricati, V.V.; Martins, G.D.G.; Kirihara, I.K.; Barbugli, B.C.; Enumo, S.R.F.; De Micheli, D. Validity and reliability of the Brazilian version of the Smartphone Addiction Scale-Short Version for university students and adult population. *Estudos de Psicologia (Campinas)* **2020**, *37*, e190117. [CrossRef]
31. Akın, A.; Altundağ, Y.; Turan, M.E.; Akın, U. The validity and reliability of the turkish version of the smart phone addiction scale-short form for adolescent. *Procedia Soc. Behav. Sci.* **2014**, *152*, 74–77. [CrossRef]
32. Kennedy, O.; Healy, S. Japanese Validation of the Smartphone Addiction Scale. *AI Mach. Learn. Lang. Education* **2019**, *2019*, 75–88.
33. Vintilă, M.; Tudorel, O.I.; Goian, C.; Bărbat, C. Determining the structure of Smartphone Addiction Scale: A bifactor model analysis. *Curr. Psychol.* **2018**, 1–8. [CrossRef]
34. Areeudomwong, P.; Ruanjai, T.; Srimalee, P. Reliability of a Thai Version of Smartphone Addiction Scale in Thai Adolescents. *J. Med Technol. Phys. Ther.* **2019**, *31*, 391–400.
35. Ching, S.M.; Yee, A.; Ramachandran, V.; Lim, S.M.S.; Sulaiman, W.A.W.; Foo, Y.L.; Kee Hoo, F. Validation of a Malay version of the smartphone addiction scale among medical students in Malaysia. *PLoS ONE* **2015**, *10*, e0139337. [CrossRef]
36. Brown, T.A. *Confirmatory Factor Analysis for Applied Research*; The Guilford Press: New York, NY, USA, 2015.
37. Muthén, L.K.; Muthén, B.O. *Mplus User's Guide*, 8th ed.; Muthén & Muthén: Los Angeles, CA, USA, 2017.

38. Rosseel, Y. lavaan: An R Package for Structural Equation Modeling. *J. Stat. Softw.* **2012**, *48*, 1–36. [CrossRef]
39. R Core Team. *R: A Language and Environment for Statistical Computing*; R Foundation for Statistical Computing: Vienna, Austria, 2020.
40. Hair, J.F., Jr.; Black, W.C.; Babin, B.J.; Anderson, R.E. *Multivariate Data Analysis*, 7th ed.; Prentice Hall: Upper Saddle River, NJ, USA, 2010.
41. Chong Guan, N.; Isa, S.M.; Hashim, A.H.; Pillai, S.K.; Harbajan Singh, M.K. Validity of the Malay version of the Internet Addiction Test: A study on a group of medical students in Malaysia. *Asia Pac. J. Public Health* **2015**, *27*, NP2210–NP2219. [CrossRef] [PubMed]
42. Jorgensen, T.D.; Pornprasertmanit, S.; Schoemann, A.M.; Rosseel, Y. *semTools: Useful Tools for Structural Equation Modeling*, R Package Version 0.5-1; 2018. Available online: https://CRAN.R-project.org/package=semTools (accessed on 5 September 2019).
43. Raykov, T. Estimation of congeneric scale reliability using covariance structure analysis with nonlinear constraints. *Br. J. Math. Stat. Psychol.* **2001**, *54*, 315–323. [CrossRef] [PubMed]
44. Colton, T. *Statistics in Medicine*, 1st ed.; Little, Brown, and Company: Boston, MA, USA, 1974.

11

Development and Validation of the Parental Smartphone Use Management Scale (PSUMS): Parents' Perceived Self-Efficacy with Adolescents with Attention Deficit Hyperactivity Disorder

Yi-Ping Hsieh [1], Cheng-Fang Yen [2,*] and Wen-Jiun Chou [3,*]

1 Department of Social Work, College of Nursing and Professional Disciplines, University of North Dakota, Grand Forks, ND 58202, USA; yiping66@gmail.com
2 Department of Psychiatry, School of Medicine, and Graduate Institute of Medicine, College of Medicine, Kaohsiung Medical University, Kaohsiung 807, Taiwan
3 Department of Child and Adolescent Psychiatry, Chang Gung Memorial Hospital, Kaohsiung Medical Center and College of Medicine, Chang Gung University, Kaohsiung 833, Taiwan
* Correspondence: chfaye@cc.kmu.edu.tw (C.-F.Y.); wjchou@cgmh.org.tw (W.-J.C.)

Abstract: The psychometric properties of the Parental Smartphone Use Management Scale (PSUMS) and its prospective relationships with symptoms of smartphone addiction and attention deficit hyperactivity disorder (ADHD) were studies in a sample of parents of adolescents with ADHD. This is a scale to measure parents' perceived self-efficacy on managing their children's smartphone use. Construct validity (exploratory factor analysis and confirmatory factor analysis), criterion-related validity (known-group validity and concurrent validity), and reliability (Cronbach's alpha) were performed for data analyses. The results showed that the PSUMS had good factorials validity and high reliabilities, with Cronbach's alphas ranging between 0.93 and 0.95. The 17-item PSUMS accounted for 78.58% of the total variance and contains three theoretically and statistically appropriate subscales: reactive management, proactive management, and monitoring. Strong relationships were found between parental smartphone use management and symptoms of smartphone addiction and ADHD in expected directions. Moreover, parents of children with smartphone addiction yielded lower scores on all three PSUMS subscales than parents of children without smartphone addiction. The PSUMS is considered a valuable and reliable tool in the study of parental management on their adolescent children's smartphone use, while providing us with important targets for intervention.

Keywords: smartphone use; parental management; scale validation; attention deficit hyperactivity disorder (ADHD); smartphone addiction

---

1. Introduction

Rapid and continuing growth in the ownership of smartphones means they have now become a central gateway to online services and information. In Taiwan, approximately 73.4% of people own a smartphone, compared with 71.8% in Singapore, 70.4% in South Korea, 63.9% in the United States, and 43.8% in China [1]. In terms of age, smartphone ownership is highest among younger adults aged 18–29 (85%) [1]. The ownership of smartphones among teenagers has also surged. For instance, Adestra [2] found that approximately 87% of teenagers aged 14–18 years have smartphones, compared with 92% of adults aged 19–34 years and 65% of adults aged 56–67 years. In Taiwan, smartphone ownership among adolescents (aged 12–17 years) ranges from 78.8% to 93.3% and is 48.7% among children (aged 6–11 years) [3]. Although half (51.3%) of elementary school children do not own a smartphone, 38.8% of these children often use a family member's smartphone. Among adolescents, smartphones are the most widely used computing devices (87%), followed by laptops (83%), tablets (51%), and desktop computers (43%) [2]. Adolescents often used a smartphone after school (82%), during class recess (74%), while taking transportation (63%), while eating food (57%), and in class (16%) [4].

Compared with adults, adolescents are more vulnerable to smartphone addiction because of the developmental stage of their brains and because they tend to have lower levels of self-control over their impulses to pursue pleasure [5,6]. A 2015 study by the Taiwan Ministry of Education reported that the prevalence of smartphone addiction among adolescents in Taiwan ranges from 13.9% to 25.7% and is even more prevalent than Internet addiction (12.6–19.5%). Smartphone addiction is associated with health problems and negative social, psychological, and behavioral effects such as sleep disturbance, depression, anxiety, low emotional intelligence, poor academic performance, risky behaviors (using a smartphone while driving or walking), and problematic behaviors [7–10]. Adolescent smartphone addiction is therefore considered a serious problem that warrants prevention and intervention.

Aside from smartphone addiction, online safety is also a major parental worry as an increasing number of children and teenagers gain access to the Internet through smartphones and tablets [11,12]. Among the common concerns that parents have about their children's Internet and smartphone use are Internet and smartphone addiction, cyberbullying, online solicitation, sexting, cyberstalking, online friendships, online reputation, and privacy issues [12,13]. Cyberbullying and sexting, for example, are associated with psychological and behavioral health problems among adolescents [14,15] and have even been linked to suicide ideation and attempts [16,17].

Erikson's theory of stages of development suggests that adolescents and young adults (in the fidelity and love stage) are eager to establish friendships and intimate relationships online and to blend their identities with those of their friends; they are also concerned about how they appear to others [18,19]. However, online environments may create a false sense of intimacy and intention. Cyber-stalkers may simulate ideal personas that lead adolescents to misjudge the intentions behind their messages; thereafter, cyber-stalkers may engage in obsessive relational intrusion which can be defined as "the repeated and unwanted pursuit of intimacy through violation of physical and/or symbolic privacy" [20]. An adolescent's stage of cognitive development and their lack of life experience, along with the anonymity of the online environment, leads to greater risk-taking behavior which puts them at risk and compromises their online safety. Given the potential risks of cybercrime and problematic Internet and smartphone use, it is essential for parents to manage, educate, and communicate with their adolescent children and guide their use of digital technology.

Attention deficit hyperactivity disorder (ADHD) is the most common psychiatric disorder among adolescents with an Internet addiction [21]. ADHD has been found to be associated with Internet addiction in both cross-sectional [22] and longitudinal studies [23]. The symptoms and characteristics of ADHD include a tendency to be bored, impaired inhibition, and low achievement, and it is associated with a higher risk of Internet addiction [24] and higher levels of parent–child conflict [25]. Parents should be able to educate their adolescent children and communicate with them about online behavior and safety, as well as executing plans to manage their adolescents' Internet and smartphone use. Therefore, a reliable metric is needed to assess self-perceived parents' self-efficacy regarding management of their ADHD adolescent children's smartphone use. The Parental Smartphone Use Management Scale (PSUMS) was therefore developed and validated in this study. In sum, this study tends to understand parents' self-efficacy and engagement in managing children's smartphone use, explore the useful parenting strategies to prevent children's smartphone addiction and victimization, and develops a reliable and valid scale.

2. Materials and Methods

2.1. Participants and Procedure

Parents of adolescents aged between 11 and 18 years who had received a diagnosis of ADHD according to the diagnostic criteria in the Diagnostic and Statistical Manual of Mental Disorders, Fifth Edition (DSM-5) [26] were recruited for this study between August 2014 and July 2015 from the child and adolescent psychiatric outpatient clinics of two medical centers in Kaohsiung, Taiwan. Two child psychiatrists conducted diagnostic interviews with the parents and made ADHD diagnoses based on the criteria in the DSM-5. Multiple data sources—including clinical observation of each adolescent's behavior and parental ratings of ADHD symptoms on the short version of the Swanson, Nolan, and Pelham, Version IV, Scale—Chinese version (SNAP-IV) [27,28]—were used to support each diagnosis. Adolescents who had an intellectual disability or autism spectrum disorder with difficulties in communication were excluded. Parents who had an intellectual disability, schizophrenia, bipolar disorder, or any cognitive deficits that resulted in significant communication difficulties were also excluded. A total of 237 parents of adolescents with an ADHD diagnosis were invited to participate in the study. Of these, six (2.5%) declined to participate and 20 (8.4%) reported that their children had not used smartphones in the previous month. Thus, 211 (89.0%) of the invited parents participated in the study and were interviewed by research assistants using the research questionnaire—the PSUMS, the Problematic Cellular Phone Use Questionnaire (PCPU-Q), and the short version of the SNAP-IV Chinese version. The Institutional Review Boards (IRBs) of Kaohsiung Medical University and Chang Gung Memorial Hospital, Kaohsiung Medical Center, approved the study (KMUHIRB-20130131). All participants were fully informed about the study and provided informed consent.

2.2. Measures

2.2.1. Parental Smartphone Use Management Scale (PSUMS)

Prior to developing the PSUMS, an item pool was established by conducting a literature review and a focus group. The item pool contained 20 items. A 7-point Likert scale was used to rate the level of agreement with items, ranging from 0 (no efficacy at all) to 6 (very strong efficacy). To ensure the face validity of the scale, psychiatrists, psychologists, and parenting specialists were consulted about the content. In response to their opinions and criticism, the scale was revised to use culture-sensitive wording and remove irrelevant content. Parents were then asked to rate their self-perceived efficacy in managing their children's smartphone use over the previous month. High PSUMS scores indicate high levels of self-efficacy.

2.2.2. Problematic Cellular Phone Use Questionnaire (PCPU-Q)

The PCPU-Q was used to assess the criterion-related validity of the PSUMS. This scale measures adolescents' problematic smartphone use [29] and comprises 12 items, each of which is rated on a 4-point Likert scale. It was developed according to the taxonomies of substance dependence classified in the Diagnostic and Statistical Manual of Mental Disorders, Fourth Edition (DSM-4) (Text Revision) [30] and modified according to the taxonomies of substance use disorder classified in the DSM-5 [26]. The PCPU-Q comprises two subscales—symptoms of problematic cellular phone use (CPU) and functional impairment caused by CPU. The first eight items address symptoms of problematic CPU among adolescents in the preceding month, including tolerance, withdrawal, CPU for longer periods of time or at higher frequencies than intended, persistent desire or unsuccessful attempts to reduce CPU, excessive time spent on CPU, giving up or reducing the number of important social, academic, or recreational activities because of CPU, continued heavy CPU despite knowledge of the physical or psychological problems caused, and an urge to use the cellular phone. The five remaining items gauge the functional impairment exhibited by an adolescent in the preceding month as a result of CPU. Higher overall scores indicate more severe levels of problematic CPU symptoms and CPU-related functional impairments. The internal reliability (Cronbach's α) of the PCPU-Q subscales was 0.92 and 0.92, respectively. According to the scale developers, when participants report four out of eight problematic CPU symptoms and at least one functional impairment, they were categorized into the cellarer-phone-addiction group for screening and analysis purposes.

2.2.3. ADHD Symptoms

The short version of the SNAP-IV (Chinese version) was used to assess the severity of ADHD symptoms exhibited in the preceding month. This version comprises 26-items encompassing the core DSM-4-derived ADHD subscales of inattention, hyperactivity and impulsivity, and the oppositional symptoms of oppositional defiant disorder [27,28]. Each item is rated on a 4-point Likert scale ranging from 0 (not at all) to 3 (very much). The Cronbach's α for inattention, hyperactivity and impulsivity, and oppositional behavior were 0.91, 0.90, and 0.93, respectively, indicating very high internal consistency.

2.3. *Analysis*

The PSUMS was administered to the 211 study participants to determine its psychometric characteristics. Construct validity was determined by using factor analysis. Specifically, 211 participants were randomly divided into two subsamples using the RANDBETWEEN function in EXCEL. The first subsample ($n = 103$) was then used for exploratory factor analysis (EFA) and the second sample ($n = 108$) was used for confirmatory factor analysis (CFA). The EFA was conducted using SPSS 24 statistical software (SPSS Inc., Chicago, IL, USA). Based on the assumption that the factors are correlated, principal axis analysis was carried out with Promax rotation, after which the Kaiser–Mayer–Olkin (KMO) measure of sampling adequacy and Bartlett testing were applied. A KMO value of >0.60 and significant statistics from Bartlett testing suggested the data was suitable for factor analysis [31]. The amount of variance accounted for indicates how well a relevant notion or construct can be measured [32].

Since the multivariate skewness (4929.18) and multivariate kurtosis (40.25) indicate the non-normal distribution for the CFA subsample, maximum likelihood with Satorra-Bentler correction was performed to determine whether the model data fit with the item-factor structures obtained from the EFA. The CFA was conducted using LAVAAN package in the R software [33]. In general, the results indicate a good fit when the standardized root mean squared residual (SRMR) below 0.08 [34,35], root mean square error of approximation (RMSEA) below 0.08 [36,37], comparative fit index (CFI) and non-normed fit index (NNFI) above 0.9 [38,39], and a normed chi-square (i.e., chi-square/df) less than 2 [31] or less than 5 [40].

Two approaches for testing criterion-related validity were applied: known-group validity and concurrent validity. Known-group validity was determined by performing independent sample t test between the smartphone-addiction group and non-smartphone-addiction group. The concurrent validity of the PSUMS was determined by examining the correlation between the PSUMS and the PCPU-Q. Internal consistency was tested to assess the reliability of the scale.

3. Results

The preliminary analysis indicated that none of the study variables were skewed or kurtotic. The sociodemographic characteristics of parents and adolescents, adolescents' ADHD symptoms, and smartphone-addiction symptoms are presented in Table 1. Descriptive statistics along with both the EFA and CFA factor loadings of the PSUMS items are presented in Table 2.

Table 1. Sociodemographic characteristics of parents and adolescents and the ADHD symptoms.

Variables	*n* (%)	Mean (*SD*)	Range
Sex of parents			
Female	175 (82.9%)		
Male	36 (17.1%)		
Sex of adolescents			
Female	28 (13.3%)		
Male	183 (86.7%)		
Age of parents (years)		43.5 (5.9)	32–64
Age of adolescents (years)		13.7 (1.8)	11–18
Marriage status of parents			
Intact	170 (80.6%)		
Not intact	41 (19.4%)		
Education duration of parents (years)		13.6 (2.8)	6–28
SNAP-IV symptoms of adolescents			
Inattention		12.8 (6.1)	0–27
Hyperactivity/impulsivity		8.9 (6.0)	0–27
Oppositional defiant		9.9 (5.7)	0–24
PCPU-Q			
Smartphone addiction	40 (19%)		
No smartphone addiction	171 (81%)		

Note: SNAP-IV: Short version of the Swanson, Nolan, and Pelham Version IV Scale—Chinese version. PCPU-Q: Problematic Cellular Phone Use Questionnaire. *SD* = standard deviation.

Table 2. Means, standard deviations, Cronbach's α, and factor loadings for the items in the PSUMS.

Items	Mean (*SD*) (*n* = 211)	EFA *n* = 103	CFA *n* = 108
Reactive Management (α = 0.93)			
I manage my child's smartphone use to prevent it from negatively affecting his/her daily life	4.35 (1.43)	0.73	0.89
I manage how and to what extent my child spends money on his/her smartphone	4.64 (1.44)	0.66	0.81
I don't allow my child to use a smartphone while doing homework	4.42 (1.48)	0.59	0.86
I manage my child's smartphone use outside of the house	3.74 (1.76)	0.59	0.80
I effectively manage when my child can and cannot use a smartphone	4.18 (1.61)	0.57	0.88
I manage my child's activities to prevent him/her from breaking laws	4.30 (1.49)	0.53	0.83
When my child is spending too much time on a smartphone, I manage his/her smartphone use effectively	4.38 (1.40)	0.52	0.90
Proactive Management (α = 0.95)			
I don't distress my child when communicating with him/her about smartphone use	3.72 (1.58)	0.93	0.91
I don't create family tension as a result of enforcing smartphone use guidelines for my child	3.81 (1.55)	0.82	0.93
I discuss and reason with my child	4.11 (1.37)	0.80	0.93
I don't get angry when I manage my child's smartphone use	3.53 (1.61)	0.72	0.83
I communicate with my child effectively and explain why I manage his/her smartphone use	4.22 (1.33)	0.70	0.93
I actively learn new information and skills to manage my child's smartphone use	4.14 (1.44)	0.55	0.82
Monitoring (α = 0.93)			
I know who my child talks with and what they talk about when using a smartphone	3.81 (1.69)	0.91	0.96
I know what my child does on the smartphone	3.86 (1.64)	0.84	0.95
I monitor which apps my child uses	3.79 (1.69)	0.72	0.88
I restrict the type of websites my child is allowed to visit on the smartphone	3.91 (1.69)	0.63	0.85

Note: EFA = exploratory factor analysis; CFA = confirmatory factor analysis; *SD* = standard deviation.

3.1. Construct Validity

3.1.1. Exploratory Factor Analysis (EFA)

An EFA was conducted on a sample of 211 parents of children with ADHD. The KMO coefficient of sampling adequacy was 0.90 which lies within the excellent range. Bartlett's Test of Sphericity, which assesses whether a matrix differs from the identity matrix, yielded significant results, indicating that the matrix did not resemble the identity matrix; this also supported the presence of factors within the data.

Principal axis factor analysis was conducted and the Promax rotation method, which assumes factors are correlated and rotates the factor structure, was used to determine the factor solutions. The initial result confirmed the proposed three-factor solution for all 20 items. After eliminating three items with cross-loadings, a factor analysis was run once more on the remaining 17 items. The results supported a three-factor solution that explained 78.58% of the total variance. The items and factor loadings for the subscales are presented in Table 2. The three-factor solution fits with the theoretical factors used to devise the measurement tool. The first factor, "reactive management" ($\alpha = 0.93$) includes seven items with factor loadings of 0.52–0.73; the items reflect parents' reactive management of children's smartphone use through rule-setting practices, responding to and controlling this use to avoid negative impacts on children's daily-life functioning. The second subscale, "proactive management" ($\alpha = 0.95$) includes 6 items with factor loadings of 0.55–0.93; the items reflect parents' perceived efficacy of their proactive management and active mediation of children's smartphone use through positive communication and reasoning. The third factor, "monitoring" ($\alpha = 0.93$) includes 4 items with factor loadings of 0.63–0.91; the items reflect parents' behavior in monitoring what their children do on their smartphones, whom they talk with, what applications they use, and the websites they visit. The score for each subscale was calculated by its mean. Pearson's correlations among the dimensions of the PSUMS are presented in Table 3.

Table 3. Correlation among the dimensions of the PSUMS.

PSUMS Dimensions	Reactive Management	Proactive Management	Monitoring
Reactive management	-		
Proactive management	0.79 **	-	
Monitoring	0.77 **	0.68 **	-

Note: ** $p < 0.01$.

3.1.2. Confirmatory Factor Analysis

The CFA fit indices were acceptable: $CFI = 0.934$, $NNFI = 0.923$, $RMSEA = 0.077$, and $SRMR = 0.053$, normed chi-square = 1.64; except for the significant chi-square test (chi-square = 189.68, $df = 116$; $p < 0.001$). Moreover, the factor loadings were strong in each factor: loadings = 0.80 to 0.90 in Reactive Management; 0.82 to 0.93 in Proactive Management; and 0.85 to 0.96 in Monitoring. Overall, the current model showed an acceptable fit to the data.

3.2. Criterion Validity

The PCPU-Q was used to determine the criterion-related validity of the PSUMS. After checking the equality of the variance, independent sample *t* test results provided strong evidence for known-groups validity, a subtype of criterion-related validity. We compared the PSUMS results between the parents of children with and without smartphone addiction. The results showed that parents of children with smartphone addiction yielded lower scores on all three PSUMS subscales than parents of children without smartphone addiction (Table 4). The correlation coefficients between three subscales of the PSUMS and two subscales of the PCPU-Q were also calculated. The results of the Pearson's correlation provided strong evidence for concurrent validity (Table 5). The PSUMS was found to be significantly correlated with the PCPU-Q (all $p < 0.001$).

Table 4. Parental smartphone use management among children with and without smartphone addiction.

PSUMS Dimensions	Have Smartphone Addiction (n = 40) Mean (SD)	No Smartphone Addiction (n = 171) Mean (SD)	t	p
Reactive management	3.30 (1.46)	4.52 (1.14)	4.93	<0.001
Proactive management	2.90 (1.39)	4.11 (1.27)	5.34	<0.001
Monitoring	2.94 (1.56)	4.05 (1.47)	4.25	<0.001

Note: *SD*: Standard Deviation.

Table 5. Correlation between Parental Smartphone Use Management Scale (PSUMS) and PCPU-Q.

PCPU-Q Dimensions	Parental Smartphone Use Management (PSUMS)		
	Reactive Management	Proactive Management	Monitoring
	r	r	r
Smartphone addiction symptoms	−0.35 **	−0.40 **	−0.33 **
Functional impairments	−0.37 **	−0.33 **	−0.26 **

Note: ** $p < 0.01$. PCPU-Q: Problematic Cellular Phone Use Questionnaire.

3.3. Reliability

The internal consistency coefficient (Cronbach's α) of the PSUMS was 0.96. As shown in Table 2, the internal consistency coefficients in the sub-dimensions of the PSUMS were 0.93 for Reactive management, 0.95 for Proactive management, and 0.93 for Monitoring.

4. Discussion

In this study we developed and validated the PSUMS to measure parents' perceived efficacy in managing the smartphone use of adolescents with ADHD. The final version of the 17-item PSUMS accounted for 78.58% of the total variance and contains three theoretically and statistically appropriate subscales: reactive management, proactive management, and monitoring. The three-factor hypothesis was supported by the scale's psychometric properties, including its construct validity (confirmed using EFA and CFA), criterion-related validity (known-group validity and concurrent validity), and reliability (internal consistency measured using Cronbach's alpha). The PSUMS adhered to psychometric standards and was shown to be a concise and promising measure of whether parents of adolescents with ADHD have the knowledge and skills required to successfully manage their children's smartphone use.

The PSUMS consists of three scales. With a rating scale from 0 to 6, an increase in scores corresponds to an increase in parents' efficacy in managing their children's smartphone use. The three smartphone-management items parents feel most confident about were in the sub-dimension "reactive management". These were: "I manage how and to what extent my child spends money on his/her smartphone", "I don't allow my child to use a smartphone while doing homework", and "when my child is spending too much time on a smartphone, I stop his/her smartphone use effectively". The two smartphone-management items they felt least confident about were in the sub-dimension "proactive management", which involved positive communication and reasoning. These were: "I don't get angry when I manage my child's smartphone use", and "I don't distress my child when communicating with him/her about smartphone use". Moreover, parents also produced low scores in regard to managing children's smartphone use outside of the house.

In terms of criterion-related validity, the subscales of the PSUMS were significantly correlated in the expected direction with the PCPU-Q. The first subscale, reactive management, concerns parental intervention in adolescents' smartphone overuse, money spending, cybercrime involvement, poor timing of use, and other smartphone behaviors that may negatively affect their daily lives. Adolescents whose parents use moderate behavioral control reported fewer problem behaviors [41,42]. Similarly, parents who set rules on media time reported that their children (aged 0–6 years) watched less television on average than other children in their age group [43]. As expected, reactive management was negatively correlated with smartphone addiction and functional impairments. Parents who scored lower on reactive management were more likely to have children with a smartphone addiction and functional impairments. The second subscale, proactive management, addresses parents' positive communication, affection toward, and reasoning with adolescents about their smartphone use. Research has shown that adolescents who exhibit the symptoms and characteristics of ADHD are more likely than other children to experience relatively high levels of parent–child conflict [25]. In our study, effective communication, high levels of affection, and reasoning around smartphone use behaviors with adolescents with ADHD was found to be a key element in the successful prevention of problematic smartphone use. Proactive management enables adolescents to discuss their feelings, negotiate rules, and communicate in a safe and caring environment. This type of parenting practice has been linked to prosocial behavior, less externalizing behavior, good mental health, and higher achievement [44–47]. As expected, proactive management was negatively correlated with smartphone addiction and functional impairments. Finally, the third subscale, parental monitoring, was defined as "a set of correlated parenting behaviors involving attention to and tracking of the child's whereabouts, activities, and adaptations" on their smartphone [48]. Parental monitoring has been associated with lower levels of alcohol and substance use [49,50]. Similarly, lower levels of parental monitoring have been found to correlate with a higher percentage of time spent on nonacademic computer use [51]. In this study, parental monitoring was negatively associated with smartphone addiction and functional impairment. The PSUMS was significantly correlated in the expected direction with the PCPU-Q, which confirmed its concurrent validity.

The PSUMS conceptualized and measured parents' self-efficacy regarding their management of the smartphone use of adolescents with ADHD. However, this research had some limitations that need to be addressed. The sample sizes used for EFA and CFA were relatively small (i.e., 103 for EFA and 108 for CFA, total of 211). However, we believed that our contribution adds on the current literature because it is hard to collect more than a hundred adolescents with diagnosed ADHD. Furthermore, studies have shown that our sample sizes were acceptable for both EFA and CFA. For EFA, a rule of thumb to calculate the sample size is using an item-participant ratio of 5 [52]. Given that the original item number of the PSUMS is 20, 100 was a sufficient number for conducting EFA. Regarding CFA, although the consensus is that 200 is a preferable sample size, Iacobucci argue that sample size at 50 is sufficient [53]. Anderson and Gerbing [54] and Kline [55] agree that using a sample size of 100 could be the minimum criterion for doing CFA. Therefore, we tentatively concluded that our sample sizes were acceptable in both EFA and CFA [56]. Nevertheless, future studies are warranted to collect a larger sample size to corroborate our findings. Although construct validity, known-groups validity and concurrent validity were supported by the results, another limitation is that all subscales of PSUMS are significantly correlated with all subscales of PCPU-Q (the criterion scale), which indicated that subscales of PSUMS may not be distinguished. However, when performing the calculation for the test of the differences between two dependent correlations with one variable in common [57], we found a significant difference between two correlations of PSUMS subscales (reactive management and monitoring) with one subscale of PCPU-Q (functional impairment) in common as criterion ($z = 2.49$, $p < 0.01$). This limitation maybe because of the nature of smartphone addiction (PCPU-Q) is related to parental smartphone use management (PSUMS), thus subscales of PSUMS cannot be fully distinguished. Future studies may use monitoring scales as criterion in testing discriminant validity in PSUMS. Despite these limitations, the overall results showed that the PSUMS has good reliability and adequate validity. The reliability and validity of the scale mean it can be used to test different samples. Furthermore, the PSUMS could also be used as a tool for developing smartphone-addiction prevention programs for adolescents.

5. Conclusions

The PSUMS is considered a valuable and reliable tool in the study of parental management on their adolescent children's smartphone use, while providing us with important targets for intervention.

This study provides a foundation for future research in education, family science, and technology science by examining the multidimensional factors associated with parents' efficacy in managing adolescents' smartphone use in the digital age. Because Internet and smartphone are widely used and become an important part of our daily life, it is essential to enhance the traditional parenting and educational programs with consideration of the management on children/adolescents' smartphone use, strength parents' efficacy in doing so, and prepare parents with right tools to face this new challenge in parenting.

Author Contributions: Conceptualization, Y.-P.H., C.-F.Y. and W.-J.C.; methodology, Y.-P.H.; software, Y.-P.H.; validation, Y.-P.H., C.-F.Y. and W.-J.C.; formal analysis, Y.-P.H.; investigation, C.-F.Y. and W.-J.C.; resources, Y.-P.H., C.-F.Y. and W.-J.C.; data curation, Y.-P.H, C.-F.Y. and W.-J.C.; writing—original draft preparation, Y.-P.H.; writing—review and editing, Y.-P.H., C.-F.Y. and W.-J.C.; visualization, Y.-P.H.; supervision, C.-F.Y. and W.-J.C.; project administration, C.-F.Y. and W.-J.C.; funding acquisition, C.-F.Y. and W.-J.C.

References

1. Pew Research Center. A Portrait of Smartphone Ownership. Available online: http://www.pewinternet.org/2015/04/01/chapter-one-a-portrait-of-smartphone-ownership/ (accessed on 4 March 2019).
2. Adestra. Consumer Adoption & Usage Study. Available online: http://www.adestra.com/resources/2016-consumer-adoption-usage-study/ (accessed on 4 March 2019).
3. Taiwan Ministry of Education. 2015 Student Network Usage Survey Report. Available online: https://www.edu.tw/News_Content.aspx?n=0217161130F0B192&s=F1AA06D56E8D6B20 (accessed on 4 March 2019).
4. Yang, S.Y.; Chen, M.D.; Huang, Y.C.; Lin, C.Y.; Chang, J.H. Association between smartphone use and musculoskeletal discomfort in adolescent students. *J. Community Health* **2017**, *42*, 423–430. [CrossRef]
5. Chóliz, M. Mobile-phone addiction in adolescence: The Test of Mobile Phone Dependence (TMD). *Prog. Health Sci.* **2012**, *2*, 33–45.
6. Steinbeis, N.; Haushofer, J.; Fehr, E.; Singer, T. Development of behavioral control and associated vmPFC–DLPFC connectivity explains children's increased resistance to temptation in intertemporal choice. *Cereb. Cortex* **2014**, *26*, 32–42. [CrossRef] [PubMed]
7. Choa, K.-S.; Lee, J.-M. Influence of smartphone addiction proneness of young children on problematic behaviors and emotional intelligence: Mediating self-assessment effects of parents using smartphones. *Comput. Hum. Behav.* **2017**, *66*, 303–311. [CrossRef]
8. Hawi, N.S.; Samaha, M. To excel or not to excel: Strong evidence on the adverse effect of smartphone addiction on academic performance. *Comput. Educ.* **2016**, *98*, 81–89. [CrossRef]
9. Thomée, S.; Härenstam, A.; Hagberg, M. Mobile phone use and stress, sleep disturbances, and symptoms of depression among young adults—A prospective cohort study. *BMC Public Health* **2011**, *11*, 1–11. [CrossRef] [PubMed]
10. White, M.P.; Eiser, J.R.; Hagberg, M. Risk perceptions of mobile phone use while driving. *Risk Anal. Int. J.* **2004**, *24*, 323–334. [CrossRef] [PubMed]
11. Boyd, D.; Hargittai, E. Connected and concerned: Variation in parents' online safety concerns. *Policy Internet* **2013**, *5*, 245–269. [CrossRef]
12. Madden, M.; Cortesi, S.; Gasser, U.; Lenhart, A.; Duggan, M. Parents, Teens, and Online Privacy (Pew Internet & American Life Project). Available online: http://pewinternet.org/Reports/2012/Teens-and-Privacy.aspx (accessed on 19 April 2019).
13. George, M.J.; Odgers, C.L. Seven fears and the science of how mobile technologies may be influencing adolescents in the digital age. *Perspect. Psychol. Sci.* **2015**, *10*, 832–851. [CrossRef]
14. Gámez-Guadix, M.; Orue, I.; Smith, P.K.; Calvete, E. Longitudinal and reciprocal relations of cyberbullying with depression, substance use, and problematic internet use among adolescents. *J. Adolesc. Health* **2013**, *53*, 446–452. [CrossRef] [PubMed]

15. Gordon-Messer, D.; Arturo Bauermeister, J.; Grodzinski, A.; Zimmerman, M. Sexting among young adults. *J. Adolesc. Health* **2012**, *52*, 301–306. [CrossRef]
16. Curnutt, H. Flashing your phone: Sexting and the remediation of teen sexuality. *Commun. Q.* **2012**, *60*, 353–369. [CrossRef]
17. Gini, G.; Espelage, D.L. Peer victimization, cyberbullying, and suicide risk in children and adolescents. *JAMA* **2014**, *312*, 545–546. [CrossRef] [PubMed]
18. Subrahmanyam, K.; Greenfield, P.M.; Tynes, B. Constructing sexuality and identity in an online teen chat room. *J. Appl. Dev. Psychol.* **2004**, *25*, 651–666. [CrossRef]
19. Subrahmanyam, K.; Smahel, D.; Greenfield, P. Connecting developmental constructions to the Internet: Identity presentation and sexual exploration in online teen chat rooms. *Dev. Psychol.* **2006**, *42*, 395–406. [CrossRef] [PubMed]
20. Cupach, W.R.; Spitzberg, B.H. *The Dark Side of Relationship Pursuit: From Attraction to Obsession and Stalking*; Lawrence Erlbaum Associates: Mahwah, NJ, USA, 2014.
21. Bozkurt, H.; Coskun, M.; Ayaydin, H.; Adak, I.; Zoroglu, S.S. Prevalence and patterns of psychiatric disorders in referred adolescents with Internet addiction. *Psychiatry Clin. Neurosci.* **2013**, *67*, 352–359. [CrossRef]
22. Yen, J.Y.; Ko, C.H.; Yen, C.F.; Wu, H.Y.; Yang, M.J. The comorbid psychiatric symptoms of Internet addiction: Attention deficit and hyperactivity disorder (ADHD), depression, social phobia, and hostility. *J. Adolesc. Health* **2007**, *41*, 93–98. [CrossRef]
23. Chen, Y.L.; Chen, S.H.; Gau, S.S.F. ADHD and autistic traits, family function, parenting style, and social adjustment for Internet addiction among children and adolescents in Taiwan: A longitudinal study. *Res. Dev. Disabil.* **2015**, *39*, 20–31. [CrossRef]
24. Ko, C.H.; Yen, J.Y.; Yen, C.F.; Chen, C.S.; Chen, C.C. The association between Internet addiction and psychiatric disorder: A review of the literature. *Eur. Psychiatry* **2012**, *27*, 1–8. [CrossRef] [PubMed]
25. Edwards, G.; Barkley, R.A.; Laneri, M.; Fletcher, K.; Metevia, L. Parent–adolescent conflict in teenagers with ADHD and ODD. *J. Abnorm. Child Psychol* **2001**, *29*, 557–572. [CrossRef]
26. American Psychiatric Association. *Diagnostic and Statistical Manual of Mental Disorders (DSM-5®)*; American Psychiatric Association: Washington, DC, USA, 2013.
27. Gau, S.S.F.; Shang, C.Y.; Liu, S.K.; Lin, C.H.; Swanson, J.M.; Liu, Y.C.; Tu, C.L. Psychometric properties of the Chinese version of the Swanson, Nolan, and Pelham, version IV scale–parent form. *Int. J. Methods Psychiatr. Res.* **2008**, *17*, 35–44. [CrossRef]
28. Swanson, J.M.; Kraemer, H.C.; Hinshaw, S.P.; Arnold, L.E.; Conners, C.K.; Abikoff, H.B.; Clevenger, W.; Davies, M.; Elliott, G.R.; Greenhill, L.L.; et al. Clinical relevance of the primary findings of the MTA: Success rates based on severity of ADHD and ODD symptoms at the end of treatment. *J. Am. Acad. Child Adolesc. Psychiatry* **2001**, *40*, 168–179. [CrossRef] [PubMed]
29. Yen, C.F.; Tang, T.C.; Yen, J.Y.; Lin, H.C.; Huang, C.F.; Liu, S.C.; Ko, C.H. Symptoms of problematic cellular phone use, functional impairment and its association with depression among adolescents in Southern Taiwan. *J. Adolesc.* **2009**, *32*, 863–873. [CrossRef]
30. American Psychiatric Association. *Diagnostic and Statistical Manual of Mental Disorders*, 4th ed.; American Psychiatric Association: Washington, DC, USA, 2000.
31. Tabachnick, B.G.; Fidell, L.S. *Using Multivariate Statistics*, 5th ed.; Allyn and Bacon: New York, NY, USA, 2007.
32. Hardy, M.; Bryman, A. *Handbook of Data Analysis*; Sage: Thousand Oaks, CA, USA, 2004.
33. Rosseel, Y. lavaan: An R Package for Structural Equation Modeling. *J. Stat. Softw.* **2012**, *48*, 1–36. Available online: http://www.jstatsoft.org/v48/i02/ (accessed on 6 April 2019). [CrossRef]
34. Hu, L.T.; Bentler, P.M. Fit indices in covariance structure modeling: Sensitivity to under-parameterized model misspecification. *Psychol. Methods* **1998**, *3*, 424–453. [CrossRef]
35. Chang, C.-C.; Su, J.-A.; Chang, K.-C.; Lin, C.-Y.; Koschorke, M.; Thornicroft, G. Perceived stigma of caregivers: Psychometric evaluation for Devaluation of Consumer Families Scale. *Int. J. Clin. Health Psychol* **2018**, *18*, 170–178. [CrossRef] [PubMed]
36. MacCallum, R.C.; Browne, M.W.; Sugawara, H.M. Power analysis and determination of sample size for covariance structure modeling. *Psychol. Methods* **1996**, *1*, 130–149. [CrossRef]
37. Wu, T.-H.; Chang, C.-C.; Chen, C.-Y.; Wang, J.-D.; Lin, C.-Y. Further psychometric evaluation of the Self-Stigma Scale-Short: Measurement invariance across mental illness and gender. *PLoS ONE* **2015**, *10*, e0117592. [CrossRef] [PubMed]

38. Bentler, P.M.; Bonnet, D.C. Significance Tests and Goodness of Fit in the Analysis of Covariance Structures. *Psychol. Bull.* **1980**, *88*, 588–606. [CrossRef]
39. Lin, C.-Y.; Luh, W.-M.; Cheng, C.-P.; Yang, A.-L.; Ma, H.-I. Evaluating the wording effect and psychometric properties of the Kid-KINDL: Using the multitrait-multimethod approach. *Eur. J. Psychol. Assess.* **2014**, *30*, 100–109. [CrossRef]
40. Wheaton, B.; Muthen, B.; Alwin, D.F.; Summers, G. Assessing Reliability and Stability in Panel Models. *Sociol. Methodol.* **1977**, *8*, 84–136. [CrossRef]
41. Furstenberg, F.F.; Cook, T.D.; Eccles, J.; Elder, G.H.; Sameroff, A.; Ardelt, M.; Bartko, W.T.; Chan, W.S.; Geitz, L.M.; Harper, C.; et al. *Managing to Make It: Urban Families and Adolescent Success*; University of Chicago Press: Chicago, IL, USA, 1999.
42. Galambos, N.L.; Barker, E.T.; Almeida, D.M. Parents do matter: Trajectories of change in externalizing and internalizing problems in early adolescence. *Child Dev.* **2003**, *74*, 578–594. [CrossRef]
43. Vandewater, E.A.; Park, S.E.; Huang, X.; Wartella, E.A. "No—you can't watch that" parental rules and young children's media use. *Am. Behav. Sci.* **2005**, *48*, 608–623. [CrossRef]
44. Padilla-Walker, L.M.; Carlo, G.; Christensen, K.J.; Yorgason, J.B. Bidirectional relations between authoritative parenting and adolescents' prosocial behaviors. *J. Res. Adolesc.* **2012**, *22*, 400–408. [CrossRef]
45. Pinquart, M. Associations of parenting dimensions and styles with externalizing problems of children and adolescents: An updated meta-analysis. *Dev. Psychol.* **2017**, *53*, 873–932. [CrossRef]
46. Steinberg, L.; Lamborn, S.D.; Dornbusch, S.M.; Darling, N. Impact of parenting practices on adolescent achievement: Authoritative parenting, school involvement, and encouragement to succeed. *Child Dev.* **1992**, *63*, 1266–1281. [CrossRef] [PubMed]
47. Uji, M.; Sakamoto, A.; Adachi, K.; Kitamura, T. The impact of authoritative, authoritarian, and permissive parenting styles on children's later mental health in Japan: Focusing on parent and child gender. *J. Child Fam. Stud.* **2014**, *23*, 293–302. [CrossRef]
48. Dishion, T.J.; McMahon, R.J. Parental monitoring and the prevention of child and adolescent problem behavior: A conceptual and empirical formulation. *Clin. Child Fam. Psychol. Rev.* **1998**, *1*, 61–75. [CrossRef] [PubMed]
49. Dodge, K.A.; Malone, P.S.; Lansford, J.E.; Miller, S.; Pettit, G.S.; Bates, J.E. A dynamic cascade model of the development of substance-use onset. *Monogr. Soc. Res. Child Dev.* **2009**, *74*, vii-119. [CrossRef]
50. Kopak, A.M.; Ayers, S.; Lopez, V.; Stevenson, P. Parental monitoring, alcohol, and marijuana use among Hispanic and non-Hispanic White adolescents: Findings from the Arizona Youth Survey. *J. Drug Issues* **2011**, *41*, 461–485. [CrossRef]
51. Epstein, J.A. Factors related to adolescent computer use and electronic game use. *ISRN Public Health* **2011**, *2012*, 1–6. [CrossRef]
52. Gorusch, R.L. *Factor Analysis*, 2nd ed.; Lawrence Erlbaum Associates: Hillsdale, NJ, USA, 1983; p. 332.
53. Iacobucci, D. Structural equations modeling: Fit indices, sample size, and advanced topics. *J. Consum. Psychol.* **2010**, *20*, 90–98. [CrossRef]
54. Anderson, J.C.; Gerbing, D.W. The effect of sampling error on convergence, improper solutions, and goodness-of-fit indices for maximum likelihood confirmatory factor analysis. *Psychometrika* **1984**, *49*, 155–173. [CrossRef]
55. Kline, R.B. *Principles and Practice of Structural Equation Modeling*; Guilford: New York, NY, USA, 1998.
56. Su, C.-T.; Ng, H.-S.; Yang, A.-L.; Lin, C.-Y. Psychometric evaluation of the Short Form 36 Health Survey (SF-36) and the World Health Organization Quality of Life Scale Brief Version (WHOQOL-BREF) for patients with schizophrenia. *Psychol. Assess.* **2014**, *26*, 980–989. [CrossRef] [PubMed]
57. Lee, I.A.; Preacher, K.J. Calculation for the Test of the Difference between Two Dependent Correlations with One Variable in Common [Computer Software]. Available online: http://quantpsy.org (accessed on 7 April 2019).

12

Problematic Use of the Internet and Smartphones in University Students: 2006–2017

Xavier Carbonell [1,*], Andrés Chamarro [2,3], Ursula Oberst [1], Beatriz Rodrigo [1] and Mariona Prades [1]

[1] FPCEE Blanquerna, Universitat Ramon Llull, 08022 Barcelona, Spain; ursulao@blanquerna.url.edu (U.O.); beatrizrc2@blanquerna.url.edu (B.R.); marionapo@blanquerna.url.edu (M.P.)
[2] Departamento de Psicología, Universitat Autónoma de Barcelona, Cerdanyola del Vallès, 08193 Barcelona, Spain; andres.chamarro@uab.es
[3] Serra Hunter Program, Generalitat de Catalunya, 08029 Barcelona, Spain
* Correspondence: xaviercs@blanquerna.url.edu

Abstract: It has been more than a decade since a concern about the addictive use of the Internet and mobile phones was first expressed, and its possible inclusion into the lists of mental disorders has recently become a popular topic of scientific discussion. Thus, it seems to be a fitting moment to investigate the prevalence of this issue over time. The aim of the present study was to analyze the prevalence of the perception of problematic Internet and smartphone use in young people over the period 2006–2017. To this end, a questionnaire on Internet use habits and two questionnaires on the negative consequences of Internet and smartphone use were administered to a sample of 792 university students. The scores were then compared with the results of former studies that had used these questionnaires. The perception of problematic Internet and mobile phone use has increased over the last decade, social networks are considered responsible for this increase, and females are perceived to be more affected than males. The current study shows how strong smartphone and Internet addiction and social media overlap. Participants from 2017 report higher negative consequences of both Internet and mobile phone use than those from 2006, but long-term observations show a decrease in problematic use after a sharp increase in 2013. We conclude that the diagnosis of technological addictions is influenced by both time and social and culture changes.

Keywords: Internet addiction; mobile phone addiction; online social network; university students; technological addictions; behavioral addictions; CERI; CERM

1. Introduction

Ever since Young [1] presented *Internet Addiction: the Emergence of a New Disorder* at the Congress of the American Psychological Association in Toronto, Internet addiction has been a widely discussed disorder in the media and in scientific literature [2]. The interest in the possible addiction to the Internet, video games, online role-playing games, television, and mobile phones has given rise to a new field of study: technological addictions [3]. In fact, the DSM-5 [4] included addiction to video games in the list of disorders that should receive further research. The negative consequences of this problem include the possible increase of stress, anxiety, and/or the "paradox" of a lack of communication, despite being more connected, especially among young people and adolescents [5–7].

Internet use and Internet access habits have recently evolved. For example, in 2015, in Spain, there was a clear preference for smartphones (88.2%) over computers (78.2%) for accessing the Internet, especially in 14–19 year olds. This evolution of preference for the phone over the computer was also observed for the accessing of leisure activities, which decreases the dominance of the computer in the professional and educational spheres [8]. Because of its popularity and because it is a relatively new device (compared to the "classical" mobile phone), the smartphone has raised concerns about its potential to be addictive [9–12] as happens with other possible behavioral addictions, such as those to the Internet or to social networking sites [13].

The prevalence of smartphone addiction has been established using different self-report measures. Among the most frequently used, and actually one of the first self-report questionnaires, there was the Mobile Phone Problem Usage Scale (MPPUS) [9,14], later translated and adapted to the Spanish population [15]. The Problematic Mobile Phone Use Questionnaire (PMPUQ) [16] has also been employed in several studies [17]. Another questionnaire used in the Spanish speaking context is the *Cuestionario de Experiencias Relacionadas con el Móvil* [Questionnaire for mobile phone-related experiences] (CERM) [18], used to collect data from young people [19] and university students [20,21]. Recently, several other questionnaires were adapted to asses smartphone addiction, like the Smartphone Addiction Scale (SAS) [22], the Smartphone Addiction Inventory (SPAI) [23], or the one used in Saudi Arabia [24]. All of them have shown their usefulness and good validity and reliability, but it is difficult to assess if problematic mobile phone use has increased over the years since researchers use different measurements and instruments.

The term 'Internet addiction' or 'smartphone addiction' is not used consistently in the literature. A review shows the use of different expressions; there is, for instance, 'digital addiction' [25], 'problematic Internet use' [26], or 'Internet-use disorder' [27]. Even the same authors use different expressions in different papers [27,28]. It is not the purpose of the present article to discuss the convenience of one term or another, nor to discuss if the negative consequences can be interpreted as an addiction or not; however, we will use the term 'addiction' for the studied phenomenon, because it was one of the first terms used [1] and because in the studies that we will compare, this term has also been used from the beginning.

Added to the scientific relevance of this issue, the media tend to echo and spread negative information about the use of mobile phones. Results of these alerts are concepts such as the so-called technostress [29], smombie (a combination of "smartphone" and "zombie") [30], fear of missing out ("FoMO") [31], and nomophobia ("no-mobile-phone phobia") [32]. However, studies on the addictive consequences of both the 'old' mobile phone [9,33–36], the current smartphone [22,24,37–40], and the Internet are cross-sectional, and therefore the temporal evolution of their addictive impact on the population is still unknown. On the basis of the aforementioned research, the objectives of the current study were, first, to explore the perception of problematic Internet and smartphone use in young people in 2017 and, second, to compare these results with former those of studies that used the same measurement instruments, in order to analyze the evolution of the negative effects of Internet and mobile phone use over a period of ten years. As Internet and smartphone use has increased considerably during the past decade, we also expect negative effects to increase over the years (H1). As shown in the previous literature, also in our study women reported a greater use of social networking sites, whereas men used more videogames and adult pages (H2). We also expect women to experiment stronger negative consequences than males (H3).

2. Materials and Methods

2.1. Participants

In the present study, 792 students from Universitat Ramon Llull of Barcelona (Spain) participated in the study in May 2017. They were studying Psychology (30.7%), Physical Education and Sports Sciences (17.2%), Education (47.6%), and Speech Therapy (4.5%). The mean age was 21.6 years (SD = 3.3), and 76.5% were women.

The data on problematic Internet and mobile phone use obtained in the present study (called Cohort 6 hereinafter) was compared with data obtained from other cohorts of university students who answered the CERI and CERM questionnaires in studies conducted by our team between 2006 and 2017:

- Cohort 1: 322 students from the fields of Psychology, Physical Education, Nursing, Physiotherapy, or Communication in Universitat Ramon Llull of Barcelona. The mean age was 19.71 years (SD = 1.73), and 72.7% were women. The data were collected during the 2005–2006 academic year [18].
- Cohort 2: 318 Psychology students from the University of Illinois at Urbana-Champaign in the United States, 51% of which were women, aged between 17 and 21 years. The data were collected during the 2013–2014 academic year [20].
- Cohort 3: 425 Psychology students from the University of Illinois at Urbana-Champaign with an average age of 19.5 (SD = 1.5); 65.4% were women. The data were collected during the 2015–2016 academic year [21].
- Cohort 4: 308 Psychology students from the Universitat Ramon Llull. The mean age was 22.2 years (SD = 4.1), and 77.9% were women. The data were collected during the 2015–2016 academic year [21].
- Cohort 5: 308 psychology students from Ibagué University in Ibagué, Colombia. The mean age was 19.8 years (SD = 3.03), and 65.6% were women. The data were collected during the 2015–2016 academic year [21].

2.2. Instruments

The following instruments were used:

- Sociodemographic data and Internet use habits were assessed with an ad hoc questionnaire. This questionnaire collected sociodemographic data (age, sex, and university degree) and frequency and type of Internet use (e.g., gambling, social networks, etc.) in a five-point Likert scale. The questionnaire also included a Likert-type question about the user's degree of agreement with the statement: "I am addicted to the Internet" and one question about gender and addiction: "Do you think that girls are more Internet-addicted than boys?"
- Addictive behaviors related to the Internet were assessed with the Cuestionario de Experiencias Relacionadas con Internet (CERI) [Questionnaire on Internet-related experiences] [18]. This questionnaire consisted of 10 items about Internet use that were answered on a four-point Likert scale. Item example: "Piensas que la vida sin Internet es aburrida, vacía y triste?" (Do you think that life without the Internet is boring, empty, and sad?). The reliability (Cronbach's alpha) in the present study was 0.76; in the original study it was 0.77.
- Addictive behaviors related to the mobile phone were assessed with the Cuestionario de Experiencias Relacionadas al Móvil (CERM) (Questionnaire on experiences related to the mobile phone) (CERM) [18]. This questionnaire consisted of 10 items about mobile phone use that were answered on a four-point Likert scale. Item example: "Hasta qué punto te sientes inquieto cuando no recibes mensajes o llamadas?" (To what extent do you feel anxious when you do not receive messages or calls?). In the present study, Cronbach's alpha was 0.73. Cronbach's alpha in the original study was 0.80. Other studies have also reported reliability indexes of 0.80 [41].

For both CERI and CERM, the scores were calculated by adding up the answers to all the items, to a maximum of 40 points; cut-off points were established in a former study [42]. CERI and CERM have been used in several studies on adolescents' excessive Internet and mobile phone use [19,43].

2.3. Procedure

Eligible participants were invited to participate in the present study by means of an email containing a link to a Google Docs form. No personal information was requested, and it was not possible to connect any of the data from the questionnaires to academic records. The participants had to click on a box to give their informed consent and continue with the study. The students did not receive any monetary or academic reward for their participation. The study was approved by the Committee of Ethics and Research of the FPCEE Blanquerna, Universitat Ramon Llull.

2.4. Data Analysis

Normality checks were run on the data. Student's t-tests were run to assess gender differences in relation to: (a) the type of use they engage in on the Internet; (b) their scores on the CERI and CERM; (c) the degree of agreement that users expressed regarding the question "I'm addicted to the Internet." To check if the use of certain Internet functions is associated with negative consequences of use, correlations were calculated between the use of the Internet functions and scores on the CERI and CERM. A multiple analysis of variance for gender and year of questionnaire administration was run to test the effects of these two factors on both the CERM and CERI scores.

3. Results

3.1. Results of the Present Study

The frequencies of Internet uses are shown in Table 1. The most frequent activities on the Internet were checking emails and sending messages, participating in social networks, and listening to music. The least frequent uses were gambling and visiting adult pages. Significant gender differences were found between all uses except for online purchases, viewing of TV series, movies or videos, and administrative tasks.

Table 1. Most frequent Internet uses by university students.

Internet Uses	Men	Women	Total	t	p
	M (SD)	*M* (SD)	*M* (SD)		
Phone calls and videoconferences	2.70 (1.12)	2.98 (1.11)	2.91 (1.27)	2.97	0.003
Email/Chat	4.60 (0.66)	4.76 (0.54)	4.72 (0.58)	3.38	0.001
Social networking	4.11 (1.06)	4.34 (0.97)	4.28 (0.99)	2.69	0.007
General information	3.80 (1.04)	3.33 (1.07)	3.44 (1.08)	5.18	0.007
Shopping	2.11 (1.00)	2.11 (1.06)	2.11 (1.05)	0.01	0.987
Videogames	2.32 (1.29)	1.63 (0.93)	1.79 (1.07)	7.94	0.000
Gambling/betting	1.44 (0.85)	1.06 (0.32)	1.15 (0.53)	8.96	0.000
Videos/TV series	3.43 (1.24)	3.52 (1.21)	3.50 (1.22)	0.90	0.364
Listening to music	3.99 (1.10)	4.24 (1.01)	4.18 (1.04)	2.90	0.004
Administrative tasks	2.58 (1.20)	2.60 (1.25)	2.59 (1.24)	0.21	0.832
Adult content	2.34 (1.08)	1.25 (0.65)	1.51 (0.90)	16.07	0.000
Academic activities	3.66 (1.01)	4.03 (0.99)	3.95 (1.01)	4.46	0.000

Descriptive statistics of the Cuestionario de Experiencias Relacionadas al Móvil (CERM) and Cuestionario de Experiencias Relacionadas con Internet (CERI) scores are presented in Table 2. The mean CERI score was 18.04 (SD = 4.50), and the mean CERM score was 15.77 (SD = 3.50) for the whole cohort 6. There were no significant differences either for gender or for the different major degrees ($F(4, 787) = 1.24$; $p = 0.291$ for the CERI, and $F(4, 787) = 1.85$; $p = 0.116$ for the CERM). To the question, "Do you think girls are more addicted to the Internet than boys?" 73.2% answered affirmatively.

Table 2. Means and standard deviations of the Cuestionario de Experiencias Relacionadas con Internet (CERI) and the Cuestionario de Experiencias Relacionadas al Móvil (CERM) scores for cohort 6.

Questionnaire	Men	Women	Total	t-Tests
	M (SD)	*M* (SD)	*M* (SD)	
Cuestionario de Experiencias Relacionadas al Móvil (CERM)	15.77 (3.55) $n = 186$	15.77 (3.50) $n = 606$	15.77 (3.50) $n = 792$	$t(790) = 0.012$ ($p = 0.884$)
Cuestionario de Experiencias Relacionadas con Internet (CERI)	18.09 (4.81) $n = 186$	18.04 (4.41) $n = 606$	18.04 (4.50) $n = 792$	$t(790) = 0.146$ ($p = 0.990$)

The correlation between the CERI and the CERM was high ($r = 0.76$, $p = 0.000$). The correlations between the different online functions and the CERI and CERM were mostly significant, but low, with the most relevant correlation being between social networks and both the CERI and the CERM (see Table 3).

Table 3. Correlations between CERI or CERM and the uses of the Internet.

Internet Uses	CERI	CERM
Email/Chat	0.15 **	0.14 **
Social networking	0.23 **	0.21 **
General information	0.14 **	0.08
Shopping	0.14 **	0.12 **
Videogames	0.10 **	0.11 **
Gambling/betting	0.15 **	0.17 **
Videos/TV series	0.12 **	0.11 **
Listen music	0.18 **	0.17 **
Administration	0.03	0.04
Adult content	0.12	0.13 **
Academic activities	0.07	0.01
Phone calls/videoconferences	0.04	0.08

Note: ** $p < 0.001$.

Regarding the self-assessment of whether they considered themselves addicted to the Internet, 375 students (47.4%) either agreed or agreed strongly with this statement. Table 4 shows that people who "strongly agreed" with the statement "I am addicted to the internet" obtained significantly higher results than the rest of the participants on both the CERI and the CERM. The correlations with the CERI and CERM were 0.38 ($p < 0.001$) and 0.34 ($p < 0.001$), respectively.

Table 4. Levels of agreement with the statement "I am addicted to the Internet" with the scores in CERI and CERM.

Level of Agreement	CERI	CERM
	M (SD)	*M* (SD)
Strongly agree	21.89 (4.71) $n = 93$	18.47 (4.22) $n = 93$
Agree	19.02 (4.20) $n = 282$	16.45 (3.25) $n = 282$
Neither agree nor disagree	16.82 (3.81) $n = 275$	14.89 (3.09) $n = 275$
Disagree	15.90 (3.58) $n = 123$	14.35 (2.71) $n = 123$
Totally disagree	16.47 (6.85) $n = 19$	14.47 (4.25) $n = 19$

3.2. Comparison between Present Study and Former Studies with CERM and CERI

As shown in Table 5, the scores in the CERI and CERM grew from 2005 to 2013 and remained stable during the 2013–2014 academic year. The number of students who showed problematic Internet use went from 1.5% in 2005 to 6.4% in 2017 and from 0.6% to 3.0%, in the case of problematic mobile phone use. The correlation between CERI and CERM was "moderate" up to 2014 and increased to "high" as of 2015.

Table 5. Scores of the university student cohorts in the CERI and the CERM.

Cohort	Year of Survey	CERI M (SD)	CERM M (SD)	Correlation CERI/CERM	Problematic Use CERI (%)	Problematic Use CERM (%)
Cohort 1	2006	14.44 (4.00)	13.07 (2.90)	0.439 **	2.2%	0.9%
Cohort 2	2013	19.65 (5.06)	17.83 (4.39)	0.530 **	9.2%	8.6%
Cohort 3	2015	18.64 (5.03)	18.38 (4.09)	0.692 **	7.5%	8.1%
Cohort 4	2015	17.05 (4.06)	16.68 (3.51)	0.734 **	2.0%	3.0%
Cohort 5	2015	17.98 (5.41)	17.88 (4.98)	0.851 **	9.3%	11.5%
Cohort 6	2017	18.04 (4.50)	15.77 (3.50)	0.760 **	6.4%	3.0%

Note: ** $p < 0.001$.

Descriptive statistics for the CERM and CERI scores, separately for males and females, over the period 2006–2017 are presented in Table 6. Cohorts 3, 4, and 5 were taken together, as data collection took place in the same year. The multivariate analysis of variance for the effects of gender and year of administration on CERI and CERM showed significant effects of both factors (except for gender on CERI) and also a combined effect (see Table 7).

Table 6. Means and standard deviations (in brackets) of the CERM and the CERI scores.

Questionnaire	2006		2013		2015		2017	
	Males	Females	Males	Females	Males	Females	Males	Females
CERM	12.28 (2.62)	13.42 (2.96)	16.95 (4.34)	19.01 (4.60)	17.39 (4.40)	17.86 (4.18)	15.77 (3.55)	15.77 (3.51)
CERI	14.35 (4.05)	14.49 (3.99)	19.11 (4.97)	19.97 (5.20)	18.19 (5.11)	17.89 (4.85)	18.09 (4.81)	18.04 (4.41)

Table 7. Tests of between-subjects effects for the factors gender and year in CERM and CERI.

Source	Variable	F	p	η^2
gender	CERM	24.16	<0.001	0.010
	CERI	0.508	0.476	0.000
year	CERM	140.99	<0.001	0.146
	CERI	70.99	<0.001	0.079
Gender × year	CERM	5.29	0.001	0.006
	CERI	1.21	0.304	0.001

Women presented higher scores in the CERM, but not in the CERI. Post-hoc Bonferroni pairwise comparisons showed that scores for both CERM and CERI had increased from the first survey: there was, in fact, a significant difference between the 2006 scores and those of all the following surveys ($p < 0.001$ in all comparisons). However, between the 2013 and the following years, there was no significant difference between 2013 and 2015, and there was even a decrease of the negative effects between 2015 and 2017 ($p < 0.001$) with respect to the CERM; for the CERI, there was a decrease from 2013 to 2015 and from 2015 to 2017 ($p < 0.001$ in both cases). Figures 1 and 2 present the results separately for CERM and CERI and for both sexes. As can be seen, the increase of the perception of problematic Internet and smartphone use was stronger for females than for males, but as of 2017, both sexes had lower scores and tended to present the same degree of negative effects.

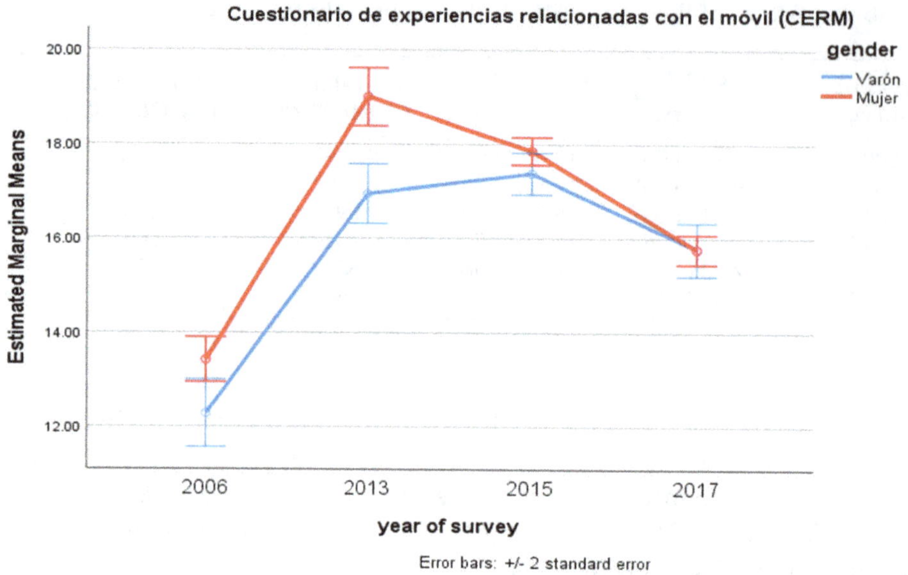

Figure 1. Estimated marginal means of Cuestionario de Experiencias Relacionadas al Móvil (CERM) for year of survey and gender.

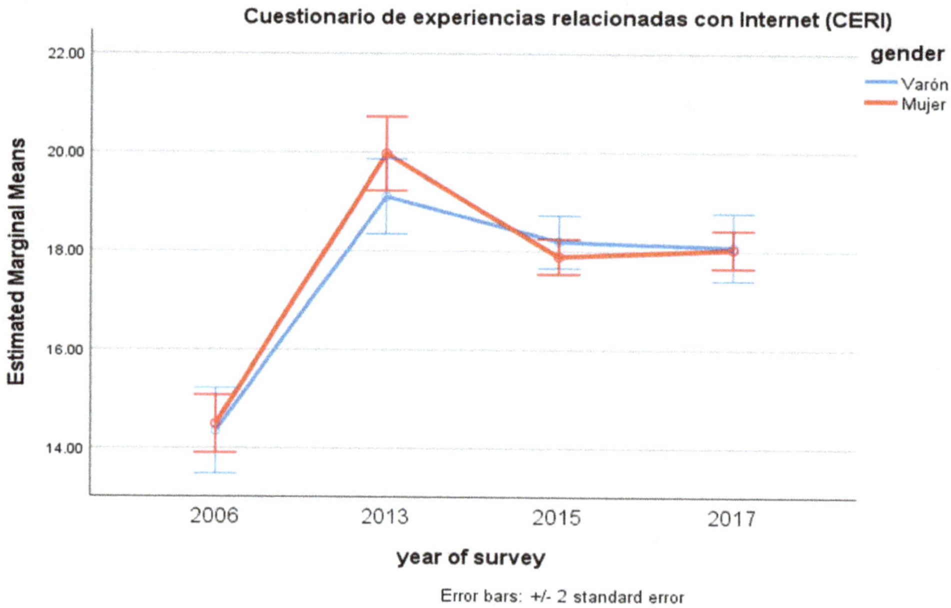

Figure 2. Estimated marginal means of the Cuestionario de Experiencias Relacionadas con Internet (CERI) for year of survey and gender.

4. Discussion

The objective of this study was to evaluate the perception of problematic Internet and mobile phone use and compare these results with those of similar cohorts from up to a decade ago. One of the problems presented by studies evaluating technological addictions to the Internet, social networks, mobile phones, and video games is the absence of longitudinal studies. It is difficult for these studies to monitor a cohort in the medium or long term because the questionnaires are administered in person or online to: (i) cohorts obtained in the general population through social networks or the like; (ii) samples of high school or university students; (iii) video gamers identified in forums. Other factors that make longitudinal studies difficult are the need for respecting the participants' anonymity and the existence of time limitations (i.e., on funding for the research projects and doctoral theses).

To overcome these difficulties, this study compared data from different cohorts of university students assessed in different moments.

Our hypotheses were partially confirmed. Taken globally, the results of the study support the idea that the perception of a problematic use of the Internet and mobile phones exists and has increased over the last decade (H1). This perception seems to go along with the growth of Internet use and all kinds of electronic devices with a screen, with which our samples became familiar during their adolescence [44]. This problematic use of the Internet is specific and not general; that is, it depends on the concrete activity that is carried out [45–47]. This can also be affirmed for mobile phones [17,48,49]. Given that the Internet applications most widely used by university students are e-mail and messaging, participating in social networks, and listening to music, we infer that the increase in the perception of problematic use is associated with the use of online social networks. The activities in which the university students invest the least time are betting games and adult pages, like in other similar samples [17,45,46] and as is expected for university students. However, despite the existence of problematic use, it seems that the term 'addiction' is an inadequate construct when used as simply "Internet addiction", because: (i) the problematic use does not depend on the mobile phone or the Internet itself, but on the activities accessed on them; (ii) the problematic use can be the symptom of other disorders, not a primary disorder in itself [10,17]; (iii) there is a risk that labeling this problematic use an addiction means pathologizing the daily life [50]. The questionnaires used make it possible to detect a concern about certain technology-based behaviors but in no case to issue a clinical diagnosis. The term 'addiction' is probably adequate when related to specific types of use, such as addiction to gaming via the Internet or to pornography via the Internet.

It is difficult to compare our data on problematic mobile use with those of other prevalence studies because of the use of different measuring instruments. A preliminary comparison shows that the range of values for problematic users or addicts ranges between 0% and 35%, with 10–20% being the most frequent values [7,10,12], although there have been reports of 48% in university students [24]. In a recent research, the percentages ranged from 3.9% in Belgium to 1% in Poland, with 1.7% addicts identified in the Spanish sample [17].

It is also not surprising that the Internet uses of young men and women are quite different from each other as there are differences in behavior and attitudes between them in the real world which are perpetuated in the network (H2). Our results show that women use social networks and academic applications more and listen to more music than men. Men play more videogames and betting games and use more adult pages than women. In any case, women's problematic use is greater (H3), probably as a consequence of their using social networks more than males and of the role that those social networks play in communication and in creating and maintaining connections [17,40,51]. Some studies suggest that there may be different thresholds for males and females with respect to these negative effects [52].

The average scores in the CERI were higher than in the CERM, as has been the case with these instruments in other studies [18,20,53]. No differences were found between men and women in the problematic use of the mobile phone despite this being a frequent result in other investigations [15,17,40,53]. Although the Internet activities of men and women were different, there were no differences found in the problematic use of the Internet [53,54]. However, the perception of our students was that women are more addicted to the Internet than men probably because of the fact that using social networks is more common than using video games. Another possible explanation is that women are more vulnerable to this type of problem because it is related to communication practices such as establishing and actively maintaining relationships, which women engage in more than men [38,40].

Social network use is the only Internet use that moderately correlated with CERI and CERM. The other correlations, in line with other studies, were low or nonexistent [17]. In fact, online social networking is considered, along with video games, to be the use with the highest risk of becoming problematic [55,56] even though there is a lack of empirical confirmation [13]. Facebook and WhatsApp (as WhatsApp could be considered a social media) could be used as a key component to understand how young people socialize through these applications [57]. A large-scale tracking of online behavior showed that the use of WhatApp over the smartphone accounted for nearly 20% of all smartphone behavior, above Facebook use [58]. The low correlation with the different Internet uses can be explained because we are talking about a population that, as a whole, bets little and consumes little pornography, which leads us to think that we would obtain higher correlations if the CERI and the CERM were applied to cohorts of people extracted from the general population, who would be more likely to bet online, consume pornography, and/or be intensive video gamers.

The correlation between the CERI and CERM was high. In fact, we wonder if it is still convenient to use both the CERI and the CERM since, at the current time, both measures may be considered equivalent in the context of young people's technology use; young people use the mobile phone more and more frequently to access the Internet [8,17,40] and tend not to distinguish between the platforms (mobile vs. computer) and the program/application. The current study confirms how strong smartphone and Internet addiction and social media overlap [47,59] and advises that the evolution of technology forces us to change and update certain research questions. For example, when we designed the CERM, the mobile phones used by the participants did not have access to the Internet, whereas at present, there is not really a distinction between mobile phones and smartphones because they are considered synonymous. We will draw upon an anecdote to illustrate this situation. When, over a decade ago, the first papers expressing concern about mobile phone addiction were published [9], they were about mobile phones without Internet access. However, last year, when we showed a fourth-year psychology student a picture of an old Nokia phone from that era, one of them asked: "But... was it possible to be addicted to that?" This question reveals to what extent the diagnosis of technological addictions is influenced by time and social and cultural change.

From our point of view, the concern over mobile phone addiction came in two distinct waves. The first was focused on the non-smart mobile phone and was mainly due to two factors: the amount of phone bills that the use led to and the high use of text messages. Phone bills were a point of concern because a flat rate did not exist, and users needed a certain learning period to understand how to manage their use so that it remained within reasonable limits. Another point of concern was the number of text messages (i.e., for women: 11 or more calls or text messages per day, see Thomee, Dellve, Harenstam, Hagberg [6]). Several studies can serve as examples [6,9,34,36]. When, thanks to new billing structures, users managed to control their phone expenses and these worries seemed to dissipate, smartphones emerged on the market. At that point, a new wave of concern started in regard to this new device, because it allowed access to the Internet and Internet-based applications such as social networks and messaging services. Several studies can serve as examples [22–24,60,61]. Here again, the influence of context and culture is crucial.

Something similar is occurring with Internet addiction. In the last decade, we have learned that it is convenient to distinguish between behavioral addictions that take place on the Internet (for example, pathological gambling), the specific uses of the Internet that can become problematic (for example, videogames and social networks), and a possible generalized Internet addiction [45,46,49]. Davis [62] offered one of the first theoretical models, which differentiates between a generalized and a specific type of Internet addiction. Later, more sophisticated models to explain the different levels of the addiction process have been developed, such as the I-PACE model [27], which is useful for understanding the development and maintenance of specific Internet-use disorders. The students who responded to the CERI 10 years ago did so thinking primarily about their connection to the Internet via their computer, whereas now they access the Internet indiscriminately from their mobile phones, other handheld devices, and home or university computer. One example of how Internet use has changed in recent years is the application WhatsApp. WhatsApp is a telephone messaging service but it shares many features with social networks and, as of 2016, it can be accessed from the computer. Therefore, students can use WhatsApp on their mobile phones or from their laptop when they are in the classroom and they create class groups on both WhatsApp and Facebook indiscriminately. Another example of the merging of lines between phone applications and Internet applications is the difficulty in distinguishing between how much time is dedicated to each application or program, since it is so common to work in multi-screen mode. Students can write an academic paper, answer emails, and have a conversation on WhatsApp, all at the same time.

The results of the comparison between the present and former studies with the CERM and the CERI show that the negative effects of Internet and mobile phone use are considerably stronger now that at the first survey in 2006. However, this is due mainly to the first period, between 2006 and 2013. Apparently, there is a downward tendency in the perception of negative consequences in the recent years, which may correspond to a progressive normalization and integration of these new technologies into our daily life.

Although we have already mentioned the limitations of the CERI and CERM (they were created in the cell phone era before the existence of the smartphone and they are self-report measures), they are easy to use and to score, thereby inviting us to continue using them when possible in order to study the evolution of the perception of the problematic use of the Internet and mobile phones. They indicate, not so much the prevalence of an addiction, but the perception of a problem by the respondents. Although the correlation of the CERI and CERM with the statement "I am addicted to the internet" was moderate, the participants who were "very much in agreement" and "agreed" with this statement obtained significantly higher results than the rest in both the CERI and the CERM. This indicates that it might be possible to use this single question to detect the perception of problematic mobile phone use of individuals, as has already been suggested [46,63]. It is highlighted that our students seem to have a perception about their Internet addiction more in line with the data obtained through the questionnaires than the participants in the study done by Pontes, Szabo, and Griffiths [46], in which 51.9% of the participants identified themselves as Internet addicts.

This study is not without limitations. Firstly, university students have a higher than average level of academic development and their use of the Internet and mobile phones is not necessarily representative of the use that other young people engage in. Secondly, a problematic use of these technologies does not correspond to any diagnostic entity and may be a reflection of their social impact. Thirdly, both the CERI and the CERM should be updated, like other mobile addiction instruments (see, Kuss, Harkin, Kanjo and Billieux [64]), because a general use of the Internet is no longer conceivable; rather, a specific one is, and more so because of the new and expanded uses of smartphones. The terms "internet addiction" and "smartphone addiction" could be 'misnomers' [49] which we might not want to use anymore. Finally, it is possible that some differences found in this study were more influenced by the cultural differences between the samples than by the temporal differences.

5. Conclusions

Although men and women use the Internet differently, their problematic use of the Internet and mobile phones are quite similar. In university students, the use of social networks is the main factor responsible for the perception of problematic use; a casuistry that has increased in the decade 2006–2016. Despite the limitations of the CERI and CERM, estimating the prevalence at different points in time offers valuable information about the evolution of the perception of problematic Internet and mobile phone use. It is convenient to repeat the studies using the same instrument in order to understand the perception of problematic Internet and mobile phone use even if it lacks clinical significance. The degree of agreement with the statement "I am addicted to the Internet" might be used as a screening question for the problematic use. Young people are worried about the phenomenon, and it is convenient to keep track of their perception on the issue in order to design, if necessary, educational campaigns for an adequate use of these technologies.

Acknowledgments: We would like to thank Marta Beranuy, Tayana Panova, Diana-Ximena Puerta, Meritxell Puértolas, and Blanca Sánchez for the transfer of their databases.

Author Contributions: Xavier Carbonell designed the study. Beatriz Rodrigo and Mariona Prades acquired the data. Andres Chamarro, Ursula Oberst and Beatriz Rodrigo did the statistical analysis. Xavier Carbonell,

Andres Chamarro, and Ursula Oberst interpreted the results. Xavier Carbonell and Ursula Oberst wrote the initial draft of the article. All authors reviewed the initial draft, participated in the writing of the final draft, and approved the final version of the manuscript.

References

1. Young, K.S. Internet Addiction: The emergence of a new clinical disorder. *Cyberpsychol. Behav.* **1998**, *1*, 237–244. [CrossRef]
2. Carbonell, X.; Guardiola, E.; Beranuy, M.; Bellés, A. A bibliometric analysis of the scientific literature on Internet, video games, and cell phone addiction. *J. Med. Libr. Assoc.* **2009**, *97*, 102–107. [CrossRef] [PubMed]
3. Griffiths, M.D. Technological addictions. *Clin. Psychol. Forum* **1995**, *76*, 14–19.
4. American Psychiatric Association. *Diagnostic and Statistical Manual of Mental Disorders (DSM-5)*; American Psychiatric Association: Arlington, VA, USA, 2013.
5. Lepp, A.; Li, J.; Barkley, J.E.; Salehi-Esfahani, S. Exploring the relationships between college students' cell phone use, personality and leisure. *Comput. Hum. Behav.* **2015**, *43*, 210–219. [CrossRef]
6. Thomée, S.; Härenstam, A.; Hagberg, M. Mobile phone use and stress, sleep disturbances, and symptoms of depression among young adults—A prospective cohort study. *BMC Public Health* **2011**, *11*, 66. [CrossRef] [PubMed]
7. Carbonell, X.; Fuster, H.; Chamarro, A.; Oberst, U. Internet and mobile phone addiction: A review of empirical Spanish studies. *Papeles Psicol.* **2012**, *33*, 82–89.
8. Fundación Telefónica. *La Sociedad de la Información en España 2016*; Fundación Telefónica: Barcelona, Spain, 2016.
9. Bianchi, A.; Phillips, J.G. Psychological predictors of problem mobile phone use. *Cyberpsychol. Behav.* **2005**, *8*, 39–51. [CrossRef] [PubMed]
10. Billieux, J.; Maurage, P.; Lopez-Fernandez, O.; Kuss, D.J.; Griffiths, M.D. Can disordered mobile phone use be considered a behavioral addiction? An update on current evidence and a comprehensive model for future research. *Curr. Addict. Rep.* **2015**, *2*, 156–162. [CrossRef]
11. Chóliz, M. Mobile phone addiction: A point of issue. *Addiction* **2010**, *105*, 373–374. [CrossRef] [PubMed]
12. Pedrero, E.J.; Rodríguez, M.T.; Ruiz, J.M. Adicción o abuso del teléfono móvil. Revisión de la literatura. *Adicciones* **2012**, *24*, 139–152. [CrossRef]
13. Carbonell, X.; Panova, T. A critical consideration of social networking sites' addiction potential. *Addict. Res. Theory* **2017**, *25*, 48–57. [CrossRef]
14. Lopez-Fernandez, O.; Honrubia-Serrano, M.L.; Gibson, W.; Griffiths, M.D. Problematic Internet use in British adolescents: An exploration of the addictive symptomatology. *Comput. Hum. Behav.* **2014**, *35*, 224–233. [CrossRef]
15. Lopez-Fernandez, O.; Losada-Lopez, J.L.; Honrubia-Serrano, M.L. Predictors of problematic Internet and mobile phone usage in adolescents. *Aloma* **2015**, *33*, 49–58.
16. Billieux, J.; Van der Linden, M.; Rochat, L. The role of impulsivity in actual and problematic use of the mobile phone. *Appl. Cogn. Psychol.* **2008**, *22*, 1195–1210. [CrossRef]
17. Lopez-Fernandez, O.; Kuss, D.; Romo, L.; Morvan, Y.; Kern, L.; Graziani, P.; Rousseau, A.; Rumpf, H.J.; Bischof, A.; Gässler, A.K.; et al. Self-reported dependence on mobile phones in young adults: A European cross-cultural empirical survey. *J. Behav. Addict.* **2017**, *6*, 168–177. [CrossRef] [PubMed]
18. Beranuy, M.; Chamarro, A.; Graner, C.; Carbonell, X. Validación de dos escalas breves para evaluar la adicción a Internet y el abuso de móvil. *Psicothema* **2009**, *21*, 480–485.
19. Muñoz-Miralles, R.; Ortega-González, R.; López-Morón, M.R.; Batalla-Martínez, C.; Manresa, J.M.; Montellà-Jordana, N.; Chamarro, A.; Carbonell, X.; Torán-Monserrat, P. The problematic use of Information and Communication Technologies (ICT) in adolescents by the cross sectional JOITIC study. *BMC Pediatr.* **2016**, *16*, 140. [CrossRef] [PubMed]
20. Panova, T.; Lleras, A. Avoidance or boredom: Negative mental health outcomes associated with use of Information and Communication Technologies depend on users' motivations. *Comput. Hum. Behav.* **2016**, *58*, 249–258. [CrossRef]

21. Panova, T.; Carbonell, X.; Chamarro, A. Uses and gratifications in smartphone use and its relationship with anxiety and depression: A multicultural perspective. *Comput. Hum. Behav.* **2018**. submitted.
22. Kwon, M.; Lee, J.Y.; Won, W.Y.; Park, J.W.; Min, J.A.; Hahn, C.; Gu, X.; Choi, J.H.; Kim, D.J. Development and validation of a Smartphone Addiction Scale (SAS). *PLoS ONE* **2013**, *8*, e56936. [CrossRef] [PubMed]
23. Lin, Y.H.; Chang, L.R.; Lee, Y.H.; Tseng, H.W.; Kuo, T.B.J.; Chen, S.H. Development and validation of the Smartphone Addiction Inventory (SPAI). *PLoS ONE* **2014**, *9*, e98312. [CrossRef] [PubMed]
24. Aljomaa, S.S.; Mohammad, M.F.; Albursan, I.S.; Bakhiet, S.F.; Abduljabbar, A.S. Smartphone addiction among university students in the light of some variables. *Comput. Hum. Behav.* **2016**, *61*, 155–164. [CrossRef]
25. Montag, C.; Walla, P. Carpe diem instead of losing your social mind: Beyond digital addiction and why we all suffer from digital overuse. *Cogent Psychol.* **2016**, *3*, 1157281. [CrossRef]
26. Anderson, E.L.; Steen, E.; Stavropoulos, V. Internet use and Problematic Internet Use: A systematic review of longitudinal research trends in adolescence and emergent adulthood. *Int. J. Adolesc. Youth* **2017**, *22*, 430–454. [CrossRef]
27. Brand, M.; Young, K.S.; Laier, C.; Wölfling, K.; Potenza, M.N. Integrating psychological and neurobiological considerations regarding the development and maintenance of specific Internet-use disorders: An Interaction of Person-Affect-Cognition-Execution (I-PACE) model. *Neurosci. Biobehav. Rev.* **2016**, *71*, 252–266. [CrossRef] [PubMed]
28. Brand, M.; Young, K.S.; Laier, C. Prefrontal control and internet addiction: A theoretical model and review of neuropsychological and neuroimaging findings. *Front. Hum. Neurosci.* **2014**, *8*, 357. [CrossRef] [PubMed]
29. Sayre, S.A.; Brod, C. *Technostress—The Human Cost of the Computer Revolution*; Addison-Wesley: Reading, MA, USA, 1984.
30. Butler, H. *Teens Pick "Smombie" as Hippest German Word*; The Local: Stockholm, Sweden, 2015.
31. Przybylski, A.K.; Murayama, K.; Dehaan, C.R.; Gladwell, V. Motivational, emotional, and behavioral correlates of fear of missing out. *Comput. Hum. Behav.* **2013**, *29*, 1841–1848. [CrossRef]
32. King, A.L.; Valença, A.M.; Nardi, A.E.; Valenca, A.M.; Nardi, A.E. Nomophobia: The mobile phone in panic disorder with agoraphobia: Reducing phobias or worsening of dependence? *Cogn. Behav. Neurol.* **2010**, *23*, 52–54. [CrossRef] [PubMed]
33. Ha, J.H.; Chin, B.; Park, D.-H.; Ryu, S.-H.; Yu, J. Characteristics of excessive cellular phone use in Korean adolescents. *Cyberpsychol. Behav.* **2008**, *11*, 783–784. [CrossRef] [PubMed]
34. Jenaro, C.; Flores, N.; Gómez-Vela, M.; González-Gil, F.; Caballo, C. Problematic internet and cell-phone use: Psychological, behavioral, and health correlates. *Addict. Res. Theory* **2007**, *15*, 309–320. [CrossRef]
35. Labrador, F.J.; Villadangos, S.M. Menores y nuevas tecnologías: Conductas indicadoras de posible problema de adicción. *Psicothema* **2010**, *22*, 180–188.
36. Sánchez-Martínez, M.; Otero, A. Factors associated with cell phone use in adolescents in the community of Madrid (Spain). *Cyberpsychol. Behav.* **2009**, *12*, 131–137. [CrossRef] [PubMed]
37. Bian, M.; Leung, L. Linking loneliness, shyness, smartphone addiction symptoms, and patterns of smartphone use to social capital. *Soc. Sci. Comput. Rev.* **2015**, *33*, 61–79. [CrossRef]
38. Gökçearslan, Ş.; Mumcu, F.K.; Haşlaman, T.; Çevik, Y.D. Modelling smartphone addiction: The role of smartphone usage, self-regulation, general self-efficacy and cyberloafing in university students. *Comput. Hum. Behav.* **2016**, *63*, 639–649. [CrossRef]
39. Lin, Y.-H.; Lin, Y.-C.; Lee, Y.-H.; Lin, P.H.; Lin, S.H.; Chang, L.R.; Tseng, H.W.; Yen, L.Y.; Yang, C.C.; Kuo, T.B. Time distortion associated with smartphone addiction: Identifying smartphone addiction via a mobile application (App). *J. Psychiatr. Res.* **2015**, *65*, 139–145. [CrossRef] [PubMed]
40. Van Deursen, A.J.A.M.; Bolle, C.L.; Hegner, S.M.; Kommers, P.A.M. Modeling habitual and addictive smartphone behavior. The role of smartphone usage types, emotional intelligence, social stress, self-regulation, age, and gender. *Comput. Hum. Behav.* **2015**, *45*, 411–420. [CrossRef]
41. Oberst, U.; Wegmann, E.; Stodt, B.; Brand, M.; Chamarro, A. Negative consequences from heavy social networking in adolescents: The mediating role of fear of missing out. *J. Adolesc.* **2017**, *55*, 51–60. [CrossRef] [PubMed]
42. Carbonell, X.; Chamarro, A.; Griffiths, M.D.; Oberst, U.; Cladellas, R.; Talarn, A. Problematic Internet and cell phone use in Spanish teenagers and young students. *Ann. Psychol.* **2012**, *28*, 789–796.
43. García-Oliva, C.; Piqueras, J.A. Experiential Avoidance and Technological Addictions in Adolescents. *J. Behav. Addict.* **2016**, *5*, 293–303. [CrossRef] [PubMed]

44. Martínez De Morentin, J.I.; Cortés, A.; Medrano, C.; Apodaca, P. Internet use and parental mediation: A cross-cultural study. *Comput. Educ.* **2014**, *70*, 212–221. [CrossRef]

45. Griffiths, M.D.; Szabo, A. Is excessive online usage a function of medium or activity? *J. Behav. Addict.* **2014**, *3*, 74–77. [CrossRef] [PubMed]

46. Pontes, H.M.; Szabo, A.; Griffiths, M.D. The impact of Internet-based specific activities on the perceptions of Internet addiction, quality of life, and excessive usage: A cross-sectional study. *Addict. Behav. Rep.* **2015**, *1*, 19–25. [CrossRef]

47. Montag, C.; Bey, K.; Sha, P.; Li, M.; Chen, Y.F.; Liu, W.Y.; Zhu, Y.K.; Li, C.B.; Markett, S.; Keiper, J. Is it meaningful to distinguish between generalized and specific Internet addiction? Evidence from a cross-cultural study from Germany, Sweden, Taiwan and China. *Asia-Pac. Psychiatry* **2015**, *7*, 20–26. [CrossRef] [PubMed]

48. Jeong, S.H.; Kim, H.; Yum, J.Y.; Hwang, Y. What type of content are smartphone users addicted to? SNS vs. games. *Comput. Hum. Behav.* **2016**, *54*, 10–17. [CrossRef]

49. Griffiths, M.D. Conceptual issues concerning Internet addiction and Internet gaming disorder: Further critique on Ryding and Kaye (2107). *Int. J. Ment. Health Addict.* **2018**, *16*, 233–239. [CrossRef] [PubMed]
50. Billieux, J.; Schimmenti, A.; Khazaal, Y.; Maurage, P.; Heeren, A. Are we overpathologizing everyday life? A tenable blueprint for behavioral addiction research. *J. Behav. Addict.* **2015**, *4*, 119–123. [CrossRef] [PubMed]
51. Sapacz, M.; Rockman, G.; Clark, J. Are we addicted to our cell phones? *Comput. Hum. Behav.* **2016**, *57*, 153–159. [CrossRef]
52. Lachmann, B.; Sariyska, R.; Kannen, C.; Cooper, A.; Montag, C. Life satisfaction and problematic Internet use: Evidence for gender specific effects. *Psychiatry Res.* **2016**, *238*, 363–367. [CrossRef] [PubMed]
53. Beranuy, M.; Oberst, U.; Carbonell, X.; Chamarro, A. Problematic Internet and mobile phone use and clinical symptoms in college students: The role of emotional intelligence. *Comput. Hum. Behav.* **2009**, *25*, 1182–1187. [CrossRef]
54. Casas, J.A.; Ruiz-Olivares, R.; Ortega-Ruiz, R. Validation of the Internet and Social Networking Experiences Questionnaire in Spanish adolescents. *Int. J. Clin. Health Psychol.* **2013**, *13*, 40–48. [CrossRef]
55. Kuss, D.J.; Griffiths, M.D. Online social networking and addiction—A review of the psychological literature. *Int. J. Environ. Res. Public Health* **2011**, *8*, 3528–3552. [CrossRef] [PubMed]
56. Ryan, T.; Chester, A.; Reece, J.; Xenos, S. The uses and abuses of Facebook: A review of Facebook addiction. *J. Behav. Addict.* **2014**, *3*, 133–148. [CrossRef] [PubMed]
57. O'Hara, K.P.; Massimi, M.; Harper, R.; Rubens, S.; Morris, J. Everyday dwelling with WhatsApp. In Proceedings of the 17th ACM Conference on Computer Supported Cooperative Work & Social Computing—CSCW'14, Baltimore, MD, USA, 15–19 February 2014; pp. 1131–1143.
58. Montag, C.; Błaszkiewicz, K.; Sariyska, R.; Lachmann, B.; Andone, I.; Trendafilov, B.; Eibes, M.; Markowetz, A. Smartphone usage in the 21st century: Who is active on WhatsApp? *BMC Res. Notes* **2015**, *8*, 331. [CrossRef] [PubMed]
59. Kittinger, R.; Correia, C.J.; Irons, J.G. Relationship between Facebook use and problematic Internet use among college students. *Cyberpsychol. Behav. Soc. Netw.* **2012**, *15*, 324–327. [CrossRef] [PubMed]
60. Haug, S.; Castro, R.P.; Kwon, M.; Filler, A.; Kowatsch, T.; Schaub, M.P. Smartphone use and smartphone addiction among young people in Switzerland. *J. Behav. Addict.* **2015**, *4*, 299–307. [CrossRef] [PubMed]
61. Darcin, A.E.; Kose, S.; Noyan, C.O.; Nurmedov, S.; Yılmaz, O.; Dilbaz, N. Smartphone addiction and its relationship with social anxiety and loneliness. *Behav. Inf. Technol.* **2016**, *35*, 520–525. [CrossRef]
62. Davis, R.A. A cognitive-behavioral model of pathological Internet use. *Comput. Hum. Behav.* **2001**, *17*, 187–195. [CrossRef]
63. Widyanto, L.; Griffiths, M.D.; Brunsden, V. A psychometric comparison of the Internet Addiction Test, the Internet-Related Problem Scale, and self-diagnosis. *Cyberpsychol. Behav. Soc. Netw.* **2011**, *14*, 141–149. [CrossRef] [PubMed]
64. Kuss, D.; Harkin, L.; Kanjo, E.; Billieux, J. Problematic smartphone use: Investigating contemporary experiences using a convergent design. *Int. J. Environ. Res. Public Health* **2018**, *15*, 142. [CrossRef] [PubMed]

13

Analysis of Gambling in the Media Related to Screens: Immersion as a Predictor of Excessive Use?

Jean-Jacques Rémond * and Lucia Romo *

Psychology Department, Laboratory EA CLIPSYD 4430, Paris Nanterre University, 92000 Nanterre, France
* Correspondance: jack-storm@orange.fr (J.-J.R.); romodesprez@gmail.com (L.R.)

Abstract: This study investigates the intricacies between the player interface proposed by the screens, (in particular on smartphone applications or in video games) and gambling. Recent research indicates connections between "immersion" and excessive screen practice. We want to understand the causal-effects between online gambling and the "immersion" variable and understand their relationship and its contingencies. This article empirically investigates whether and how it is possible to observe immersion with its sub-dimensions in gambling on different screens. The objective of this study was to analyze: (1) the costs and benefits associated with gambling practice on screens (2) the link between gambling practice and screen practice (video game, Internet, mobile screen); (3) to observe the propensity to immersion for individuals practicing gambling on screens; and (4) to examine the comorbidities and cognitive factors associated with the practice of gambling on screen. A total of 432 adults (212 men, 220 women), recruited from Ile-de-France (France), responded to a battery of questionnaires. Our study suggests that immersion variables make it possible to understand the cognitive participation of individuals towards screens in general, the practice of gambling on screens and the excessive practice of screens.

Keywords: gambling; video-game addiction; screen addiction; immersion; problematic Internet use; comorbidity; cognitive distortion

---

1. Introduction

This innovative study is an extension of previous studies based on gamblers commitment to screens on slot machine operated electronically [1–4]. The notion of "gambler" for its part, is understood very broadly and includes any person who would bet on chance [5].

In this study, we consider the practice of the lottery, bingo, sports betting, card games, dice games and electronic slot machines. These practices may include the virtual format.

1.1. Gambling

Through the literature, it is easily recognized that these practices have a high participation rate in Western cultures [6–8]. The excessive practice of gambling can generate problems that affect all spheres of a person's life. The negative consequences can be significant and include financial debts, bankruptcy, family disputes and dissolution, criminal behavior and suicidal acts [9–13]. Gambling addiction has recently been reclassified in the DSM-5 [14] in the category of "substance-related addictions and behavioral addictions". As such, excessive gambling and gambling practice are recognized [15]. Gambling practice exists on a continuum ranging from casual, recreational, problematic and excessive gambling.

Epidemiological research on problematic gambling practice has revealed predominant risk factors, including age, whereby young people are more prone to these risks; living in urban areas than rural areas; socially and economically disadvantaged and with easy access to gambling [16].

Some authors [17–20] have argued that well-established risk factors are age, gender, cognitive distortions (misperceptions, illusion of control), sensory characteristics, schedules, comorbidities (personality disorder), AD/HD, substance use, depression, anxiety and illegal acts. The difficulty in regulating emotions is also a risk factor. Authors have found that low self-control, emotional dysregulation, a need to change mood, fill an existential or emotional void (lack of social interaction, relieve boredom), need for approval and avoid difficulties, increased the severity of gambling problems [21–23].

The distinction in gender composition for the practice of gambling has been particularly studied in the literature [24–28]. The practice of gambling has traditionally been regarded as an essentially masculine activity, but studies have shown a significant prevalence of women [25,26,29]. Men are more likely to play for excitement or sensation seeking, while for women, gambling can be related to emotional regulation. Women also begin gambling practice at a later age than men and generally have a faster rate of gambling than men [30]. The distinction between the reasons for gambling practice between men and women may reflect differential comorbidities between the gender.

Concerning comorbidities, a number of studies have revealed that pathological gamblers are more likely to experience problems of psychiatric comorbidity [9,31,32], among adults and teenagers [33–38]. The most common comorbidities found are depression, anxiety, alcoholism and obsessive-compulsive behavior. Studies also report that compulsive gamblers are more likely to report mood disorders, attention deficit disorders with or without hyperactivity [39–44]. Clarke found that pathological gamblers were more depressed than gamblers with no gambling problems [45]. This is reflected in recent studies [36]. Pathological gamblers may also experience cognitive distortions, such as denial, superstition, overconfidence, sense of control, etc. [46,47]. Irrational beliefs would be reinforced when the player reaches a high level of immersion while playing on the Internet or on electronic machines [48–53].

Even before practicing gambling on modern screens through the Internet, the first interactive mediation with gambling involved electronic slot machines. The first studies on immersion and gambling were based on the interactive format of these machines. They show lower rates of engagement of the general population, in contrast to traditional gambling, but studies show that they are more closely associated with problematic use [48]. Studies describe a gambling trajectory, going as far as problematic practice, more accelerated for players playing on an electronic slot machine (on average one year), in contrast to traditional gambling players (on average three and a half years) [54]. These gambling practices on the screens, within casinos, are also more strongly related to psychological distress than other forms of gambling [55]. This acceleration of short-term commitment to gambling by these media can be explained by the immersive and continuous audiovisual experience that can stimulate the pursuit of the game phases [48,56]. These devices also use a faster play rate compared to other traditional forms of gambling. These variables can be found in gambling formats on the Internet via modern screens.

Individual differences in the tendency to be immersed in gambling via electronic machines can contribute to the development of behaviors towards gambling. Individuals in a state of excessive immersion may no longer be able to perceive external stimuli outside the game [57], future appointments or physiological evidence (such as the need for food or to urinate). Just like the traditional gambling, players report relieving chronic stress or negative emotions [44,57]. If positive reinforcement (earning money) is the motivation, the most common among players, negative reinforcement (avoidance) is a significant predictor of gambling and its severity [58]. An avoidance copying style revolves around leaving or avoiding the stressful situation. Typically, this includes distraction via specific tasks or social engagement. Based on the pathways model, individuals who are emotionally vulnerable endorse an escape pattern of gambling where the primary motivation for gambling is avoidance of negative emotions and situations. Although few empirical studies have observed the "immersion" variable on gambling's electronic machines, Schull argues that for some players, this mental state of avoidance may be the consequence of gaming behavior on electronic machines [57].

1.2. Gambling on Screens

When the mobile game is discussed in research, it was often included under the aegis of "Internet games" [6,59–63], regardless of the different platforms and user behavior. It is essential to distinguish the behavior of a gamer of Internet with elements of gambling according to whether a gamer practices this activity on a fixed screen, or on a mobile screen, or on software dedicated to gambling, or on platforms Video games integrating these gambling forms. Studies have already shown that mobile gambling is associated with a high risk of problem gambling [64].

Gambling software or applications on mobile monitors and screens such as smartphones offer greater interactivity [65,66]. The advent of gambling practice on a smartphone increased the practice of betting and lottery playing [67]. Players now have instant access to their favorite game type. To understand the immersion variable of the gambling player on the mobile screen, it is necessary to understand the playful modality of the media proposed for the player on this screen, as well as the playful mode of the related technology. Numerous studies have examined these two modalities [68–71].

Gambling on mobile phones includes several ways to access gambling. This can be through an application, an optimized site, a game on the phone, or written messages. The status of these activities as gambling remains uncertain in a regulatory and legislative framework. Gainsbury et al. [59] give an online gambling taxonomy that separates different activities depending on whether the payment is mandatory or optional, depending on luck or skill, the platform on which the game is played and the proposed theme in connection with gambling. In Gainsbury's taxonomy, the term "online gambling" refers to "gambling on the Internet" where the notions of virtual gambling and gambling are integrated into a gaming format of video games, so the gambler on the Internet will spend the money via the game for a reward and the appearance will be likened to a gambling, but also a wider range of activities such as multiplayer casino video games, practice games, competitions or tournaments based on gambling (for example, poker).

The study also investigate if any model of research on video games on mobile screens can't get closer to models on gambling when it has concealed a financial incentive and chance. The visual, sound and hedonic appeal would thus could thus to influence the player. Immersion theories largely contribute to explain an individual's commitment to the screen [72–75].

1.3. Immersion and Gambling

If we consider studying gambling-related immersion, then we have to consider the notion of the player's commitment and desire to play the game on the screen. Immersion can be defined as "the physical experience of being immersed (...) the sensation of being surrounded by a completely different reality, (...), the whole of our perceptive apparatus" [76]. Immersion also comes from the Latin term "immergo" meaning to be damaged in the sense of a complete absorption that can harm the individual.

The immersion uses the flow principles based on the Csikszentmihalyi theory [77,78]. "Flow is the term given to a constellation of subjective experiences reported by people engaged in fulfilling activities" [72]. The flow experience is multifaceted. First, it involves the attenuation of the different attentional processes; Csikszentmihalyi argues for a definition that would be the fusion of action and sensations, a decrease in the perception of time and a distortion of consciousness [77]. Csikszentmihalyi refers, on several occasions, to flow as a state representing "the highest level of well-being" [77]. However, this assumption is based on the assumption that the activity from which the immersion is derived would be positive or without consequences for excessive use. If gambling activities on screens with their fast pace of play can provide an immersive experience, gamers may unconsciously pursue gambling activities until this results in significant financial losses. If the individual is directed toward a specific goal, evaluative thinking is mitigated during the immersion phase, individuals may be less able to discern whether the accumulated financial losses exceed the expected limits. This conception of immersion related to gambling on screens or on electronic gambling machines has been the subject of few studies. Dixon et al. [79] have shown that the introduction of "concealed losses into victories" in modern media such as electronic machines or screens favors a model of empowering the experience [57]. As it was, the losses still permitted to acquire points of experience or even multiple losses made it possible to obtain all the same credits to replay. Indeed, this function creates a continuous stream of small victories, as opposed to large occasional gains separated by long phases of losses. In the study by Dixon et al. [79], network participants reported an increase in sensation related to immersion. There is a limit to the assessment and interpretation of immersion degree on electronic slot machines. Indeed, few studies assess immersion in relation to excessive practice and propose a holistic model of excessive behaviors related to the cognitive processes in interaction during the phases of viewing and practice of gambling.

For this study, we distinguish the processes of suggestibility to immersion, cognitive processes related to the quality of immersion, as demonstrated by Psotka and Davison [80]. Thus, self-awareness, concentration, attention, self-control are variables belonging to the domain of suggestibility processes of immersion, while sensory skills, the search for new experimentation, persistence of the object, distractibility are processes related to the quality of immersion. A dissociative state could help players cope with stressors and provide relief from aversive states like anxiety, depression or boredom. A number of studies [81–86] have shown a link between pathological gambling and the dissociation experiment during gambling phases. Cartmill et al. studied the relationship between anxiety state, dissociation states and gambling problems depending on the severity of gambling problems [81].

Recent studies support the idea that basic attention is disrupted in problem gamblers. Similarly, studies have shown that gambling-related stimuli create interference in the processing of information. In these studies, pathological gamblers had to perform the Stroop test [87,88]. In the Diskin and Hodgins studies, the pathological gambler group responded significantly more slowly to the objectives presented than the casual gamblers. This difference in latency was interpreted as an attentional narrowing resulting from the fact that pathological gamblers overvalued the visual stimuli of the game to the detriment of peripheral events.

In addition to attentional bias and visual processing deficits, studies have shown that players have distractibility [89]. Distractibility can interfere with the processing of affective information, which reduces the empathic analysis of pain stimuli (Kam, Xu, and Handy [90]). It is possible to consider that players with mood disorders pre-existing in the practice of gambling may seek, in the gambling on the screens, a form of escape. These perceptual deficits can cause functional impairment. The elderly present a high risk of idiopathy and report a higher frequency of distractibility. This suggests that distractibility can lead to physiological consequences via a reduction in the processing of environmental information [91].

This study focuses on the immersion process during the phases of cast projection of the screen and gambling stimuli on the screens can be modulated in order to adapt prevention messages during the phases of game on the screens to the gambling players [92], in particular for the new media related to screens that encourage a first gambling experience [93].

2. Objectives and Hypothesis

Our study focuses on the link between gambling and the new medias related to screens, with "immersion" as a moderator variable. By examining the costs and degree of gambling practice on the screens, we may presume, on the one hand, the importance of evaluating the practices on the screens as a priority, and on the other hand, to consider evaluating the immersion variable and its sub-dimensions. In order to show the interest of studying the immersion variable, we have to consider that the immersion degree is higher for people at risk of excessive use of screens and even higher for people practicing excessively screens and having a problematic practice of gambling.

Hypothesis

Following the examination of previous researches in the field, five hypotheses have been formulated:

Hypothesis 1 (H1). *The economic costs of purchasing applications or gambling games on the screens are more important in gamblers with problem gambling than non-problem gamblers.*

Hypothesis 2 (H2). *Individuals with problem gambling practice have higher scores on scales assessing excessive gambling practices.*

Hypothesis 3 (H3). *The propensity to immersion scores are higher: for people with gambling addiction [1], than for those with no problem gambling practice; And for people with gambling addiction and high scores on scales evaluating practice on screens [2].*

Hypothesis 4 (H4). *Individuals with problem gambling and high scores on scales assessing screen practices, unlike those with only a problem gambling practice, have higher scores on scales assessing anxiety and depression; On the scale assessing impulsivity; To scale assessing emotional regulation; On the scale assessing cognitive distortions.*

Hypothesis 5 (H5). *Individuals with very high scores on the immersion scale (QPI) and low scores at the ICJP scale had significantly lower scores at scales assessing screen practices.*

3. Methods

3.1. Data Collection and Sampling

According to the criteria of the Helsinki Declaration on Consent to Research and Clinical Practice, a paper and online protocol was proposed to a French adult population on a voluntary and anonymous basis. The paper version of the protocol has been distributed mainly to students from universities in Île-de-France region of France (bachelor degree) (n = 222; 51.27%) and to those coming from various socio-professional categories (n = 211; 48.73%). The online questionnaire was distributed to various social media. No financial incentives were offered. The online questionnaire was filled out on different types of screens (computer, tablet, and smartphone). Four hundred thirty-three questionnaires were collected. The final sample (n = 432) comprised 212 men (49%) and 220 women (51%), with an average age of 21.94 years (SD = 5.51).

3.2. Scales Related to Games of Gambling

The Canadian Problem Gambling Index (ICJE) is a measure of the severity of gambling problems over the past 6 months. This instrument, developed in English and French, has nine questions rated 0–3 (never, sometimes, most of the time, always). A comparison between the CPGI and another questionnaire commonly used in prevalence studies of pathological gambling, the South Oaks Gambling Screen (SOGS, Lesieur and Blume, [94]) reveals that the two instruments generate identical rates (Ladouceur, Jacques, Chevalier, Sévigny, and Hamel, [95]).

The Gambling Related Cognition Scale (GRCS) is a translated and validated tool of the Gambling Related Cognitions Scale (GRCS). The ECJ has a good psychometric quality and has 23 items on a seven-point Lickert scale that identify a variety of game-related cognitions. It identifies the gambler's expectations of the game, his control illusions, the predictive power he believes to have on the game, his perception of his ability to resist a desire to play, and the interpretations gained through motivating its continuation of the game.

3.3. Immersion

The Questionnaire on the Propensity to Immersion (QPI) (Bouchard et al. [96,97]). The French QPI scale, initially named ITQ, consists of 18 items, on a seven-point Lickert scale, and is a self-questionnaire measuring the propensity for immersion. With a Cronbach α of 0.88, the scale proposes to evaluate the total propensity to immersion and contain four variables (focus, implication, play, and emotion).

3.4. Scales Assessing Screen Practices

The Problematic Internet Use Questionnaire (PIUQ) scale has been chosen to evaluate the excessive use of the Internet, validated in French by Kern and Acier [98]). The version used consists of twelve items, on a six-point Lickert scale, and four dimensions (self-control, negative consequences, psychological weaning and Internet concerns). The Cronbach alpha of the overall score is between 0.87 and 0.91 according to the studies of Demrovics, Szeredi and Razsa, [99].

The Smartphone Addiction Scale (SAS) of Kwon et al. [100] was chosen to evaluate smartphone practices. The internal consistency and concurrent validity were analyzed with a Cronbach alpha of 0.97. This scale consists of 34 items on a six-point Lickert scale and was constructed from the Y-scale (scale assessing Internet addiction), a visual analog scale and the diagnostic criteria for abuse and of the psychoactive substance dependence of DSM-IV-TR. A more recent Belgian-French version (Smartphone Addiction Scale Short version or SAS-SV, Psychological Sciences Research Institute, Louvain-la-Neuve, Belgium) (Lopez-Fernandez [101])) exists for adolescents with ten items with a Cronbach alpha of 0.90.

The Video Game Addiction Test was selected to assess the excessive use of video games (Van Rooij et al. [102]). The scale consists of 14 items, on a five-point Lickert scale, where five variables (loss of control, preoccupation, withdrawal symptoms, adjustment/mood modification, conflict) can be visualized. It has good internal consistency with a 0.93 Cronbach alpha.

Additional items were added to the initial protocol to glimpse the different modes of screen-related practices, as well as the financial costs associated with screen practices.

3.5. *Impulsiveness*

"Impulsivity" variable was measured using the UPPS Impulsive Behavior Scale (UPPS, Whiteside, Lynam, Miller and Reynolds, [103]). This evaluation questionnaire was validated in the French version by Van der Linden et al. [104]. The French scale includes 20 items on a four-point Lickert scale and has good psychometric qualities with a Cronbach α of 0.70 to 0.84 for the internal consistency of the different subscales.

3.6. *Symptomatology*

Data on anxiety and depression were collected using Hospital Anxiety and Depression (HAD), a self-rated scale for anxiety-depressive disorders in non-psychiatric populations. The HAD (Zigmond and Snaith, [105]) contains 14 items, divided into two factors (depression: seven items, and anxiety: seven items). The internal consistency varies from 0.68 to 0.93 (mean 0.83) for anxiety, and from 0.67 to 0.90 (mean 0.82) for depression. This scale shows good sensitivity, and specificity for identifying anxiety-depressive disorders.

3.7. *Emotion*

The Emotional Regulation Questionnaire (ERQ) scale was developed by Gross and John [106]). It consists of ten items on a seven-point Lickert scale with two variables (cognitive re-evaluation and cognitive repression). Internal validity has a Cronbach alpha of 0.79 for re-evaluation and 0.73 for cognitive repression.

4. Results

Correlations analyses were made between the combinations of variables considered in this study. In order to test the aforementioned hypotheses, statistical analyzes were carried out using the Statistica software (v.13.2, StatSoft society, Tulsa, OK, USA). Descriptive statistics helped to identify the characteristics of the population in our sample. An analysis of variance and correlations (Chi2 and Student's *t*-tests) were performed. Finally, a multiple regression models and a principal component analysis (PCA) were proposed.

4.1. *Descriptive Statistics*

The average individual in our sample is a French male (M = 1.5), aged 22 (M = 21.9), with no children (M = 0.2), who has at least a bachelor level, and is predominantly student. On average, they spend between

2 and 4 h on the computer, 1–2 h on the tablets, 1–2 h on game consoles and 2–4 h on smartphones. In our sample, 54.04% reported feeling dependent on the computer, 6.7% on tablets, 4.6% on game consoles and 58.66% on smartphones. The costs and wagers according to the gambling practice on the screens were analyzed (Table 1). We also estimated excessive media practices related to screens (Table 2).

Table 1. Costs and prevalence of gambling.

Cost Buying by Material	Total (n = 432)		ICJP NPb (n = 397) (A)		ICJP Ar (n = 19) (B)		CPGI Path (n = 8) (C)		T p A vs. B	T p A vs. C	T p B vs. C
	M (€)	SD (€)									
(Total sample, Mean) Mobile Application	n = 56, 12.93%		n = 37, 9.32%		n = 5, 26.32%		n = 1, 12.5%		0.27	0.33	0.93
	12.23	38.04	12.95	40.92	9	8.94	2	/	0.78	0.73	0.37
Cost buying Bets	n = 35, 8.08%		n = 31, 7.81%		n = 8, 42.11%		/		3.45	0.27	0.51
	0.91	3.74	1.03	3.96	15.5	35.36	/	/	<0.001	0.78	0.62
(Total sample, Mean) Computer	n = 58, 13.39%		n = 40, 10.08%		n = 6, 31.58%		n = 2, 25%		3.21	1.75	0.23
	55.31	88.07	45.12	60.74	113.33	192.94	85	91.92	0.001	0.08	0.82
Cost buying Bets	n = 34, 7.85%		n = 29, 7.3%		n = 4, 21.05		n = 1, 12.5%		3.88	6.6	0.21
	21.03	86.1	3.1	9.58	143.75	239.21	50	/	<0.001	<0.001	0.84
(Total sample, Mean) Game console	n = 34, 7.85%		n = 22, 5.54%		n = 3, 15.79%		n = 2, 0.46%		1.66	0.43	1.21
	118.33	141.79	112.5	142.59	200	180.28	60	56.57	0.1	0.66	0.24
Cost buying Bets	n = 19, 4.39%		n = 16, 4.03%		/		/				
	1.05	3.15	1.25	3.42	/	/	/	/			

CPGI: Canadian Pathological Game Index, (NPb): Non-problematic; (Ar): At risk; (Path): Pathological.

Table 2. Scores of the intensity of the practices on the screens (PIUQ, SAS, VAT) for gambling players (ICJP).

Scales	ICJP NPb (n = 397)		ICJP Ar (n = 19)		ICJP Path (n = 8)		Anova 1		Anova 2	
PIUQ practices	total sample (n)	Mean (%)	n	M (%)	n	M (%)				
PIUQ NP	131	33	/		/					
PIUQ a little	239	62.2	10	52.63	3	37.5				
PIUQ Prob	27	6.8	9	47.37	5	62.5				
PIUQ PrSign	9	2.27	/		/					
	M.	ET.	M.	ET.	M.	ET.	F	p	F	p
PIUQ Tot	28.93	9.99	41.16	7.68	44.63	5.53	21.1	0.001	11.9	0.001
AC	2.89	1.17	3.44	1.01	4	0.56	5.41	0.004	4.28	0.02
CN	2.59	0.99	3.58	0.77	3.63	0.98	13.05	0.001	7.59	0.001
SP	2.09	1.1	3.47	1.25	3.5	0.76	20.34	0.001	5.8	0.005
P	2.11	0.89	2.89	0.99	3.75	0.64	19.81	0.001	6.92	0.002
DT	2.41	0.83	3.35	0.64	3.72	0.46	21.04	0.001	11.99	0.001
SAS practices	Total Sample (n)	Mean (%)	Total Sample (n)	Mean (%)	Total Sample (n)	Mean (%)				
SAS NP	392	98.74	16	84.21	6	75				
SAS Dp	11	2.77	2	10.53	2	25				
SAS Abus	3	0.76	1	5.26	/					
	M.	ET.	M.	ET.	M.	ET.	F	p	F	p
SAS Tot	69.43	28.69	90.26	32.55	103.88	25.52	10.04	0.001	5.45	0.007
PVQ	9.46	4.59	12.42	5.29	16.13	4.52	11.57	0.001	8.49	0.001
AP	15.98	7.82	20.26	9.1	23.38	7.19	5.97	0.002	2.8	0.07
RS	12.15	6.15	15.21	6.36	19.38	3.89	7.49	0.001	2.98	0.05
ROC	13.63	6.48	17.68	8.23	21.25	5.7	8.52	0.001	3.12	0.05
SU	10.75	4.97	14.11	5.04	12.75	3.58	4.7	0.009	4.13	0.02
T	7.45	4.24	10.58	4.27	11	4.78	7.41	0.001	3.32	0.04
VAT practices	Total Sample (n)	Mean (%)	Total Sample (n)	Mean (%)	Total Sample (n)	Mean (%)				
VAT NP	353	88.92	8	42.11	3	37.5				
VAT Path	53	13.35	11	57.89	5	62.5				
	M.	ET.	M.	ET.	M.	ET.	F	p	F	p
VAT Tot	23.11	11.43	36	10.37	35.38	15.95	15.49	0.001	3.87	0.03
PC	7.28	3.81	10.89	3.41	9.88	5.25	9.65	0.001	5.2	0.009
Pré	4.81	2.67	7.47	2.74	7.75	3.81	13.13	0.001	2.3	0.11
SS	1.69	1.11	2.47	1.43	2.63	1.6	6.85	0.001	0.65	0.65
AMH	3.14	1.8	5.11	2.08	5.75	2.66	17.89	0.001	1.09	0.34
C	6.19	3.41	10.05	3.24	9.38	4.72	14.51	0.001	5.44	0.007

Table 2: CPGI: Canadian Pathological Game Index, (NPb): Non-problematic; (Ar): At risk; (Path): Pathological; PIUQ: Problematic Internet Use Questionnaire, (NP): Non pathological; (Little): little risk; Prob: Problems; PrSign: significant problem; (SC): Self-checking; (NC): Negative consequences; (PW): Psychological weaning; (C): concern; (TD): Total dimension. SAS: Smartphone Addiction Scale, (NP): Non-pathological; (PD): Probable dependence;

(Abuse): excessive abuse with repercussions on daily life; (DDL): Disruption of daily life; (PA): Positive Anticipation; (WS): Withdrawal Social; (COR): Cyberspace-oriented relationship; (OU): Over-use; (T): Tolerance. VAT: Video Game Addiction Test, (NP): Non-pathological; (Path): Pathological; (LoC): Loss of Control; (C): Concern; (WS): Weaning syndrome; (AMM): Adaptation/Modification of Mood; (C): Conflicts. Anova 2 with variable control "gambling players playing on at least one of the three screen types" (smartphone/touch pad, computer, console). The significance threshold is the threshold $p < 0.05$.

Analysis of the correlations on the total sample allowed us to see that the intensity of the gambling practice was positively correlated with the expenses related to the purchase of applications, computer games, video games, and consoles, as well as bets offered on applications, on the computer, and in video games; To the set of cognitive distortions described in the GRCS scale; The intensity of Internet practice (PIUQ); The positive and negative UPPS urgency; The intensity of impulsivity (UPPS); To all the variables making up the intensity of the practice of mobile screens (SAS); To the set of variables of the intensity of the practice of video games; Psychological distress including depression (HAD-D); and to the "game" variable of the immersion scale.

4.2. Costs and Prevalence of Gambling/Gambling on Screens

The maximum bet amount differs significantly depending on the intensity of the gambler's practice. The difference is significant for computerization between non-pathological gamblers and pathological gamblers ($t = 6.6$, $p < 0.001$). The use of mobile and computer screens between non-pathological gamblers and problem gamblers is also significant ($t = 3.45$, $p = 0.001$ for mobile screens and $t = 3.88$, $p = 0.001$). The purchase of computer games is also significant between non-pathological gamblers and problem gamblers ($t = 3.22$; $p = 0.001$). For gambling players on the computer, bets between non-pathological and pathological gambler's are significantly different ($t = 2.97$, $p = 0.01$) (Table 1). Linked to the screens, players' bets are also significantly different. Individuals with a problematic practice have higher gambling bets than those with moderate Internet practice ($t = 2.95$; $p = 0.003$). Similarly, those with problem gambling practice are more likely than non-pathologists ($t = 2.14$, $p = 0.03$).

Table 2 illustrates the different practices related to gambling on screens and the intensity of this practice. Anova analysis revealed a significant difference between the different groups representing the intensity of Internet practice (PIUQ) and the score obtained at the ICJP scale ($F = 23.91$, $p < 0.001$). Similarly, we observed a significant difference between the groups representing the intensity of the practice of the mobile screens (SAS) and the scores obtained at the ICJP scale ($F = 12.27$, $p < 0.001$). This significant difference is found in the weighting variables "gambling gamblers on mobile screen applications" ($F = 11.02$, $p < 0.001$), "gambling players on computers" ($F = 36.24$, $p < 0.001$) and "gambling players on mobile, console and computer applications" ($F = 83.05$, $p < 0.001$). Finally, there was a significant difference between the groups representing the intensity of the video games practice and the score obtained at the ICJP scale ($F = 39.45$, $p < 0.001$). The difference is significant only with the weighting variable "players with a gambling practice on mobile screen applications" ($F = 7.26$, $p = 0.01$).

4.3. Gambling on Screens and Comorbidities

For gambling on screens, the first elaborated multiple linear regression models consists of 34 variables ($F = 2.42$, $p < 0.01$). These included comorbidities (impulsivity, depression, emotional regulation), cognitive distortions, and scaling variables that evaluated excessive screen-related practices. The variable to be predicted is the practical variable of gambling on the screens with the ICJP scale and the positive variable to play the games of gambling on a screen. This model accounts for 78% of the total variance.

The variable perturbation of daily life (of the SAS scale) ($p = 0.004$) is the best predictor of pathological gambling on screens and especially on mobile screens. Other variables have a predictive value, although lower such as the "lack of premeditation" variable (from the UPPS scale) ($p = 0.04$);

The variable "game expectations" ($p = 0.01$) and the "inability to abstain from playing" variable ($p = 0.01$) (from the GRCS scale). The second linear regression model, with 13 closest variables, accounts for 64% of the total variance. The variable "lack of premeditation" ($p = 0.004$), "sensation seeking" ($p = 0.02$), "expectation of the game" ($p = 0.08$), and the total dimensions of the PIUQ ($p = 0.03$) are the predictors of pathological gambling on the screens (Table 3).

Table 3. Comorbidities and gambling on screens.

Scales and Sub-Dimensions	CPGI NPb (n = 397)		CPGI Ar (n = 19)		CPGI Path (n = 8)		Anova 1 Traditional Gambling		Anova 2 Gambling on Console and Mobile Screen		Anova 3 Gambling on Computer		Anova 4 Gambling on All Media Together	
	M.	SD.	M.	SD.	M.	SD.	F	p	F	p	F	p	F	p
							2.07	0.001	2.37	0.33	2.04	0.006	53.21	0.02
GRCS	43.61	26.08	50.75	33.69	93.5	12.5	4.07	0.02	3.98	0.14	6.51	0.003	1.11	0.37
- ALJ	8.67	5.23	10.75	7.44	14.75	3.77	1.41	0.25	7.1	0.07	2.54	0.09	1.47	0.28
- IC	6.13	4.05	18.5	3.87	5.38	4.69	8.32	0.001	0.85	0.5	17.12	0.001	1.35	0.31
- PP	12.43	8.5	13.38	8.21	26	3.74	4.3	0.01	15.32	0.02	4.94	0.01	1.1	0.37
- IA	9.02	6.77	12.13	9.4	16.75	5.38	2.46	0.09	3.05	0.19	2.61	0.08	1.51	0.27
- IF	7.35	4.73	9.13	7.4	17.5	1.91	5.64	0.003	3.22	0.18	7.56	0.001	1.43	0.29
UPPS	46.76	8.9	51.75	11.34	/		0.02	0.89	2.34	0.24	1.04	0.36	2.94	0.1
- UN	9.46	3.42	10.63	2.88	/		0.22	0.64	1.52	0.35	0.48	0.62	0.45	12.82
- UP	11.26	3.01	11	2.45	/		1.5	0.22	0.52	0.64	0.22	0.8	1.31	0.32
- RS	11.37	2.82	12	2.73	/		0.64	0.43	5.75	0.09	0.79	0.46	1.51	0.27
- MPer	7.22	2.8	9.38	2.67	/		5.06	0.03	1.97	0.28	2.21	0.13	6.17	0.02
- MPré	7.46	2.36	8.75	2.71	/		4.08	0.04	1.96	0.29	1.48	0.24	7.88	1.17
ERQ	4.28	1.11	4.13	1.1	4.93	0.74	1.39	0.25	5.2	0.11	0.76	0.47	0.3	0.75
- RC	4.34	1.42	4.29	1.5	4.96	0.94	1.96	0.14	3.41	0.17	0.37	0.69	0.1	0.91
- RE	4.21	1.24	3.88	1.19	4.88	1.09	0.35	0.7	8.78	0.06	0.89	0.42	0.88	0.17
HAD	11.23	5.4	10.2	1.08	16.5	8	4.09	0.02	32.03	0.009	3.82	0.03	3.67	0.07
Anxiety	6.54	3.38	5	3.21	9	3.37	0.29	0.75	5.55	0.09	1.91	0.16	1.83	0.21
Depression	4.02	2.92	3	1.6	7.75	6.24	0.82	0.44	8.07	0.06	3.36	0.04	5.08	0.03

CPGI: Canadian Pathological Game Index, (NPb): Non-problematic; (Ar): At risk; (Path): Pathological; HAD: Hospital Anxiety and Depression; GRCS: Gambling Related Cognition Scale; IF: Interpretation Favorable; IC: Illusion of Control; PP: Predictive power; ERG: Expectations Related to the Game; AI: Inability to Stop Playing; ERQ: Emotion Relationship Questionnaire; CR: Cognitive reassessment; ER: Expressive repression; UPPS: Impulsive Behavior Scale; NU: Negative urgency; PE: Positive Emergency; SS: Sensation Seeking; LPe: Lack of perseverance; LPr: Lack of premedication. The Anova for the UPPS concerned only problematic and non-pathological gamblers. Anova 2 with control of the variable "practice of gambling on console and mobile screens". Anova 3 with control of the variable "practice of gambling on a computer". Anova 4 with control of the variable "practice of gambling all confused screens". The significance threshold is the threshold $p < 0.05$.

In the case of comorbidities (anxiety, depression, emotional regulation, impulsivity, cognitive distortions), the only predictive variable for pathological gambling on the screens was "control illusion" ($p = 0.03$). The 14 variables accounted for 78% of the total variance.

Conversely, the linear regression model suggests that the predictors of excessive use of the Internet shows that 30 variables explain 54% of the total variance, six variables were significant. The variables of gambling practice ($p = 0.001$), tolerance ($p < 0.001$), preoccupation ($p = 0.003$), focus ($p = 0.01$), perturbation of daily life, ($p = 0.04$) and implication ($p = 0.04$) were predictive of excessive use of the Internet.

It is also noted that the predictive variables of excessive video gaming practice when we gamble regularly are different from the excessive practice of pure video gaming practice. For example, the variables "lack of perseverance" (UPPS), "lack of premeditation" (UPPS), the "game" variable of the immersion scale (QPI), the "inability to abstain from playing" GRCS) and "tolerance" (SAS) are predictive of the excessive gambling practice associated with regular gambling (82% of the total variance with 31 variables) (Table 3).

4.4. Immersion, Gambling on Screens and Comorbidities

I was observed that immersion scores were significantly higher for people with gambling addiction (Table 4). A Student test was carried out to glimpse the link between immersion and the use of screens. The scores for the VAT, PIUQ and SAS scales are significantly different according to the three immersion thresholds (low, moderate, high), respectively for the PIUQ scale ($t = 2.51$, $p = 0.01$), for the scale SAS ($t = 3.26$, $p = 0.001$) for the VAT scale ($t = 4.03$, $p = 0.001$). The surface analysis of the responses shows that, starting from a high immersion threshold, the individual is less likely to have a high score on scales assessing the intensity of Internet practice and on the scale evaluating the intensity of gambling practice.

Table 4. Scores related to propensity to immersion according to the intensity of gambling alone/ gambling on screens.

Immersion Variables	CPGI NPb (n = 397)		CPGI Ar (n = 19)		CPGI Path (n = 8)		Anova 1 Traditional Gambling		Anova 2 Gambling on Console and Mobile Screen		Anova 3 Gambling on Computer		Anova 4 Gambling on All Media Together	
	M.	SD.	M.	SD.	M.	SD.	F	p	F	p	F	p	F	p
Immersion (QPI)	53.46	18.22	55.16	19.17	63.5	11.98	2.26	0.01	34.84	0.001	24.85	0.001	80.10	0.001
Focus	17.88	6.53	16.37	6.61	18.38	3.54	0.52	0.59	21.47	0.001	45.65	0.001	26.86	0.001
Implication	14.66	6.58	15.37	6.19	17	3.63	0.6	0.55	12.5	0.001	10.85	0.001	31.53	0.001
Emotion	11.96	5.84	11.47	4.34	14.13	3.36	0.63	0.53	23.69	0.001	25.98	0.001	26.45	0.001
Game	5.61	4.23	8.47	4.25	10.25	2.87	8.68	0.001	286.94	0.001	142.33	0.001	760.52	0.001

CPGI: Canadian Pathological Game Index, (NPb): Non-problematic; (Ar): At risk; (Path): Pathological; QPI: Immersion propensity questionnaire. Anova 2 with control of the variable "Intensity of practices on the Internet". Anova 3 with control of the variable "Intensity of the practices of video games". Anova 4 with control of the variable "Intensity of practices on mobile screens". The significance threshold is the threshold $p < 0.05$.

Multiple linear regression analysis was used to analize the predictive power of immersion for the practice of gambling on screens in relation with comorbidities. In our model, 14 variables were integrated which explained 48% of the variance ($F = 2.84$, $p = 0.004$) with impulsivity, emotional regulation, anxious and depressive comorbidities and cognitive distortions. Predictors of immersion in the practice of games of chance on the screens are positive urgency (UPPS), anxiety (HAD), predictive power (GRCS), inability to Refraining from Playing (GRCS) and Interpretation for Game Continuation (GRCS).

A principal component analysis (PCA) was carried out to study the relationship between immersion according to the intensity of the gambling practice on the screens and the other variables of our study. Three axes were selected, representing 52.92% of the total variance. The first axis ($\lambda = 26.51\%$) is characterized and particularly correlated, on the negative side, by all cognitive distortions (GRCS); By the variables implication, emotion, game and total dimensions of immersion; The practice of mobile displays (SAS); The Negative Emergency and the Positive Urgency of Impulsivity (UPPS), and Internet Practice (PIUQ). This axis is a "size" factor, ordering individuals according to their scores on all scales. The two axis ($\lambda = 14.98\%$) is characterized by anxiety (HAD), all variables of immersion on the positive side and the inability to abstain from playing (GRCS) Impulsivity (UPPS), including sensation seeking (UPPS) and negative urgency (UPPS). The three-axis ($\lambda = 11.43\%$) is characterized by negative urgency (UPPS), positive urgency (UPPS) and sensation seeking (UPPS), total impulsivity (UPPS) and the illusion of control and interpretation favorable to the pursuit of the game on the negative side.

5. Discussion

The objective of this study was to assess the practice of gambling on screens, and to understand the impact of the perceived intensity of immersion by an individual on the practice of screens and gambling on the screens, as well as determining the associated comorbidities. The results obtained in this study highlight certain psychological and psychopathological specificities of gamblers on screens related to immersion.

First, the prevalence of problematic practices is consistent with the literature, particularly for Internet practice (2.27% versus 1–3.2% in the literature for European countries including France and Germany) [107–109], particularly for the practice of gambling (i.e., 1.85% in our study against 0.2–3% according to the estimate of the prevalence studies in France) [107–110], for the practice of video games (13.35% for our study against 14% for the most recent French study) and for the practice of mobile screens (2.77% lower for our study unlike the study Validation of the SAS scale which was at 9.6%) (Tablets, smartphones) [111].

The results of our study confirmed that pathological and problematic gamblers are more prone to spend more money than non-pathological gamblers and also significantly different depending on the interface chosen, whether it is a fixed screen or mobile, via a console or a computer. These increased costs can be explained by the ease of access, the possibility of betting during uninterrupted periods and the immersive interactivity of gambling software on the Internet [3,112–114]. Our first hypothesis is confirmed.

We also showed that individuals who were tending to excessive gambling had significantly higher scores on scales assessing fixed-screen and mobile screens (whose behaviors had been assessed by a recent scale that focused solely on self-action directed to a mobile display, including the smartphone or touchpad) (Table 2). The practice of gambling could thus participate in the propensity of excessive practices related to screens. It is important, however, to see the same cognitive distortions found in these different types of excessive practices [115,116]. The intensity of immersion would therefore be a predominant factor in the detection of the excessive practice related to the screen. This confirms the high level of commitment generated during excessive practice phases, as well as the role of the dissociation contained in the "focus" variable [117,118].

Our fourth hypothesis is only partially confirmed. Concerning, the practice of gambling on mobile screens, the only cognitive distortion variable, "predictive power" was significantly different according to the three groups. Regarding only the practice of computer gambling, the set of cognitive distortion scores, with the exception of gambling expectations, were significantly different between the groups. Concerning the practice of gambling on all the screens combined, the variable cognitive distortion was not significant. However, depressive variables (HAD) and lack of perseverance (UPPS) were significantly different across groups. Although the literature demonstrates that cognitive distortions can predict future commitment to excessive gambling, gaming expectations differ according to the interface used, and cognitive distortions are much less pronounced in practice on mobile screens [47,119,120].

The analysis of the area of responses between three variables (PIUQ, ICJP and QPI) showed that, starting from a high immersion threshold, the individual is less likely to have a high score at the scales evaluating the "Intensity of Internet and gambling practice". Immersion could thus be perceived as a protection factor from a certain threshold.

Finally, variables explaining pathological gambling on the screens allow us to adjust the prevention modalities for the gambling on the screens. Indeed, taking into account the format of the screen (for mobile or fixed purposes), daily life disruption (SAS) variables, lack of premeditation (UPPS), sensation seeking (GRCS), expectations related to the (GRCS) and impulsivity (total PIUQ sums) were predictive of excessive gambling.

There are limitations to this study. The research was constructed from self-assessment, dealing with general behavioral behavior with respect to screens and the Internet and not only on immersion experienced during a main task (a task that would be delimited by a specific action on a continuum within a virtual universe of gambling). This may be a bias in assessing the prevalence of excessive screen-related practices in this population. The average age of our population is also low, our sample could have been enlarged by older people. Also, we could have chosen scales assessing anxiety-depression disorders regularly used in clinical practice such as "Generalized Anxiety Disorder scale (GAD-7) or Patient Health Questionnaire (PHQ). Finally, the distribution of practices according to their intensities is heterogeneous. Better distribution of groups would have been preferable.

Neurophysiological measurements and longitudinal analysis would allow a more precise glimpse of the cognitive processes related to immersion variables.

6. Conclusions

This study explored the involvement of gambling gamblers in the screens. It also showed the implication of the immersion variable in relation to the intensity of the practice of gambling on the screens. Immersion thus plays a mediating role between cognitive resources and the impact on screen practices.

The practice of gambling begins in adolescence. Studies also indicate that those who gamble during childhood will be more likely to become compulsive gamblers later in life [85,121,122]. It would therefore be essential to reinforce our understanding of the negative consequences of gambling-related behaviors on the screens and also to increase the methods of prevention and intervention [123].

The interest is also to be able to modulate the variables of immersion in the therapeutic management of excessive practice or, upstream, to improve prevention by proposing prevention messages at precise level thresholds Immersion according to the variables composing it [124]. It is also a possibility for game developers to modulate cognitive factors related to immersion leading to excessive practice and thus avoid future problems of excessive and impulsive behavior.

Acknowledgments: No funding was associated with this research. The laboratory of Paris-Nanterre University (Paris, FRANCE) financially supported this research both in the costs related to research and those related to publication.

Author Contributions: Lucia Romo and Jean-Jacques Rémond have conceived and designed the experimentation and more specifically participated in the recruitment of study participants. Jean-Jacques Rémond analyzed the data; Jean-Jacques Rémond and Lucia Romo wrote the paper.

References

1. Griffiths, M. Behavioural addiction: An issue for everybody? *Empl. Counc. Today* **1996**, *8*, 19–25. [CrossRef]
2. Maclin, O.H.; Dixon, M.R.; Hayes, L.J. A computerized slot machine simulation to investigate the variables involved in gambling behavior. *Behav. Res. Methods Instrum. Comput.* **1999**, *31*, 731–734. [CrossRef] [PubMed]
3. Gainsbury, S.M.; King, D.L.; Russell, A.M.; Delfabbro, P.; Derevensky, J.; Hing, N. Exposure to and engagement with gambling marketing in social media: Reported impacts on moderate-risk and problem gamblers. *Psychol. Addict. Behav.* **2016**, *30*, 270. [CrossRef] [PubMed]
4. Adams, P.J.; Wiles, J. Gambling machine annexes as enabling spaces for addictive engagement. *Health Place* **2017**, *43*, 1–7. [CrossRef] [PubMed]
5. Bolen, D.W.; Boyd, W.H. Gambling and the gambler: A review and preliminary findings. *Arch. Gen. Psychiatry* **1968**, *18*, 617–630. [CrossRef] [PubMed]
6. Kairouz, S.; Paradis, C.; Nadeau, L.; Tovar, M.-L.; Pousset, M. A cross-cultural comparison of population gambling patterns and regulatory frameworks: France and Québec. *J. Public Health Policy* **2016**, *37*, 467–482. [CrossRef] [PubMed]
7. Kessler, R.C.; Hwang, I.; LaBrie, R.; Petukhova, M.; Sampson, N.A.; Winters, K.C.; Shaffer, H.J. DSM-IV pathological gambling in the National Comorbidity Survey Replication. *Psychol. Med.* **2008**, *38*, 1351–1360. [CrossRef] [PubMed]
8. Volberg, R.A. Fifteen years of problem gambling prevalence research: What do we know? Where do we go? *J. Gambl. Issues* **2004**. [CrossRef]
9. Shaffer, H.J.; Martin, R. Disordered gambling: Etiology, trajectory, and clinical considerations. *Annu. Rev. Clin. Psychol.* **2011**, *7*, 483–510. [CrossRef] [PubMed]
10. Bouju, G.; Grall-Bronnec, M.; Landreat-Guillou, M.; Venisse, J.-L. Jeu pathologique: Facteurs impliqués. *L'Encéphale* **2011**, *37*, 322–331. (In French) [CrossRef] [PubMed]

11. Schmit, S.; Chauchard, E.; Chabrol, H.; Sejourne, N. Évaluation des caractéristiques sociales, des stratégies de coping, de l'estime de soi et de la symptomatologie dépressive en relation avec la dépendance aux jeux vidéo en ligne chez les adolescents et les jeunes adultes. *L'Encéphale* **2011**, *37*, 217–223. (In French) [CrossRef] [PubMed]
12. Chan, C.C.; Li, W.W.L.; Leung, E.C.I. The Etiology of Problem Gambling. In *Problem Gambling in Hong Kong and Macao*; Springer: New York, NY, USA, 2016; pp. 75–94.
13. Husky, M.M.; Michel, G.; Richard, J.-B.; Guignard, R.; Beck, F. Gender differences in the associations of gambling activities and suicidal behaviors with problem gambling in a nationally representative French sample. *Addict. Behav.* **2015**, *45*, 45–50. [CrossRef] [PubMed]
14. American Psychiatric Association. *Diagnostic and Statistical Manual of Mental Disorders (DSM-5®)*; American Psychiatric Pub.: Washington, DC, USA, 2013.
15. Clark, L. Disordered gambling: The evolving concept of behavioral addiction. *Ann. N. Y. Acad. Sci.* **2014**, *1327*, 46–61. [CrossRef] [PubMed]
16. Dowling, N.A.; Merkouris, S.S.; Greenwood, C.J.; Oldenhof, E.; Toumbourou, J.W.; Youssef, G.J. Early risk and protective factors for problem gambling: A systematic review and meta-analysis of longitudinal studies. *Clin. Psychol. Rev.* **2016**, *51*, 109–124. [CrossRef] [PubMed]
17. Griffiths, M.; Wood, R.T. Risk factors in adolescence: The case of gambling, videogame playing, and the Internet. *J. Gambl. Stud.* **2000**, *16*, 99–225.
18. Hing, N.; Russell, A.; Tolchard, B.; Nower, L. Risk factors for gambling problems: An analysis by gender. *J. Gambl. Stud.* **2016**, *32*, 511–534. [CrossRef] [PubMed]
19. Welte, J.W.; Barnes, G.M.; Wieczorek, W.F.; Tidwell, M.-C.O.; Parker, J.C. Risk factors for pathological gambling. *Addict. Behav.* **2004**, *29*, 323–335. [CrossRef] [PubMed]
20. Johansson, A.; Grant, J.E.; Kim, S.W.; Odlaug, B.L.; Götestam, K.G. Risk factors for problematic gambling: A critical literature review. *J. Gambl. Stud.* **2009**, *25*, 67–92. [CrossRef] [PubMed]
21. Maniaci, G.; Picone, F.; van Holst, R.J.; Bolloni, C.; Scardina, S.; Cannizzaro, C. Alterations in the emotional regulation process in gambling addiction: The role of anger and alexithymia. *J. Gambl. Stud.* **2017**, *33*, 633–647. [CrossRef] [PubMed]
22. Navas, J.F.; Perandres-Gomez, A.; Perales, J.C. OR-78: Associations between adaptive emotion regulation strategies and gambling-related cognitive biases in gambling disorder patients. *J. Behav. Addict.* **2016**, *5*, 32–34. [CrossRef] [PubMed]
23. Jauregui, P.; Estevez, A.; Urbiola, I. Pathological gambling and associated drug and alcohol abuse, emotion regulation, and anxious-depressive symptomatology. *J. Behav. Addict.* **2016**, *5*, 251–260. [CrossRef] [PubMed]
24. Potenza, M.N.; Steinberg, M.A.; McLaughlin, S.D.; Wu, R.; Rounsaville, B.J.; O'Malley, S.S. Gender-related differences in the characteristics of problem gamblers using a gambling helpline. *Am. J. Psychiatry* **2001**, *158*, 1500–1505. [CrossRef] [PubMed]
25. González-Ortega, I.; Echeburúa, E.; de Corral, P.; Polo-López, R. Pathological gambling: Clinical gender differences. In *Psychopathology in Women*; Springer: New York, NY, USA, 2015; pp. 713–726.
26. McCormack, A.; Shorter, G.W.; Griffiths, M.D. An empirical study of gender differences in online gambling. *J. Gambl. Stud.* **2014**, *30*, 71–88. [CrossRef] [PubMed]
27. Grant, J.E.; Kim, S.W. Gender differences in pathological gamblers seeking medication treatment. *Compr. Psychiatry* **2002**, *43*, 56–62. [CrossRef] [PubMed]
28. Merkouris, S.S.; Thomas, A.C.; Shandley, K.A.; Rodda, S.N.; Oldenhof, E.; Dowling, N.A. An update on gender differences in the characteristics associated with problem gambling: A systematic review. *Curr. Addict. Rep.* **2016**, *3*, 254–267. [CrossRef]
29. Casey, E. *Women, Pleasure and the Gambling Experience*; Routledge: Abingdon, UK, 2016.
30. Wenzel, H.G.; Dahl, A.A. Female pathological gamblers—A critical review of the clinical findings. *Int. J. Ment. Health Addict.* **2009**, *7*, 190–202. [CrossRef]
31. Crockford, D.N.; El-Guebaly, N. Psychiatric comorbidity in pathological gambling: A critical review. *Can. J. Psychiatry* **1998**, *43*, 43–50. [CrossRef] [PubMed]
32. Hartmann, M.; Blaszczynski, A. The longitudinal relationships between psychiatric disorders and gambling disorders. *Int. J. Ment. Health Addict.* **2016**, 1–29. [CrossRef]
33. Griffiths, M.; Sutherland, I. Adolescent gambling and drug use. *J. Community Appl. Soc. Psychol.* **1998**, *8*, 423–427. [CrossRef]

34. Van Rooij, A.J.; Kuss, D.J.; Griffiths, M.D.; Shorter, G.W.; Schoenmakers, T.M.; Van de Mheen, D. The (co-)occurrence of problematic video gaming, substance use, and psychosocial problems in adolescents. *J. Behav. Addict.* **2014**, *3*, 157–165. [CrossRef] [PubMed]
35. Carbonneau, R.; Vitaro, F.; Brendgen, M.; Tremblay, R.E. Trajectories of gambling problems from mid-adolescence to age 30 in a general population cohort. *Psychol. Addict. Behav.* **2015**, *29*, 1012–1021. [CrossRef] [PubMed]
36. Dussault, F.; Brendgen, M.; Vitaro, F.; Carbonneau, R.; Boivin, M.; Tremblay, R.E. Co-morbidity between gambling problems and depressive symptoms: A longitudinal perspective of risk and protective factors. *J. Gambl. Stud.* **2016**, *32*, 547–565. [CrossRef] [PubMed]
37. Cook, S.; Turner, N.E.; Ballon, B.; Paglia-Boak, A.; Murray, R.; Adlaf, E.M.; Ilie, G.; den Dunnen, W.; Mann, R.E. Problem gambling among Ontario students: Associations with substance abuse, mental health problems, suicide attempts, and delinquent behaviours. *J. Gambl. Stud.* **2015**, *31*, 1121–1134. [CrossRef] [PubMed]
38. Palaiologou, A.; Kotzia, D.; Anagnostopoulos, D.C.; Lazaratou, H. Risk factors and comorbidity of pathological gambling in adolescence. *J. Adolesc. Psychol. Psychiatry* **2015**, *2015*, 3. [CrossRef]
39. Fatseas, M.; Alexandre, J.-M.; Vénisse, J.-L.; Romo, L.; Valleur, M.; Magalon, D.; Chéreau-Boudet, I.; Luquiens, A.; Guilleux, A.; Groupe, J.E.U.; et al. Gambling behaviors and psychopathology related to Attention-Deficit/Hyperactivity Disorder (ADHD) in problem and non-problem adult gamblers. *Psychiatry Res.* **2016**, *239*, 232–238. [CrossRef] [PubMed]
40. Porteret, R.; Bouchez, J.; Baylé, F.J.; Varescon, I. ADH/D and impulsiveness: Prevalence of impulse control disorders and other comorbidities, in 81 adults with attention deficit/hyperactivity disorder (ADH/D). *L'Encephale* **2016**, *42*, 130–137. [CrossRef] [PubMed]
41. Romo, L.; Rémond, J.J.; Coeffec, A.; Kotbagi, G.; Plantey, S.; Boz, F.; Kern, L. Gambling and attention deficit hyperactivity disorders (ADHD) in a population of french students. *J. Gambl. Stud.* **2015**, *31*, 1261–1272. [CrossRef] [PubMed]
42. Romo, L.; Legauffre, C.; Guilleux, A.; Valleur, M.; Magalon, D.; Fatséas, M.; Chéreau-Boudet, I.; Luquiens, A.; Vénisse, J.L.; JEU Group; et al. Cognitive distortions and ADHD in pathological gambling: A national longitudinal case-control cohort study. *J. Behav. Addict.* **2016**, *5*, 649–657. [CrossRef] [PubMed]
43. American Psychiatric Association. *DSM-IV-TR: Diagnostic and Statistical Manual of Mental Disorders, Text Revision*; American Psychiatric Association: Washington, DC, USA, 2000; p. 75.
44. Lister, J.J.; Milosevic, A.; Ledgerwood, D.M. Psychological characteristics of problem gamblers with and without mood disorder. *Can. J. Psychiatry* **2015**, *60*, 369–376. [CrossRef] [PubMed]
45. Clarke, D. Impulsivity as a mediator in the relationship between depression and problem gambling. *Personal. Individ. Differ.* **2006**, *40*, 5–15. [CrossRef]
46. Taylor, R.N.; Parker, J.D.; Keefer, K.V.; Kloosterman, P.H.; Summerfeldt, L.J. Gambling related cognitive distortions in adolescence: Relationships with gambling problems in typically developing and special needs students. *J. Gambl. Stud.* **2015**, *31*, 1417–1429. [CrossRef] [PubMed]
47. Griffiths, M.D. The role of cognitive bias and skill in fruit machine gambling. *Br. J. Psychol.* **1994**, *85*, 351–369. [CrossRef]
48. MacLaren, V.; Ellery, M.; Knoll, T. Personality, gambling motives and cognitive distortions in electronic gambling machine players. *Personal. Individ. Differ.* **2015**, *73*, 24–28. [CrossRef]
49. Harrigan, K.; MacLaren, V.; Brown, D.; Dixon, M.J.; Livingstone, C. Games of chance or masters of illusion: Multiline slots design may promote cognitive distortions. *Int. Gambl. Stud.* **2014**, *14*, 301–317. [CrossRef]
50. Ladouceur, R.; Mayrand, M.; Dussault, R.; Letarte, A.; Tremblay, J. Illusion of control: Effects of participation and involvement. *J. Psychol.* **1984**, *117*, 47–52. [CrossRef]
51. Ladouceur, R.; Mayrand, M. Evaluation of the "illusion of control": Type of feedback, outcome sequence, and number of trials among regular and occasional gamblers. *J. Psychol.* **1984**, *117*, 37–46. [CrossRef]
52. Ladouceur, R.; Walker, M. A cognitive perspective on gambling. *Trends Cogn. Behav. Ther.* **1996**, *5*, 89–120.
53. Ladouceur, R.; Sévigny, S. Structural characteristics of video lotteries: Effects of a stopping device on illusion of control and gambling persistence. *J. Gambl. Stud.* **2005**, *21*, 117–131. [CrossRef] [PubMed]
54. Breen, R.B.; Zimmerman, M. Rapid onset of pathological gambling in machine gamblers. *J. Gambl. Stud.* **2002**, *18*, 31–43. [CrossRef] [PubMed]

55. Khanbhai, Y.; Smith, D.; Battersby, M. Gender by preferred gambling activity in treatment seeking problem gamblers: A comparison of subgroup characteristics and treatment outcomes. *J. Gambl. Stud.* **2017**, *33*, 99–113. [CrossRef] [PubMed]
56. Murch, W.S.; Clark, L. Games in the brain neural substrates of gambling addiction. *Neuroscientist* **2016**, *22*, 534–545. [CrossRef] [PubMed]
57. Schüll, N.D. *Addiction by Design: Machine Gambling in Las Vegas*; Princeton University Press: Princeton, NJ, USA, 2012.
58. Cookman, M.L.; Weatherly, J.N. Investigating possible effects of ethnicity and age on gambling as an escape. *J. Gambl. Stud.* **2016**, *32*, 499–509. [CrossRef] [PubMed]
59. Gainsbury, S.M.; Hing, N.; Delfabbro, P.H.; King, D.L. A taxonomy of gambling and casino games via social media and online technologies. *Int. Gambl. Stud.* **2014**, *14*, 196–213. [CrossRef]
60. Gainsbury, S.; Wood, R.; Russell, A.; Hing, N.; Blaszczynski, A. A digital revolution: Comparison of demographic profiles, attitudes and gambling behavior of Internet and non-Internet gamblers. *Comput. Hum. Behav.* **2012**, *28*, 1388–1398. [CrossRef]
61. Kairouz, S.; Nadeau, L.; Paradis, C. *Portrait of Gambling in Quebec: Prevalence, Incidence and Trajectories over Four Years*; Concordia University: Montréal, QC, Canada, 2011.
62. Williams, R.J.; Wood, R.T.; Parke, J. *Routledge International Handbook of Internet Gambling*; Routledge: Abingdon, UK, 2012.
63. Yani-de-Soriano, M.; Javed, U.; Yousafzai, S. Can an industry be socially responsible if its products harm consumers? The case of online gambling. *J. Bus. Ethics* **2012**, *110*, 481–497. [CrossRef]
64. Gainsbury, S.M.; Delfabbro, P.; King, D.L.; Hing, N. An exploratory study of gambling operators' use of social media and the latent messages conveyed. *J. Gambl. Stud.* **2016**, *32*, 125–141. [CrossRef] [PubMed]
65. Allen, J.L.; Massing, S.A.; Moyles, B.P.; Pacey, L.J.; Ward, M.J. Mobile Device Applications for Casinos. U.S. Patent 20140045586 A1, 13 February 2014.
66. Hing, N.; Gainsbury, S.; Blaszczynski, A.; Wood, R.; Lubman, D.; Russel, A. *Interactive Gambling*; Australian Gambling Research Centre, Australian Institute of Family Studies: Melbourne, Australia, 2014.
67. Griffiths, M. Mobile phone gambling. In *Encyclopedia of Mobile Computing and Commerce*; IGI Global: Hershey, PA, USA, 2007; pp. 553–556.
68. Korhonen, H.; Koivisto, E.M. Playability heuristics for mobile games. In Proceedings of the 8th Conference on Human-Computer Interaction with Mobile Devices and Services, Helsinki, Finland, 12–25 September 2006; ACM: New York, NY, USA, 2006; pp. 9–16.
69. Wakefield, R.L.; Whitten, D. Mobile computing: A user study on hedonic/utilitarian mobile device usage. *Eur. J. Inf. Syst.* **2006**, *15*, 292–300. [CrossRef]
70. Turel, O.; Serenko, A.; Bontis, N. User acceptance of hedonic digital artifacts: A theory of consumption values perspective. *Inf. Manag.* **2010**, *47*, 53–59. [CrossRef]
71. Wunnava, S. Mobile commerce usage: Application of theory of reasoned action (TRA) and technology acceptance model (TAM). *World J. Soc. Sci.* **2015**, *5*, 41–50.
72. Csikszentmihalyi, M. *Flow: The Psychology of Optimal Experience*; Harper & Row: New York, NY, USA, 1990; 303p.
73. Csikszentmihalyi, M.; Csikszentmihalyi, I.S. *Optimal Experience: Psychological Studies of Flow in Consciousness*; Cambridge University Press: Cambridge, UK, 1992.
74. Csikszentmihalyi, M.; Asakawa, K. Universal and cultural dimensions of optimal experiences. *Jpn. Psychol. Res.* **2016**, *58*, 4–13. [CrossRef]
75. Csikszentmihalyi, M.; Khosla, S.; Nakamura, J. Flow at Work. In *The Wiley Blackwell Handbook of the Psychology of Positivity and Strengths-Based Approaches at Work*; Oades, L.G., Steger, M.F., Fave, A.D., Passmore, J., Eds.; John Wiley & Sons, Ltd.: Hoboken, NJ, USA, 2016; pp. 99–109.
76. Randolph, L.; Murray, J.; Lanham, R. Hamlet on the holodeck: The future of narrative in cyberspace. *JSTOR* **1998**, *72*, 187–190.
77. Csikszentmihalyi, M. Toward a psychology of optimal experience. In *Flow and the Foundations of Positive Psychology*; Springer: New York, NY, USA, 2014; pp. 209–226.
78. Nakamura, J.; Csikszentmihalyi, M. The concept of flow. In *Flow and the Foundations of Positive Psychology*; Springer: New York, NY, USA, 2014; pp. 239–263.
79. Dixon, M.J.; Graydon, C.; Harrigan, K.A.; Wojtowicz, L.; Siu, V.; Fugelsang, J.A. The allure of multi-line games in modern slot machines. *Addiction* **2014**, *109*, 1920–1928. [CrossRef] [PubMed]

80. Psotka, J.; Davison, S. *Cognitive Factors Associated with Immersion in Virtual Environments*; Army Research Institute: Alexandria, VA, USA, 1993.
81. Cartmill, T.; Slatter, T.; Wilkie, B. The role of anxiety and dissociation in young Australian gamblers. *J. Gambl. Stud.* **2015**, *31*, 1215–1226. [CrossRef] [PubMed]
82. Diskin, K.M.; Hodgins, D.C. Narrowing of attention and dissociation in pathological video lottery gamblers. *J. Gambl. Stud.* **1999**, *15*, 17–28. [CrossRef] [PubMed]
83. Diskin, K.M.; Hodgins, D.C. Narrowed focus and dissociative experiences in a community sample of experienced video lottery gamblers. *Can. J. Behav. Sci. Can. Sci. Comport.* **2001**, *33*, 58–64. [CrossRef]
84. Diskin, K.M.; Hodgins, D.C. Psychophysiological and subjective arousal during gambling in pathological and non-pathological video lottery gamblers. *Int. Gambl. Stud.* **2003**, *3*, 37–51. [CrossRef]
85. Gupta, R.; Derevensky, J.L. Adolescent gambling behavior: A prevalence study and examination of the correlates associated with problem gambling. *J. Gambl. Stud.* **1998**, *14*, 319–345. [CrossRef] [PubMed]
86. Wood, R.T.; Griffiths, M.D. The acquisition, development and maintenance of lottery and scratchcard gambling in adolescence. *J. Adolesc.* **1998**, *21*, 265–273. [CrossRef] [PubMed]
87. Boyer, M.; Dickerson, M. Attentional bias and addictive behaviour: Automaticity in a gambling-specific modified Stroop task. *Addiction* **2003**, *98*, 61–70. [CrossRef] [PubMed]
88. McCusker, C.G.; Gettings, B. Automaticity of cognitive biases in addictive behaviours: Further evidence with gamblers. *Br. J. Clin. Psychol.* **1997**, *36*, 543–554. [CrossRef] [PubMed]
89. Handy, T.C.; Kam, J.W. Mind wandering and selective attention to the external world. *Can. J. Exp. Psychol.* **2015**, *69*, 183. [CrossRef] [PubMed]
90. Kam, J.W.; Xu, J.; Handy, T.C. I don't feel your pain (as much): The desensitizing effect of mind wandering on the perception of others' discomfort. *Cogn. Affect. Behav. Neurosci.* **2014**, *14*, 286–296. [CrossRef] [PubMed]
91. Nagamatsu, L.S.; Kam, J.W.; Liu-Ambrose, T.; Chan, A.; Handy, T.C. Mind-wandering and falls risk in older adults. *Psychol. Aging* **2013**, *28*, 685–691. [CrossRef] [PubMed]
92. Harris, A.; Parke, A.; Griffiths, M.D. The case for using personally relevant and emotionally stimulating gambling messages as a gambling harm-minimisation strategy. *Int. J. Ment. Health Addict.* **2016**, 1–10. [CrossRef]
93. Savard, A.-C.; Turcotte, D.; Tremblay, J. <<La première fois que j'ai joué...>>: L'expérience d'adolescents considérés comme ayant des difficultés avec les jeux de hasard et d'argent. *J. Gambl. Issues* **2016**, 44–67. (In French) [CrossRef]
94. Lesieur, H.R.; Blume, S.B. The South Oaks Gambling Screen (SOGS): A new instrument for the identification of pathological gamblers. *Am. J. Psychiatry* **1987**, *144*, 9.
95. Ladouceur, R.; Jacques, C.; Chevalier, S.; Sévigny, S.; Hamel, D. Prevalence of pathological gambling in Quebec in 2002. *Can. J. Psychiatry* **2005**, *50*, 451–456. [CrossRef] [PubMed]
96. Bouchard, S.; Robillard, G.; Renaud, P. *Questionnaire sur la Propension à L'immersion. Lab Cyberpsychologie L'UQO*; Laboratoire de Cyberpsychologie de l'UQO: Outaouais, QC, Canada, 2002.
97. Robillard, G.; Bouchard, S.; Renaud, P.; Cournoyer, L.G. Validation canadienne-française de deux mesures importantes en réalité virtuelle: l'Immersive Tendencies Questionnaire et le Presence Questionnaire. Presented at the 25e Congrès Annu Société Québécoise Pour Rech En Psychol SQRP, Trois-Rivières, QC, Canada, 1–3 November 2002.
98. Kern, L.; Acier, D. Adaptation française de l'échelle problematic internet use questionnaire. *Lévolution psychiatr.* **2013**, *78*, 357–371. [CrossRef]
99. Demetrovics, Z.; Szeredi, B.; Rózsa, S. The three-factor model of Internet addiction: The development of the Problematic Internet Use Questionnaire. *Behav. Res. Methods* **2008**, *40*, 563–574. [CrossRef] [PubMed]
100. Kwon, M.; Lee, J.-Y.; Won, W.-Y.; Park, J.-W.; Min, J.-A.; Hahn, C.; Gu, X.; Choi, J.-H.; Kim, D.-J. Development and validation of a smartphone addiction scale (SAS). *PLoS ONE* **2013**, *82*, e56936. [CrossRef] [PubMed]
101. Lopez-Fernandez, O. Short version of the smartphone addiction scale adapted to Spanish and French: Towards a cross-cultural research in problematic mobile phone use. *Addict. Behav.* **2017**, *64*, 275–280. [CrossRef] [PubMed]
102. Van Rooij, A.J.; Schoenmakers, T.M.; Van den Eijnden, R.J.; Vermulst, A.A.; van de Mheen, D. Video game addiction test: Validity and psychometric characteristics. *Cyberpsychol. Behav. Soc. Netw.* **2012**, *15*, 507–511. [CrossRef] [PubMed]
103. Whiteside, S.P.; Lynam, D.R.; Miller, J.D.; Reynolds, S.K. Validation of the UPPS impulsive behaviour scale: A four-factor model of impulsivity. *Eur. J. Personal.* **2005**, *19*, 559–574. [CrossRef]

104. Van der Linden, M.; d'Acremont, M.; Zermatten, A.; Jermann, F.; Larøi, F.; Willems, S.; Juillerat, A.-C.; Bechara, A. A French adaptation of the UPPS impulsive behavior scale. *Eur. J. Psychol. Assess.* **2006**, *22*, 38–42. [CrossRef]
105. Zigmond, A.S.; Snaith, R.P. The hospital anxiety and depression scale. *Acta Psychiatr. Scand.* **1983**, *67*, 361–370. [CrossRef] [PubMed]
106. Gross, J.J.; John, O.P. Individual differences in two emotion regulation processes: Implications for affect, relationships, and well-being. *J. Pers. Soc. Psychol.* **2003**, *85*, 348. [CrossRef] [PubMed]
107. Planzer, S.; Gray, H.M.; Shaffer, H.J. Associations between national gambling policies and disordered gambling prevalence rates within Europe. *Int. J. Law Psychiatry* **2014**, *37*, 217–229. [CrossRef] [PubMed]
108. Costes, J.-M.; Pousset, M.; Eroukmanoff, V.; Le Nezet, O.; Richard, J.-B.; Guignard, R.; Beck, F.; Arwidson, P. Les niveaux et pratiques des jeux de hasard et d'argent en 2010. *Tendances* **2011**, *77*, 8.
109. Costes, J.-M.; Kairouz, S.; Eroukmanoff, V.; Monson, E. Gambling patterns and problems of gamblers on licensed and unlicensed sites in France. *J. Gambl. Stud.* **2016**, *32*, 79–91. [CrossRef] [PubMed]
110. Grall-Bronnec, M.; Bouju, G.; Landréat-Guillou, M.; Vénisse, J.-L. Évaluation sociodémographique, clinique et du parcours de jeu d'un échantillon de joueurs pathologiques français. *L'Encéphale* **2010**, *36*, 452–460. (In French) [CrossRef] [PubMed]
111. Patesson, R. Enquête sur L'addiction des Jeunes aux Smartphones. In *XIe Colloque du Réseau International et Interdisciplinaire Pour les Enjeux et Usages des Technologies de L'information et de la Communication (EUTIC) «Les Ecosystèmes Numériques et la Démocratisation Informationnelle: Intelligence Collective, Développement Durable, Interculturalité, Transfert de Connaissances»*. 2015. Available online: https://hal-uag.archives-ouvertes.fr/hal-01375819/ (accessed on 14 February 2017).
112. Monaghan, S. Responsible gambling strategies for internet gambling: The theoretical and empirical base of using pop-up messages to encourage self-awareness. *Comput. Hum. Behav.* **2009**, *25*, 202–207. [CrossRef]
113. Gainsbury, S.M.; Russell, A.; Wood, R.; Hing, N.; Blaszczynski, A. How risky is Internet gambling? A comparison of subgroups of Internet gamblers based on problem gambling status. *New Media Soc.* **2015**, *17*, 861–879. [CrossRef]
114. Schull, N.D. Digital Gambling: The coincidence of desire and design. *Ann. Am. Acad. Political Soc. Sci.* **2005**, *597*, 65–81. [CrossRef]
115. McBride, J.; Derevensky, J. Gambling and video game playing among youth. *J. Gambl. Issues* **2016**, 156–178. [CrossRef]
116. Forrest, C.J.; King, D.L.; Delfabbro, P.H. The measurement of maladaptive cognitions underlying problematic video-game playing among adults. *Comput. Hum. Behav.* **2016**, *55*, 399–405. [CrossRef]
117. Mazzoni, E.; Cannata, D.; Baiocco, L. Focused, not lost: The mediating role of temporal dissociation and focused immersion on problematic internet use. *Behav. Inf. Technol.* **2017**, *36*, 11–20. [CrossRef]
118. Lehenbauer-Baum, M.; Klaps, A.; Kovacovsky, Z.; Witzmann, K.; Zahlbruckner, R.; Stetina, B.U. Addiction and engagement: An explorative study toward classification criteria for internet gaming disorder. *Cyberpsychol. Behav. Soc. Netw.* **2015**, *18*, 343–349. [CrossRef] [PubMed]
119. King, D.L.; Delfabbro, P.H. Is preoccupation an oversimplification? A call to examine cognitive factors underlying internet gaming disorder. *Addiction* **2014**, *109*, 1566–1567. [CrossRef] [PubMed]
120. Yakovenko, I.; Hodgins, D.C.; El-Guebaly, N.; Casey, D.M.; Currie, S.R.; Smith, G.J.; Williams, R.J.; Schopflocher, D.P. Cognitive distortions predict future gambling involvement. *Int. Gambl. Stud.* **2016**, *16*, 175–192. [CrossRef]
121. Griffiths, M. *Adolescent Gambling*; Psychology Press: Hove, UK, 1995.
122. King, D.L.; Delfabbro, P.H. Early exposure to digital simulated gambling: A review and conceptual model. *Comput. Hum. Behav.* **2016**, *55*, 198–206. [CrossRef]
123. St-Pierre, R.; Derevensky, J.L. Youth gambling behavior: Novel approaches to prevention and intervention. *Curr. Addict. Rep.* **2016**, *3*, 157–165. [CrossRef]
124. Davies, B.; Blake, E. Evaluating existing strategies to limit video game playing time. *IEEE Comput. Graph. Appl.* **2016**, *36*, 47–57. [CrossRef] [PubMed]

14

The Associations between Family-Related Factors and Excessive Internet Use in Adolescents

Anna Faltýnková [1], Lukas Blinka [1,*], Anna Ševčíková [1] and Daniela Husarova [2]

[1] Faculty of Social Studies, Masaryk University, Brno 601 77, Czech Republic; anafaltynkova@gmail.com (A.F.); asevciko@fss.muni.cz (A.Š.)

[2] Department of Health Psychology and Methodology Research, Faculty of Medicine, P.J. Safarik University in Kosice, Košice 040 01, Slovakia; daniela.husarova@upjs.sk

* Correspondence: lukasblinka@gmail.com

Abstract: This study examined the relationship between Excessive Internet Use (EIU) in adolescents and their family environment, namely the family type, the family economic status, the effect of parental care, the level of parental control, the amount of parental monitoring, the quality of communication, and the time spent together. The study was based on data from an international survey, Health Behaviour in School Aged Children (HBSC), conducted in Slovakia. The sample representative for adolescents included 2547 participants (51% boys) aged 13–15. Multiple-step linear regression revealed that higher parental care and parental monitoring predicted lower EIU, while higher parental overprotection and lower socioeconomic status predicted higher EIU. The results suggest that both so-called optimal parenting (i.e., the balance of emotional warmth and protection) and the adolescent's autonomy lower the risk of EIU. Family factors explained about 14% of the variance, which suggests that aside from personal, cognitive and affective factors, a close social environment also plays an important role in adolescence EIU.

Keywords: adolescent internet use; excessive internet use; internet addiction; family factors; parenting styles

---

1. Introduction

The internet and the use of various digital devices are among the most important socialization factors and leisure activities in the lives of adolescents. The extent and intensity of internet usage has spawned research on both the benefits and the risks of online activities, including their addictive potential. This facilitated the inclusion of Internet Gaming Disorder in the International Classification of Diseases 11th Revision (ICD-11, World Health Organization). Generalized internet addiction has not reached such a consensus in the scientific community and various terms have been proposed (e.g. internet addiction, compulsive internet use [1]; pathological internet use [2]; problematic internet use [3]; internet use disorder [4]. In this paper, we work with the term Excessive Internet Use (EIU) and define it as a problem that manifests as preoccupation, mood changes, difficulties with limiting time online, and subsequent conflicts, including difficulties that belong among the symptoms of addictive behaviour. In our study, EIU represents an umbrella term for any excessive online behaviour. Although some older literature suggests the existence of generalised internet addictions [2], more current literature leans towards specific internet use disorders [4]. This has been supported by empirical findings that generalised and specific internet addiction mostly overlap [5], and that some online applications, especially online gaming [6] and social networking [7], contribute to this phenomenon more than others.

Adolescents are often shown to be the most vulnerable group in terms of developing EIU [8]. Their vulnerability stems from specific immaturity that is characteristic for the developmental period and includes increased impulsivity, impaired self-regulation, and higher tendencies toward reward-seeking behaviours [9,10]. Given the fact that the internet is a readily available tool that is thoroughly embedded in their everyday routines [11], EIU may become an issue for some adolescents. Higher levels of internet use have been linked to a range of problems, such as nervousness and irritability due to lack of sleep [12], increased depression [13], health problems caused by sedentary behaviour [14,15], and neglecting academic and other responsibilities [16,17].

Prior research has mostly investigated various individual risk factors that range from low self-esteem and self-efficacy [18,19], self-directedness [20], neuroticism [21], and loneliness [22] to attention difficulties [23]. As such, the role of social environment is neglected in models that describing both generalised and specific disordered internet use-only the role of social cognition (e.g., feelings of isolation, perceived lack of social support) is mentioned in the Interaction of Person-Affect-Cognition-Execution (I-PACE) model [4] and the Cognitive-Behavioral Model of Pathological Internet Use [2]. However, theories of problematic adolescent behaviour, e.g., the Problem Behavior Theory [24] and theories for media effects, e.g., the Differential Susceptibility to Media Effects Model [25] propose stronger consideration of the environmental influence, notably the family, which may both predictand moderate adolescent behaviour, including patterns of internet use.

The family environment is the closest social environment for adolescents and it plays an essential role in development [26]. Previous research suggests that the presence of a dysfunctional and high-conflict family environment may increase the likelihood of developing various forms of adolescent pathological behaviour, like alcohol use and gambling [27,28], as well as developing excessive online behaviour [29]. Specifically, dysfunctional parent–child communication [30], the existence of family conflict [31], and the lower emotional availability of parents [32] have been found to be associated with EIU in adolescents. More parental emotional warmth and care have been shown to be protective factors against EIU [32,33].

Parents face challenges as their adolescent grows. Adolescents develop their own individuality and learn to take responsibility for their own actions. Their needs for privacy and independence gain importance [34], but at the same time compete with needs for closeness and relatedness, which still remains significant [35]. Insufficient social support in this developmental stage can intensify feelings of loneliness or social isolation, which often appear in adolescence [36]. Indeed, the levels of social support have been found to be associated with EIU [37]. Therefore, parents have to find a balance between promoting autonomy and monitoring behaviour, which also applies to internet use. According to existing literature, restriction and control are associated with negative outcomes, while parental monitoring promotes healthy and positive psychological development [38]. With respect to internet use, the adequate monitoring of an adolescent´s whereabouts and the strategies of behavioural control have been linked to lower levels of EIU [39,40], while intrusive parental control and autonomy restriction are likely to manifest as risk factors for EIU [41].

The present overview suggests that family environmental factors might play an important role in moderating internet use in adolescence. However, to our knowledge, none of the available studies have comprehensively examined these factors in relation to EIU. Therefore, the aim of this study is to analyse the associations between EIU and an array of family-related factors—family composition, socioeconomic status, parenting strategies (e.g., care, monitoring, overprotection), quality of communication, and time spent together, while controlling for adolescent gender, age, and digital screen time. We assume that adolescents, who experience sufficient social support, care, and personal autonomy will report lower scores for EIU than those who perceive their parents as unloving, too controlling, and restrictive of their personal freedom.

2. Materials and Methods

2.1. Data Collection

We used data from the Health Behaviour in School-aged Children (HBSC) study, which was a cross-national survey conducted in Slovakia in 2014. A two-step procedure was used for data collection in order to obtain a nationally representative sample of adolescents. In the first step, 151 elementary schools were randomly selected from the register of all eligible schools in Slovakia, as provided by the Slovak Institute of Information and Prognosis for Education. In the second step, every school that agreed to participate had one randomly selected class per grade within the target group of students (i.e., fifth to ninth grades). Standardized self-reporting questionnaires were administered by trained administrators and completed by individual students during a classroom session. The study was approved by the Ethics Committee of the Medical Faculty at P.J. Safarik University in Kosice (No: 9/2012). All participation was fully voluntary and anonymous. Parental consent was obtained before administration.

2.2. Sample

A total of 10,179 Slovak adolescents aged 11–15 participated in the survey and completed the self-report questionnaire. Measures listed below were offered only to these children. Items to measure excessive internet use were included only in version A of the questionnaire, which was designed for students aged 13–15 (only 3135 adolescents were given version A). We also eliminated participants who did not provide 50% of the values for any of the variables of interest. The final sample consisted of 2547 adolescents from 13 to 15 years old ($M = 14.32$, $SD = 0.91$), with 50.9% being boys.

2.3. Measures

HBSC followed the strict methodology of the survey, which also applied to the translation process. All of the measures used in the study were translated from English to Slovak using the back-translation procedure. Moreover, back-translations are also independently checked by a translation team within the HBSC network, which was specifically established for this task.

EIU was measured using the *Excessive Internet Use* scale (EU Kids Online network; eukidsonline.net). This scale was validated in 25 European countries [42]. It consists of five items that cover five of the six factors of the components for the model of behavioural addiction [43]: salience ("I have gone without eating and sleeping because of the internet"); withdrawal symptoms ("I have felt bothered when I cannot be on the internet"); tolerance ("I have caught myself surfing when I am not really interested"); relapse ("I have tried unsuccessfully to spend less time on the internet"); and conflict ("I have spent less time than I should with either family, friends, or doing schoolwork because of the time I spend on the internet"). Using a four-point scale (ranging from 1 = "never" to 4 = "very often"), participants rated how often they had experienced the symptoms in the preceding12 months. The final variable was created as a mean of the five items, with higher numbers representing more excessive internet use. The scale was reliable. Cronbach's alpha equaled 0.79.

Digital screen time was assessed as the total time spent on the computer during an average weekday. The scale had nine options that ranged from zero hours a day to seven and more hours a day. Digital screen time was previously associated with the greater duration of internet use per week and with internet addiction [44].

Socioeconomic status was assessed by a question about the perceived financial situation of the family (1 = "our family is not at all well off" to 5 = "our family is very well off").

Family composition was constructed as a dichotomous variable, with 0 representing an incomplete family (e.g., the child lives with only one parent and/or step-parent, or with none of the parents) and 1 representing a complete family (e.g., the child lives with both parents in one household).

Parental care was assessed with a composite score that combines information from two scales that measure identical construct. Eight items were taken from the Parental Bonding Instrument: A Brief

Current Form (PBI-BC [45]) and four items came from the Multidimensional Scale of Perceived Social Support (MSPSS [46]). Items in both subscales measure parental warmth, interest, and supportive behaviour from the adolescents' perspective (e.g., "My mother/my father helps me as much as she/he can"; "My family is willing to help me make decisions."). The scale had a single-factor structure and the composite score for the variable was constructed as a mean score of 12items for the mother and father. For children who had only one parent, the mean score was computed for one parent. This allowed us to avoid reducing the statistical power because of the exclusion of children from single-parent families. The scale was reliable and Cronbach's alpha equaled 0.88.

Parental overprotection was measured with eight items from the Parental Bonding Instrument: A Brief Current Form (PBI-BC [45]). The scale is designed to measure parental control and overprotective behaviour from the perspective of the adolescent (e.g., "Mother/father likes me to make my own decisions"). Participants completed scales for mothers and fathers separately, and each item was rated on a three-point scale according to the perceived frequency of certain behaviour (1 = "never"; 2 = "sometimes"; 3 = "almost always"). The variable Parental Overprotection was constructed as a mean score of items for paternal overprotection and maternal overprotection. For children who had only one parent, the mean score was computed for one parent. The scale was reliable and Cronbach's alpha equaled 0.65.

Parental monitoring was measured with a five-item scale for how much the parents know about the following aspects of their adolescent's life: how they spend their free time; what they do after school; where they go in the evening; how they spend their money; and who their friends are. Response options were 1 = "she/he knows a lot"; 2 = "she/he knows a little"; and 3 = "she/he knows nothing". The mean score was computed from all 10items for the mother and father. For children who had only one parent, the mean score was computed for one parent. The scale was reliable and Cronbach's alpha equaled 0.88.

Time spent together was measured by eight items that assessed how often adolescents engaged in certain common activities with their parents, like playing indoor games, visiting relatives, and watching television. For each item, participants were asked to choose the most appropriate of the following five response categories: 1 = "never"; 2 = less often"; 3 = "about once a week"; 4 = "most days"; and 5 = "every day". The variable was constructed as a mean score of all eight items. The scale was reliable and Cronbach's alpha equaled 0.85.

Quality of communication with parents was measured by asking respondents how easy was for them to talk to their parents about things that bothered them (1 = "very easy" to 4 = "very difficult"). The mean score was computed from both items for the mother and father. For children with only one parent we used the single score they chose for that parent. The scale was reliable and Cronbach's alpha equaled 0.68.

Descriptive statistics and Cronbach's alpha values for all of the scales are presented in Table 1.

Table 1. Descriptive statistics for study variables.

	M	*SD*	Skewness	Kurtosis	Cronbach´s Alpha
Excessive internet use	1.62	0.61	1.37	1.95	0.79
Age	14.32	0.91	0.18	−0.46	
Incomplete family			−1.57	0.47	
Digital screen time	4.43	2.17	0.56	−0.41	
Socioeconomic status	3.84	0.83	−0.50	0.29	
Parental care	3.73	0.66	−1.04	1.18	0.88
Parental overprotection	1.64	0.35	0.24	−0.07	0.65
Parental monitoring	2.47	0.46	−0.81	0.06	0.88
Time spent together	2.82	0.79	0.30	0.05	0.85
Communication	2.81	0.81	−0.34	−0.44	0.68

2.4. Data Analysis

The data were analysed using IBM SPSS Statistics 25 software. Spearman´s correlation coefficients were calculated for all of the variables. Gender differences in the level of excessive internet use and other variables were assessed using the Mann–Whitney U-test. Nonparametric tests were used because the majority of variables were not normally distributed (values of skewness and kurtosis are presented in Table 1). To determine the associations between excessive internet use and family factors, we conducted a hierarchical multiple regression that controlled for the gender and age of the participants and for the frequency of computer use. Variables were entered into the regression in two steps with the Enter method. In the case of sufficiently large sample sizes, regression analysis provided valid results, even for non-normally distributed variables [47]. Control variables were entered in the regression in the first step. All of the family factors were entered in the second step. The assumptions of regression analysis were met: the VIF score for any variable was below 1.94 (tolerance above 0.52), indicating no problem with multicollinearity, and the residuals were uncorrelated (Durbin–Watson coefficient = 1.88) and approximately normally distributed.

3. Results

The means, standard deviations, and Spearman´s rank correlation coefficients of the studied variables are presented in Table 2. On average, participants reported relatively low scores on excessive internet use ($M = 1.62$, $SD = 0.61$). The majority of the sample obtained the minimum possible score in the EIU scale; thus, the distribution of the dependent variable was positively skewed. Excessive internet use was positively related to adolescent age, frequency of computer use, and parental overprotection, and negatively related to all other family variables.

Table 2. Spearman´s rank correlations of all study variables.

	1	2	3	4	5	6	7	8	9	10
1. Excessive internet use	-									
2. Age	0.10 **	-								
3. Digital screen time	0.23 **	0.12 **	-							
4. Socioeconomic status	−0.13 **	−0.08 **	−0.02	-						
5. Family composition	−0.03	−0.01	−0.05 *	0.14 **	-					
6. Parental care	−0.24 **	−0.10 **	−0.05 *	0.27 **	0.03	-				
7. Parental overprotection	0.23 **	−0.03	0.05 **	−0.12 **	−0.07 **	−0.34 **	-			
8. Parental monitoring	−0.28 **	−0.10 **	−0.17 **	0.17 **	0.14 **	0.52 **	−0.28 **	-		
9. Time spent together	−0.13 **	−0.16 **	−0.08 **	0.26 **	0.06 **	0.46 **	−0.11 **	0.37 **	-	
10. Parental communication	−0.17 **	−0.09 **	−0.03	0.23**	−0.01	0.51 **	−0.22 **	0.31 **	0.33 **	-

$^{*}p < 0.05$, $^{**}p < 0.01$.

A Mann–Whitney U test was conducted to compare the level of excessive internet use in boys ($M = 1.62$, $SD = 0.64$) and girls ($M = 1.62$, $SD = 0.59$). There was no significant difference ($U = 806670.5$, $p > 0.05$, $\eta^2 = 0.01$). There were also no differences between boys and girls in parental care ($U = 807552.5$, $p > 0.05$, $\eta^2 = 0.01$), parental overprotection ($U = 783925.0$, $p > 0.05$, $\eta^2 = 0.06$), parental monitoring ($U = 794794.0$, $p > 0.05$, $\eta^2 = 0.03$), communication ($U = 806933.0$, $p > 0.05$, $\eta^2 = 0.01$), time spent together ($U = 809466.5$, $p > 0.05$, $\eta^2 = 0.002$), socioeconomic status ($U = 800034.5$, $p > 0.05$, $\eta^2 = 0.02$), family composition ($U = 791531.0$, $p > 0.05$, $\eta 2 = 0.04$), and digital screen time ($U = 795816.5$, $p > 0.05$, $\eta^2 = 0.03$).

Regression coefficients for each predictor are presented in Table 3.

Table 3. Regression coefficients.

	Model 1			Model 2		
	B	*SE*	*β*	*B*	*SE*	*β*
Constant	0.65	0.19		1.01	0.23	
Age	0.05	0.01	0.07 ***	0.04	0.01	0.06 ***
Gender	0.01	0.02	0.01	0.02	0.02	0.02
Digital screen time	0.06	0.01	0.22 ***	0.05	0.01	0.18 ***
Socioeconomic status				−0.04	0.02	−0.05 *
Family composition				0.02	0.03	0.01
Parental care				−0.08	0.02	−0.08 ***
Parental overprotection				0.29	0.04	0.17 ***
Parental monitoring				−0.20	0.03	−0.15 ***
Time spent together				0.06	0.02	0.08 ***
Communication				0.01	0.02	0.01
R		0.23			0.37	
R^2		0.06			0.14	
Adjusted R^2		0.05			0.14	

* $p < 0.05$, *** $p < 0.001$.

The first model, including age, gender, and frequency of computer use, significantly predicted excessive internet use ($F(3, 2544) = 49.14$; $p < 0.001$) and accounted for 5.5% of the variance of the dependent variable. Both age ($t(2544) = 3.69$; $p < 0.001$) and digital screen time ($t(2544) = 11.09$; $p < 0.001$) significantly predicted EIU.

After entering family-related variables in the second step, the proportion of explained variance increased to 14% and this model also significantly predicted EIU ($F(10, 2537) = 41.37$; $p < 0.001$). Our analysis revealed that higher socioeconomic status ($t(2537) = -2.44$; $p < 0.05$), parental care ($t(2537) = -3.19$; $p < 0.01$), and parental monitoring ($t(2537) = -6.62$; $p < 0.001$) were significant negative predictors (i.e., protective factors) of EIU. Parental overprotection ($t(2537) = 8.14$; $p < 0.001$) and time spent together ($t(2537) = 3.75$; $p < 0.001$) significantly predicted EIU in the opposite direction, indicating that those variables figure as risk factors. The associations between family composition ($t(2537) = 0.53$; $p > 0.05$), parental communication ($t(2537) = 0.23$; $p > 0.05$), and excessive internet use were not significant. Age and frequency of computer use remained significant predictors, whereas association between gender and excessive internet use remained insignificant.

4. Discussion

This study examined family environmental factors in relation to adolescent Excessive Internet Use. The findings show that the strongest protective factor was the parental monitoring of the adolescent's activities (e.g., knowing about friends, knowing how they spend free time), followed by parental care (e.g., emotional warmth, overall support within the family environment). On the other hand, the strongest risk factor associated with a higher score of EIU was parental overprotection (e.g., parental behaviour that decreases adolescents' independence), followed by increased time spent together and lower socioeconomic status of the family.

These findings point to two important issues. First, our study supports the so-called optimal parenting that seems to be an ideal parenting strategy that is associated with lower scores for EIU [48]. Parents who use this strategy might be successful at balancing their care for their adolescents and their protection, while, at the same time, respecting their personal autonomy [49]. As the need for autonomy in adolescence increases with age, autonomy restrictions may lead to diverse problems, including lower self-esteem or self-efficacy. Sufficient support for autonomy has a protective function, which has also been shown in previous studies [50].

Second, from the perspective of associations among family environmental factors and problematic behaviour in youth, our results show a mix of similarities and dissimilarities between EIU and other traditional problematic adolescent behaviours. In the case of traditional antisocial adolescent behaviours, such as drinking alcohol and delinquency, parental monitoring and care have generally been identified as protective factors, while parenting styles that harm the confidence and independence of children were found to be risk factors [51,52]. On the other hand, antisocial behaviours were often explained decreased family monitoring and involvement [52,53]. In this respect, EIU seems to be distinct from traditional antisocial and problematic behaviours—our results showed that overprotection and increased time at home and in the family environment (in other words, decreased time in peer groups) increase EIU. The distinction between EIU and problematic adolescent behaviour is further supported by De Looze and his colleagues [54], who found that the overall trend in the decrease of substance use in recent adolescents is not related to increased use of digital media; thus, EIU is not simply a replacement for other forms of problematic behaviour. Despite the fact that some studies found an association between EIU and various conduct problems [55,56], and that problematic adolescent behaviours and EIU share some underpinnings with ADHD [57], our study points to the need for specific parenting approaches when addressing EIU and when addressing traditional problematic behaviours. The mutual relatedness of EIU and other forms of problematic behaviours should be the subject of a more thorough investigation.

It must be noted that family factors themselves explain only about 8% (14% if we include digital screen time and age) of the variance of EIU. This is in line with previous research that showed that family factors explained 6% of the variance of EIU through parental mediation strategies [58]. It is likely that the strongest influences for EIU are personality and psychological factors, like ADHD, lower self-esteem, and emotional difficulties in general [42], which is also suggested by theoretical models like the I-PACE [4], and cognitive-behavioural models [2,59]. Since environmental factors play a non-negligible role in adolescent lives and they should be incorporated into theoretical models of EIU and specific internet disorders as has been done in general media-effect models (e.g., Differential Susceptibility to Media-Effects Model [25]).

The strength of associations was rather weak in our study. Except for parental monitoring and overprotection, all other significant predictors were negligible. Whether they remained significant only due to the large sample size or because they indeed play some role in EIU should be the focus of further research. For example, lower social economic status, although correlated with EIU, lost most of its strength in the factor analysis. However, the literature has identified lower socioeconomic status as a risk factor of EIU [60]. In our research, lower socioeconomic status worked in the same direction as parental over protection, the time that the adolescent spent at home, and the time that the adolescent spent with digital devices. This may indicate that, in such families, there is a lack resources for meaningful structured afterschool activities (e.g., sports, music lessons) and that digital devices are used as cheap alternatives for filling free time. Such a hypothesis needs further investigation.

The results of this study should be considered in light of several limitations. First, since the research design is cross-sectional, causal relationships between family factors and EIU could not be inferred based on our results. In this case, longitudinal studies would better examine the direction of the observed effects. Second, the data were obtained solely from adolescent self-report questionnaires. For future studies, it would be useful to complement this method of data collection with reports from parents to provide a comparison for parent–adolescent dyads. Third, the data did not include variables to measure specific internet-related mediation strategies, so we were only able to analyse general attitudes in parenting and the atmosphere in the family. In addition, digital screen time did not measure internet use, per se. Nonetheless, prior research has clearly shown that digital screen time predominantly overlaps with time spent online [61]. And, lastly, the main variable, EIU, although used in many previous studies and validated in most European countries, consists of only five items and does not allow for an in-depth investigation of the excessive use of various applications. This may be problematic from the perspective of the ongoing discussion of generalised vs. specific internet-based disorders. In this respect, our study lacked the differentiation of the applications that contribute to EIU Also, the main variable has not been validated for discriminative purposes, and it is a continuum without differentiation between healthy and pathological internets users. Despite these limitations, the main advantages of this study are the use of the national representative sample of adolescents and a several family variables that allow for their mutual control in the regression analysis.

5. Conclusions

Our study revealed several important factors associated with adolescent Excessive Internet Use. The strongest protective factor was the parental monitoring of their adolescent's activities (i.e., parents being aware of what, where, when, and with whom their adolescent children spend their leisure time). This was supported by higher care (i.e., emotional warmth, atmosphere in the family). The main risk factor of EIU appeared to be the parental overprotection (i.e., parental behaviour that harmed the respondent's independence and confidence). Certain risk factors, although very small, were also brought by the lower socioeconomic status of the family and increased time spent at home, which were also supported by increased digital screen time. These results indicate that optimal parenting is a balance among parental care, protection, and allowing adolescents to build independence and competence. It also points to the potential role of family lifestyles associated with limited resources.

Author Contributions: A.F. conducted the statistical analysis. A.F. and L.B. conducted the literature review and wrote the draft of the article. A.Š. and D.H. helped with the interpretation of the findings and draft editing. All authors have read and agreed to the published version of the manuscript.

References

1. Van Rooij, A.J.; Schoenmakers, T.M.; van den Eijnden, R.J.; van de Mheen, D. Compulsive Internet use: The role of online gaming and other internet applications. *J. Adolesc. Health* **2010**, *47*, 51–57. [CrossRef]
2. Davis, R.A. A cognitive-behavioral model of pathological Internet use. *Comput. Hum. Behav.* **2001**, *17*, 187–195. [CrossRef]
3. Shapira, N.A.; Goldsmith, T.D.; Keck, P.E.; Khosla, U.M.; McElroy, S.L. Psychiatric features of individuals with problematic Internet use. *J. Affect. Disord.* **2000**, *57*, 267–272. [CrossRef]
4. Brand, M.; Young, K.S.; Laier, C.; Wölfling, K.; Potenza, M.N. Integrating psychological and neurobiological considerations regarding the development and maintenance of specific Internet-use disorders: An Interaction of Person-Affect-Cognition-Execution (I-PACE) model. *Neurosci. Biobehav. Rev.* **2016**, *71*, 252–266. [CrossRef] [PubMed]
5. Montag, C.; Bey, K.; Sha, P.; Li, M.; Chen, Y.F.; Liu, W.Y.; Reuter, M. Is it meaningful to distinguish between generalized and specific Internet addiction? Evidence from a cross-cultural study from Germany, Sweden, Taiwan and China. *Asia Pac. Psychiatry* **2015**, *7*, 20–26.
6. Blinka, L.; Škařupová, K.; Ševčíková, A.; Wölfing, K.; Müller, K.W.; Dreier, M. Excessive internet use in European adolescents: What determines differences in severity? *Int. J. Public Health* **2015**, *60*, 249–256. [CrossRef]
7. Lopez-Fernandez, O. Generalized Versus Specific Internet Use-Related Addiction Problems: A Mixed Methods Study on Internet, Gaming, and Social Networking Behaviours. *Int. J. Environ. Res. Public Health* **2018**, *15*, 2913. [CrossRef]
8. Kuss, D.J.; van Rooij, A.J.; Shorter, G.W.; Griffiths, M.D.; van de Mheen, D. Internet addiction in adolescents: Prevalence and risk factors. *Comput. Hum. Behav.* **2013**, *29*, 1987–1996. [CrossRef]
9. Boucher, M.; Sandhu, P. The Neurobiology of Adolescent Addiction. In *Clinical Handbook of Adolescent Addiction*; Rosner, R., Ed.; Wiley: Hoboken, NJ, USA, 2007; pp. 78–87.
10. Spear, L. The Teenage Brain: Adolescents and Alcohol. *Curr. Dir. Psychol. Sci.* **2013**, *22*, 152–157. [CrossRef]
11. Livingstone, S.; Haddon, L.; Görzig, A.; Ólafsson, K. Risk and safety on the internet: The role of online skills and internet self-efficacy. *New Media Soc.* **2011**, *12*, 309–329. [CrossRef]
12. Marino, C.; Vieno, A.; Lenzi, M.; Borraccino, A.; Lazzeri, G.; Lemma, P. Computer Use, Sleep Difficulties, and Psychological Symptoms Among School-Aged Children: The Mediation Role of Sleep Difficulties. *Int. J. Sch. Health* **2016**, *4*, 50–58. [CrossRef]

13. Ha, J.H.; Kim, S.; Bae, S.; Bae, S.; Kim, H.; Sim, M.; Lyoo, I.; Cho, S. Depression and Internet Addiction in Adolescents. *Psychopathology* **2007**, *402*, 424–430. [CrossRef] [PubMed]
14. Vandelanotte, C.; Sugiyama, T.; Gardiner, P.; Owen, N. Associations of Leisure-Time Internet and Computer Use With Overweight and Obesity, Physical Activity and Sedentary Behavior: Cross-Sectional Study. *J. Med. Internet Res.* **2009**, *11*, e28. [CrossRef] [PubMed]
15. Brindova, D.; Dankulincova Veselska, Z.; Klein, D.; Hamrik, Z.; Sigmundova, D.; van Dijk, J.P.; Reijneveld, S.A.; Madarasova Geckova, A. Is the association between screen-based behavior and health complaints among adolescents moderated by physical activity? *Int. J. Public Health* **2015**, *60*, 139–145. [CrossRef] [PubMed]
16. Kim, S.Y.; Kim, M.S.; Park, B.; Kim, J.H.; Choi, H.G. The associations between internet use time and school performance among Korean adolescents differ according to the purpose of internet use. *PLoS ONE* **2017**, *12*, e0174878. [CrossRef]
17. Camerini, A.L.; Chulz, P.J.; Jeannet, A.M. The social inequalities of Internet access, its use, and the impact on children´s academic performance: Evidence from a longitudinal study in Switzerland. *New Media Soc.* **2017**, *20*. [CrossRef]
18. De Berardis, D.; D´Albenzio, A.; Gambi, F.; Sepede, G.; Valchera, A.; Conti, C.M.; Fulcheri, M.; Cavuto, M.; Ortolani, C.; Salerno, R.M.; et al. Alexithymia and its relationships with dissociative experiences and Internet addiction in a nonclinical sample. *Cyberpsychol. Behav.* **2009**, *12*, 67–69. [CrossRef]
19. Montag, C.; Jurkiewicz, M.; Reuter, M. Low self-directedness is a better predictor for problematic internet use than high neuroticism. *Comput. Hum. Behav.* **2010**, *26*, 1531–1535. [CrossRef]
20. Servidio, R.; Gentile, A.; Boca, S. The Mediational Role of Coping Strategies in the Relationship Between Self-Esteem and Risk of Internet Addiction. *Eur. J. Psychol.* **2018**, *14*, 176–187. [CrossRef]
21. Wu, C.Y.; Lee, M.B.; Liao, S.C.; Chang, L.R. Risk Factors of Internet Addiction among Internet Users: An Online Questionnaire Survey. *PLoS ONE* **2015**, *10*, e0137506. [CrossRef]
22. Xinxin, S.; Wang, J.; Zou, H. Family Functioning and Internet Addiction among Chinese Adolescents: The Mediating Roles of Self-esteem and Loneliness. *Comp. Hum. Behav.* **2017**, *76*, 201–210.
23. Tateno, M.; Teo, A.R.; Shirasaka, T.; Tayama, M.; Watabe, M.; Kato, T.A. Internet addiction and self-evaluated attention-deficit hyperactivity disorder traits among Japanese college students. *Psychiatry Clin. Neurosci.* **2016**, *70*, 567–572. [CrossRef] [PubMed]
24. Jessor, R.; Jessor, S.L. *Problem Behavior and Psychological Development: A Longitudinal Study of Youth*; Academic Press: New York, NY, USA, 1977.
25. Valkenburg, P.M.; Peter, J. The Differential Susceptibility to Media Effects Model. *J. Commun.* **2013**, *63*, 221–243. [CrossRef]
26. Bronfenbrenner, U.; Moris, P.A. The Bioecological Model of Human Development. In *Handbook of Child Psychology*, 6th ed.; Damon, W., Lerner, R.M., Eds.; Wiley: Hoboken, NJ, USA, 2007; pp. 793–828.
27. McComb, J.L.; Sabiston, C.M. Family Influences on Adolescent Gambling Behavior: A Review of the Literature. *J. Gambl. Stud.* **2010**, *26*, 503–520. [CrossRef]
28. Swaim, R.C.; Stanley, L.R. Effects of Family Conflict and Anger on Alcohol Use among American Indian Students: Mediating Effects of Outcome Expectancies. *J. Stud. Alcohol Drugs* **2018**, *79*, 102–110. [CrossRef]
29. Schneider, L.A.; King, D.L.; Delfabbro, P.H. Family factors in adolescent problematic Internet gaming: A systematic review. *J. Behav. Addict.* **2017**, *6*, 321–333. [CrossRef]
30. Kim, Y.H.; Chong, Y.S. Parent-Child Communication, Peer-Relationship and Internet Addiction in Children. *J. Korean Home Econ. Assoc.* **2005**, *43*, 103–114. [CrossRef]
31. Wu, C.; Wong, H.T.; Yu, K.F.; Fok, K.W.; Yeung, S.M.; Lam, C.H.; Liu, K.M. Parenting approaches, family functionality, and internet addiction among Hong Kong adolescents. *BMC Pediatrics* **2016**, *16*, 130. [CrossRef]
32. Karaer, Y.; Akdemir, D. Parenting styles, perceived social support and emotion regulation in adolescents with internet addiction. *Compr. Psychiatry* **2019**, *92*, 22–27. [CrossRef]
33. Yao, M.Z.; He, J.; Ko, D.M.; Pang, K. The influence of personality, parental behaviors, and self-esteem on internet addiction: A study of Chinese college students. *Cyberpsychol. Behav. Soc. Netw.* **2014**, *17*, 104–110. [CrossRef]
34. Branje, S. Development of Parent-Adolescent Relationships: Conflict Interactions as a Mechanism of Change. *Child Dev. Perspect.* **2018**, *12*, 171–176. [CrossRef]
35. Reis, O.; Buhl, H.M. Individuation during adolescence and emerging adulthood–Five German studies. *Int. J. Behav. Dev.* **2008**, *32*, 369–371. [CrossRef]

36. Laursen, B.; Hartl, A.C. Understanding loneliness during adolescence: Developmental changes that increase the risk of perceived social isolation. *J. Adolesc.* **2013**, *36*, 1261–1268. [CrossRef] [PubMed]
37. Wang, E.S.T.; Wang, M.C.H. Social support and social interaction ties on internet addiction: Integrating online and offline contexts. *Cyberpsycholg. Behav. Soc. Netw.* **2013**, *16*, 843–849. [CrossRef] [PubMed]
38. Bleakley, A.; Ellithorpe, M.; Romer, D. The Role of Parents in Problematic Internet Use among US Adolescents. *Media Commun.* **2016**, *4*, 24–34. [CrossRef]
39. Lin, C.H.; Lin, S.L.; Wu, C.P. The effects of parental monitoring and leisure boredom on adolescents´ internet addiction. *Adolescence* **2009**, *44*, 993–1004.
40. Shek, D.T.L.; Zhu, X.; Ma, C.M.S. The Influence of Parental Control and Parent-Child Relational Qualities on Adolescent Internet Addiction: A 3-Year Longitudinal Study in Hong Kong. *Front. Psychol.* **2018**, *9*, 1–16. [CrossRef]
41. Li, C.; Dang, J.; Zhang, X.; Zhang, Q.; Guo, J. Internet addiction among Chinese adolescents: The effect of parental behavior and self-control. *Comput. Hum. Behav.* **2014**, *41*, 1–7. [CrossRef]
42. Škařupová, K.; Ólafsson, K.; Blinka, L. Excessive Internet Use and its association with negative experiences: Quasi-validation of a short scale in 25 European countries. *Comput. Hum. Behav.* **2015**, *53*, 118–123. [CrossRef]
43. Griffiths, M. A 'components' model of addiction within a biopsychosocial framework. *J. Subst. Use* **2005**, *10*, 191–197. [CrossRef]
44. Gupta, A.; Khan, A.M.; Rajoura, O.P.; Srivastava, S. Internet addiction and its mental health correlates among undergraduate college students of a university in North India. *J. Family Med. Prim. Care* **2018**, *7*, 721–727. [PubMed]
45. Klimidis, S.; Minas, I.H.; Ata, A.W. The PBI-BC: A Brief Current Form of the Parental Bonding Instrument for Adolescent Research. *Compr. Psychiatry* **1992**, *33*, 374–377. [CrossRef]
46. Zimet, G.D.; Dahlem, N.W.; Zimet, S.G.; Farley, G.K. The Multidimensional Scale of Perceived Social Support. *J. Personal. Assess.* **1988**, *52*, 30–41. [CrossRef]
47. Lumley, T.; Diehr, P.; Emerson, S.; Chen, L. The importance of the normality assumption in large public health data sets. *Annu. Rev. Public Health* **2000**, *23*, 151–169. [CrossRef]
48. Floros, G.; Siomos, K. The relationship between optimal parenting, Internet addiction and motives for social networking in adolescence. *Psychiatry Res.* **2013**, *209*, 529–534. [CrossRef]
49. Parker, G. Parental rearing style: Examining for links with personality vulnerability factors for depression. *Soc. Psychiatry Psychiatr. Epidemiol.* **1990**, *28*, 97–100. [CrossRef]
50. Shek, D.T.L.; Zhu, X.; Dou, D. Influence of Family Processes on Internet Addiction Among Late Adolescents in Hong Kong. *Front. Psychiatry* **2019**, 10. [CrossRef]
51. Baumrind, D. The influence of parenting style on adolescent competence and substance use. *J. Early Adolesc.* **1991**, *11*, 56–95. [CrossRef]
52. Ary, D.V.; Duncan, T.E.; Duncan, S.C.; Hops, H. Adolescent problem behavior: The influence of parents and peers. *Behav. Res. Ther.* **1999**, *37*, 217–230. [CrossRef]
53. Dishion, T.J.; Patterson, G.R.; Stoolmiller, M.; Skinner, M.L. Family, school, and behavioral antecedents to early adolescent involvement with antisocial peers. *Dev. Psychol.* **1991**, *27*, 172–180. [CrossRef]
54. De Looze, M.; van Dorsselaer, S.; Stevens, G.W.J.M.; Boniel-Nissim, M.; Vieno, A.; Van den Eijnden, R.J.J.M. The decline in adolescent substance use across Europe and North America in the early twenty-first century: A result of the digital revolution? *Int. J. Public Health* **2019**, *64*, 229–240. [CrossRef] [PubMed]
55. Lim, J.A.; Gwak, A.R.; Park, S.M.; Kwon, J.G.; Lee, J.Y.; Jung, H.Y.; Sohn, B.K.; Kim, J.W.; Kim, D.J.; Choi, J.S. Are adolescents with internet addiction prone to aggressive behavior? The mediating effect of clinical comorbidities on the predictability of aggression in adolescents with internet addiction. *Cyberpsychol. Behav. Soc. Netw.* **2015**, *18*, 260–267. [CrossRef] [PubMed]
56. Blinka, L.; Šmahel, D. Predictors of adolescents' excessive internet use: A comparison across European countries. In Proceedings of the 15th European Conference on Developmental Psychology, Bergen, Norway, 23–27 August 2011; pp. 337–341.
57. Wang, B.Q.; Young, K.S.; Zhou, X.; Liu, J.; Lv, Z.T. The association between attention deficit/hyperactivity disorder and internet addiction: A systematic review and meta-analysis. *BMC Psychiatry* **2017**, *17*, 260. [CrossRef] [PubMed]
58. Kalmus, V.; Blinka, L.; Ólafsson, K. Does It Matter What Mama Says: Evaluating the Role of Parental Mediation in European Adolescents' Excessive Internet Use. *Child. Soc.* **2015**, *29*, 122–133. [CrossRef]

59. Dong, G.; Potenza, M.N. A cognitive-behavioral model of Internet gaming disorder: Theoretical underpinnings and clinical implications. *J. Psychiatr. Res.* **2014**, *58*, 7–11. [CrossRef]
60. Bitto Urbanova, L.; Holubcikova, J.; Madarasova Geckova, A.; Reijneveld, S.A.; van Dijk, J.P. Does Life Satisfaction Mediate the Association between Socioeconomic Status and Excessive Internet Use? *Int. J. Environ. Res. Public Health* **2019**, *16*, 3914. [CrossRef]
61. Vaala, S.E.; Bleakley, A. Monitoring, Mediating, and Modeling: Parental Influence on Adolescent Computer and Internet Use in the United States. *J. Child. Media* **2015**, *9*, 40–57. [CrossRef]

15

Commuting, Life-Satisfaction and Internet Addiction

Bernd Lachmann [1,*], Rayna Sariyska [1], Christopher Kannen [2], Maria Stavrou [3] and Christian Montag [1,4]

1 Molecular Psychology, Institute of Psychology and Education, Ulm University, Helmholtzstrasse 8/1, 89081 Ulm, Germany; rayna.sariyska@uni-ulm.de (R.S.); christian.montag@uni-ulm.de (C.M.)
2 Department of Informatics, University of Bonn, 53012 Bonn, Germany; info@ckannen.com
3 Department of Psychology, Goldsmiths, University of London, London SE14 6NW, UK; mstav010@gold.ac.uk
4 Key Laboratory for NeuroInformation/Center for Information in Medicine, School of Life Science and Technology, University of Electronic Science and Technology of China, Chengdu 611731, China
* Correspondence: bernd.lachmann@uni-ulm.de

Abstract: The focus of the present work was on the association between commuting (business and private), life satisfaction, stress, and (over-) use of the Internet. Considering that digital devices are omnipresent in buses and trains, no study has yet investigated if commuting contributes to the development of Internet addiction. Overall, $N = 5039$ participants ($N = 3477$ females, age $M = 26.79$, $SD = 10.68$) took part in an online survey providing information regarding their commuting behavior, Internet addiction, personality, life satisfaction, and stress perception. Our findings are as follows: Personality seems to be less suitable to differentiate between commuter and non-commuter groups, which is possibly due to commuters often not having a choice but simply must accept offered job opportunities at distant locations. Second, the highest levels of satisfaction were found with income and lodging in the group commuting for business purposes. This might be related to the fact that commuting results in higher salaries (hence also better and more expensive housing style) due to having a job in another city which might exceed job opportunities at one's own living location. Third, within the business-commuters as well as in the private-commuter groups, females had significantly higher levels of stress than males. This association was not present in the non-commuter group. For females, commuting seems to be a higher burden and more stressful than for males, regardless of whether they commute for business or private reasons. Finally, we observed an association between higher stress perception (more negative attitude towards commuting) and Internet addiction. This finding suggests that some commuters try to compensate their perceived stress with increased Internet use.

Keywords: commuting; well-being; personality; gender; stress; Internet addiction

---

1. Introduction

Commuting is a wide spread occurrence with millions of people afflicted around the globe [1]. Therefore, commuting behavior has the potential to influence both well-being and life satisfaction of a great part of the population either positive [2], where people regard travelling itself as enjoyable or negative [3], where they see it as a burden. The reasons to accept extended travel times are diverse. Some individuals commute to facilitate a better housing situation or to combine family and vocational goals [4]. Other reasons to commute might include promising career perspectives or financial incentives [5].

From an economical point of view, it seems logical that the costs and benefits of commuting should be at equilibrium to achieving decent levels of life satisfaction [3]. This means that increased costs of commuting (e.g., in terms of higher stress or lower well-being) should be compensated in some way, by higher benefits of the provided job opportunity, for example. Interestingly, this equilibrium is not always met and commuters are often willing to carry higher burdens than non-commuters. This has been coined as the 'Commuting Paradox' in the literature [5].

In the commuting literature physiological issues have also been investigated. A recent study examined the relation between commuting distance, cardiorespiratory fitness, and metabolic risk factors [6]. They found a negative association between commuting distance and physical activity (doing sports on a regular basis) as well as cardiorespiratory fitness and a positive association between commuting distance and Body-Mass-Index, waist circumference, and systolic/diastolic blood pressure. Another study from Norway [7] explored the association between long commutes and subjective health complaints. Again, those who reported longer travel times had more musculoskeletal pain and gastrointestinal problems. Moreover, commuters with a travel history of more than 10 years reported significantly more health complaints than those commuting for two years or less. The perceived level of stress should also be considered [8], since the commuting situation is often difficult to control (e.g., traffic jams, delays in public transport, bad weather conditions). This in turn has the potential to contribute to higher stress levels and frustration. Taking into account the link between health and well-being [9,10] the commuting situation should be associated with well-being. Interestingly, there is evidence that females suffer more under the burden of commuting than males. A study analyzing the effects of commuting on health with regard to gender [11] revealed that females with longer commuting times did seek medical advice and called in sick more often compared to males. An association between commuting and perceived higher stress levels could only be observed in females [12,13]. Presumably, the commuting situation, ceteris paribus, has a more adverse effect on females than males.

Aside from the relation between commuting and health/perceived stress, several studies investigated the direct link between commuting and life satisfaction. Here, the findings are mixed. An early study by Stutzer & Frey [3] concluded that commuting and life satisfaction are negatively related. Moreover, they demonstrated that commuting was characterized by rather low levels of positive effect, with a simultaneous fairly high negative effect. Similar findings were observed in another study investigating the commuting situation, salary, and life satisfaction [4]. In this work, commuting was negatively associated with overall life satisfaction but had no effect on the domains of life satisfaction, work and family. Furthermore, Lyons & Chatterjee [14] reported detrimental effects of commuting on stress, fatigue, and overall dissatisfaction. However, according to the authors, overall life satisfaction could even be increased if commuters can make their own decisions on how to use their travel time. If commuters experience these choices as worthwhile, a positive impact on life satisfaction could be the result [15]. In contrast to the studies mentioned so far, a positive relationship between commuting time and life satisfaction was found by Morris [16]. The authors observed such an association between commuting time and life satisfaction more strongly in rural areas and small cities. This association was visible only to a much weaker extent in large cities, most probably due to the higher degree of traffic congestions. Usually, traffic congestions are not controllable and therefore limit the individual's self-determination. Subsequently, this could lead to a change in life satisfaction [17]. One study examined the association between life satisfaction and work commute [18]. The participants of this study reported mostly positive or neutral feelings during work commute and, consequently, a higher level of happiness. As possible reasons for this, the authors postulate that short work commutes could provide a buffer between work and private sphere, which in turn contributes to an increased level of well-being. For longer commutes, social and entertainment activities could counteract stress or boredom, as well as increase positive effects.

It is worth noting that one possible reaction to stress might be the increased use of the Internet [19]. Since smartphones offer Internet access and are more often than not in people's possession [20] it seems worthwhile to investigate the association between perceived stress (also in terms of attitude towards commuting) and Internet use [21] while commuting. If commuters show a negative attitude towards commuting and/or a high stress level one way to compensate for this could be an increased use of the Internet. As a growing number of researchers around the globe are currently investigating if problematic Internet use represents a societal problem (for an overview see Montag & Reuter [22]; Brand et al. [23]: I-PACE model; Petry & O'Brien [24]: Inclusion of Internet Gaming Disorder in Section III of DSM-5), the question arises if commuting itself also represents a vulnerability factor in becoming addicted to the Internet. Long commutes, in particular, could lead to excessive usage of digital channels. On the other hand, it is imaginable that commuting leads to less time spent on the Internet aside from commuting, because much of what needs to be done online has been already finished during the commute. In short, there is little awareness of studies investigating associations between Internet addiction and commuting. That is the reason why we also address this topic in this work. Internet addiction has been investigated for more than 20 years now [25,26] and much progress has been made to understand problematic Internet use. Although no consensus has been reached with respect to necessary symptoms of Internet addiction, symptoms such as preoccupation with the Internet, withdrawal symptoms when not being online, loss of control and problems in social/work life due to the overuse are of importance [27] Prevalence rates differ across the world, but in Germany (where the current investigated sample has been recruited) about 1% of the population is afflicted [28]. In the context of Internet addiction, it is necessary to distinguish between generalized (generalized pathological Internet use) and specific forms (e.g., excessive online gambling, shopping or social network use) of Internet addiction [29–31]. The present work focuses on unspecific tendencies towards Internet addiction in the realm of commuting.

Overall, an association between commuting and life satisfaction was found in many studies; however, the direction of this association is not trivial to understand. Moreover, it is noticeable that the reviewed research focuses on non-commuters vs. commuters, but they do not ask the question of whether people commute because of private (e.g., to see one's own partner on the weekend) or business reasons (going to work and return back home). Reasons to commute could be an important factor because commuting may not always be considered as a burden [5], but as a fulfilling activity [2]. It is, therefore, conceivable that the motivation behind commuting or personality factors have an impact on the well-being of the commuters. Furthermore, there seems to be a gender specific effect in commuting, with females showing higher stress levels than males [13]. Therefore, in the present study (i) we investigated the association between commuting and life satisfaction in three separate groups: non-commuters, business commuters, and private commuters. In this context, we also examined the underlying personality structure in these groups since several studies reported associations between personality and life satisfaction [32–35] (see Supplementary Material for analyses on the associations of personality). Moreover (ii), we intended to replicate earlier findings about higher stress perception of females in commuting situations [11–13]. This time we also wanted to extend this in the realm of being a non-commuter, business-commuters, and private commuter. Finally (iii), we investigated the association between Internet addiction, life satisfaction, and stress (in relation to commuting). We expected a positive association between a negative attitude toward commuting (and high stress perception) and high Internet addiction.

2. Materials and Methods

For the present study, we asked participants to provide information via a specific designed online questionnaire covering various aspects of commuting. The online questionnaire could be filled in using any suitable device (e.g., tablet, smartphone, personal computer) with access to the Internet.

2.1. Participants

Overall $N = 5039$ participants ($N = 3477$ females) answered the online questionnaire and provided socio-demographic information, information on personality data and life satisfaction, as well as data concerning their commuting behavior. The mean age of the sample was 26.79 ($SD = 10.68$) ranging from 11 years to 98 years. Concerning educational training within the sample, the number of school leaving certificates was distributed as follows: a total of 31.8% had no school leaving certificate, 30.8% had a secondary school leaving certificate, 14.9% had a Baccalaureate-Diploma, and 22.5% had a university degree. Participation was voluntarily and completely anonymous. There was no monetary incentive, but upon completion of the questionnaire, all participants got a brief individual feedback on their personality profiles, life satisfaction, and Internet use (Internet addiction) based on the data provided. The local ethics committee of the Ulm University, Ulm, Germany approved the study, and all participants gave electronic consent prior to participation.

2.2. Materials

The data for the present study were gathered by means of an online questionnaire. In addition to collecting data on demographics, we requested information on personality (see Supplementary Material. For further information on the used personality questionnaire please refer to Rammstedt et al. [36] and John et al. [37]), life satisfaction, and Internet addiction. Furthermore, the participants gave information on their commuting status (none, business, private) and their (emotional) attitude towards commuting, particularly stress. To assess the overall attitude towards commuting, we asked the participants four questions ("Commuting does not matter to me" (item 1, inverse coding), "Commuting deteriorates my mood" (item 2), "Commuting deteriorates my quality of life" (item 3), and "Commuting stresses me" (item 4)). All items could be rated from 1 ("I do not agree at all") to 5 ("I totally agree"). For the analyses, item 4 was analyzed both as a single item (to assess the participants stress level in relation to commuting) and also combined in the short four-item scale described above (to assess the overall 'attitude towards commuting'; ATC). The scores of the four items are simply added up, after reversing the score of item 1. Cronbach's alpha for the ATC scale was alpha = 0.85.

Life satisfaction as one distinct part of subjective well-being, aside from positive and negative effect [38], was measured via questions retrieved from the German Socio-Economic Panel (SOEP) [39]. One section of the panel covers the current life situation within several areas, contributing to overall life satisfaction. For the purpose of this survey, we asked for the degree of satisfaction in the following areas: health, job, income, lodging, leisure, and overall satisfaction with life. Following a recommendation of the SOEP, the question for overall satisfaction with life was presented at the end of the life satisfaction questionnaire. This was done to avoid possible interference with specific domains of life satisfaction. It is important to note that overall life satisfaction is not a simple composite of the various domains of life satisfaction. In fact, all life satisfaction items are considered to be distinct, but also overlap to some extent (e.g., a person more satisfied with his leisure might have, as a consequence, a higher score on overall satisfaction). The items were answered, using a Likert scale, ranging from 0 ("completely dissatisfied") to 10 ("completely satisfied").

To gather data on Internet overuse we administered a short version of the Internet Addiction Test IAT [25], the short Internet Addiction Test (s-IAT) from [40]. This inventory consists of 12 items as opposed to the original version, which contains 20 items. The psychometric quality of the s-IAT has been considered to be of good effect [40]. The Cronbach's alpha in our sample was high (alpha = 0.88). To more effectively assess the association between commuting and Internet use we asked an additional question; "because of commuting I use digital devices more often" (CMD). This could be rated from 1 ("I do not agree at all") to 5 ("I totally agree").

2.3. Procedure

Since the size of the total sample greatly relied upon the publicity of the online questionnaire, the study was introduced during interviews with several national radio and TV stations. This approach was taken to ensure high media coverage throughout Germany, and to avoid biases caused by the restriction of local samples. The audience was given a short introduction to the rationale of the study, combined with information on how to access the online questionnaire. Completed questionnaires were stored on servers and processed for further analyses.

2.4. Statistical Analysis

The statistical analyses were conducted using SPSS 22.0 for windows (IBM SPSS Statistics, Chicago, IL, USA). Differences in life satisfaction and personality variables for non-commuters, business commuters, and private commuters were investigated using ANOVAs, with the additional inclusion of gender effects. The associations between perceived stress, attitude towards commuting, Internet addiction, and life satisfaction were examined within the three groups of commuter type using Pearson correlations, as well as ANOVAs to test for gender effects.

3. Results

3.1. Data Cleaning and Descriptive Statistics

After inspection of the data, 25 participants were discovered to have provided conspicuous age information: A total of 20 participants reported an age of zero. Information on age was given using a slider ranging from 0 to 99 years, where 0 was the default value. Indicating an age of zero means that the participants did not provide any information on their age. Furthermore, we found 5 participants reporting an age between 1 and 9 years. Considering the rationale of the present study, it was uncertain as to whether or not these individuals indeed reported their real age and, if such was the case, were able to complete the questionnaire in a suitable way. Therefore, we decided to exclude these 25 participants, an overall (0.5% of the original sample; 18 commuting either for business or private plus 7 non-commuters) from the sample, which left an overall sample size of N = 5039 participants (N = 5064 before) for the analyses. Moreover, N = 409 participants reported both business-commuting and private-commuting, which forfeited their inclusion into one specific group. There were no further exclusions. We further investigated participants between 11 and 14, because at 15 years, persons are allowed to start working (with a vocational training). A closer inspection of participants with an age less than 15 showed that 28 persons (in our sample a total of 248 participants were younger than 15 years) reported to undertake business-commuting. This seems to be unusual considering the age of these participants. On the other hand, commuting to and from school (97.6% of the participants younger than 15 years reported to be still in school) is obligatory and therefore might be for some participants more connected to the term business rather than private-commuting. For that reason we did not exclude those participants from the sample. All variables were normally distributed and there were no outliers. Table 1 shows the descriptive statistics for the complete sample, and non-commuters (means, standard deviation, observed minimum and maximum values, skew and standard deviation of the skew) were calculated life satisfaction variables, Internet addiction (s-IAT), CSM ("Commuting stresses me"), and ATC (overall "attitude towards commuting").

Table 1. Means and Standard Deviation, Minimum, Maximum and Skewness for life satisfaction variables, and Internet variables for the complete sample (CS) and non-commuters (NC).

Variables	Min	Max	Mean	SD	Skewness	SD
Overall satisfaction	0	10	7.28/7.27	2.19/2.20	−1.06/−1.05	0.03/0.04
Health	0	10	6.62/6.65	2.30/2.30	−0.71/−0.69	0.03/0.04
Job (N = 4616/3401)	0	10	6.81/6.82	2.42/2.43	−0.86/−0.87	0.03/0.04
Income	0	10	5.38/5.36	2.96/3.00	−0.28/−0.26	0.03/0.04
Lodging	0	10	7.30/7.33	2.53/2.54	−1.04/−1.05	0.03/0.04
Leisure	0	10	6.55/6.58	2.38/2.37	−0.56/−0.56	0.03/0.04
Family	0	10	7.07/7.10	2.60/2.60	−0.90/−0.90	0.03/0.04
CSM (N = 1413)	1	5	2.86/2.86	1.20/1.20	−0.05	0.07
CMD	1	5	2.85/3.11	1.45/1.32	−0.02/−0.27	0.07/0.20
ATC	4	20	10.72/11.29	3.85/3.77	0.16/0.11	0.07/0.20
s-IAT	12	60	27.01/27.06	8.37/8.45	0.74/0.72	0.03/0.04

(N = 5039/3774, CS/NC), Internet use (s-IAT), CSM ("Commuting stresses me"), ATC (overall "attitude towards commuting"), and CMD ("because of commuting I use digital devices more often").

Please refer to Table 2 for the descriptive statistics of business-commuters and private commuters.

Table 2. Means and Standard Deviation, Minimum, Maximum, and Skewness for life satisfaction variables, and Internet variables for business-commuters (BC) and private commuters (PC).

Variables	Min	Max	Mean	*SD*	Skewness	*SD*
Overall satisfaction	0	10	7.43/6.97	2.08/2.52	−1.17/−1.00	0.09/0.18
Health	0	10	6.55/6.58	2.22/2.36	−0.75/−1.00	0.09/0.18
Job (N = 663/153)	0	10	6.78/6.72	2.38/2.31	−0.80/−0.79	0.10/0.20
Income	0	10	5.75/4.73	2.71/3.05	−0.43/−0.16	0.09/0.18
Lodging	0	10	7.44/6.66	2.39/2.77	−1.19/−0.76	0.09/0.18
Leisure	0	10	6.48/6.51	2.32/2.52	−0.60/−0.72	0.09/0.18
Family	0	10	7.09/6.71	2.55/2.76	−0.91/−0.78	0.09/0.18
CSM	1	5	2.86/2.86	1.19/1.23	1.19/−0.14	0.09/0.18
CMD	1	5	2.66/2.94	1.48/1.40	0.19/−0.11	0.09/0.18
ATC	4	20	10.71/10.61	3.87/3.93	0.19/0.12	0.09/0.18
s-IAT	12	60	26.30/27.77	7.71/8.49	0.75/0.68	0.09/0.18

(N = 676/180, BC/PC). Internet use (IAT), CSM ("Commuting stresses me"), ATC (overall "attitude towards commuting"), and CMD ("because of commuting I use digital devices more often").

3.2. Association between Life Satisfaction and Commuting Status

A one-way ANOVA showed a main effect of commuting status on income ($F_{(2,4627)} = 9.53$, $p < 0.001$; Levene's test: $F_{(2,4627)} = 7.40$, $p = 0.001$), lodging ($F_{(2,4627)} = 7.03$, $p = 0.001$; Levene's test: $F_{(2,4627)} = 6.00$, $p = 0.003$), and overall LS ($F_{(2,4627)} = 3.41$, $p = 0.033$; Levene's test: $F_{(2,4627)} = 4.61$, $p = 0.010$). Since Levene's test indicated the presence of heteroscedasticity, we used the Games-Howell test for post hoc analyses as recommended by Field & Miles [41]. The Games-Howell post-hoc analysis revealed significant differences between income scores of the non-commuting and business-commuting groups ($p = 0.002$; −0.39, 95% CI [−0.66, −0.12]), the non-commuting and private-commuting groups ($p = 0.020$; 0.63, 95% CI [0.08, 1.18]), and the business-commuting and private-commuting groups ($p < 0.001$; 1.02, 95% CI [0.43, 1.60]). For lodging scores, differences were found between non-commuters and private commuters ($p = 0.004$; 0.68, 95% CI [0.18, 1.18]) as well as between business-commuters and private-commuters ($p = 0.002$; 0.79, 95% CI [0.25, 1.32]). No effects on overall life satisfaction were found by post hoc analyses. To visualize our findings, please refer to Figure 1.

We also investigated these associations for gender effects. A one-way ANOVA showed a main effect of commuting status on income ($F_{(2,1420)} = 4.32$, $p = 0.014$; Levene's test: $F_{(2,1420)} = 9.06$, $p < 0.001$) for males. Again, due to a positive Levene's test, we used a Games-Howell test for the post hoc analysis and found a significant difference between non-commuting and business-commuting groups ($p = 0.005$; −0.57, 95% CI [−1.00, −0.15]) with higher income scores for the business-commuting group. For females, the analysis of variance revealed a main effect of commuting status on income ($F_{(2,3204)} = 6.00$, $p = 0.003$; Levene's test: $F_{(2,3204)} = 2.41$, $p = 0.090$),), lodging ($F_{(2,3204)} = 4.81$, $p = 0.008$; Levene's test: $F_{(2,3204)} = 3.47$, $p = 0.031$), and overall LS ($F_{(2,3204)} = 3.17$, $p = 0.042$; Levene's test: $F_{(2,3204)} = 2.17$, $p = 0.114$). A Games-Howell test revealed a significant difference for females between lodging scores of non-commuting and private-commuting groups ($p = 0.015$; 0.63, 95% CI [0.09, 1.17]) and of business-commuting and private-commuting groups ($p = 0.006$; 0.79, 95% CI [0.18, 1.40]). A generalized Tukey 2 post hoc test was used for income and overall life satisfaction since a Levene's test did not indicate unequal variances. Females showed significant differences for income scores of the non-commuting and private-commuting groups ($p = 0.007$; 0.80, 95% CI [0.17, 1.43]) as well as for the business-commuting and private-commuting groups ($p = 0.002$; 1.03, 95% CI [0.32, 1.73]). Again, overall life satisfaction showed no significant result in the post hoc analysis. An independent-sample t-test provided significantly lower scores for health ($M_{female} = 6.56$, $SD_{female} = 2.32$; $M_{male} = 6.89$, $SD_{male} = 2.25$; $t(3772) = 3.99$, $p < 0.001$) and leisure ($M_{female} = 6.50$, $SD_{female} = 2.37$; $M_{male} = 6.78$, $SD_{male} = 2.36$; $t(3772) = 3.31$, $p = 0.001$) for females compared to males, but only in the non-commuting group.

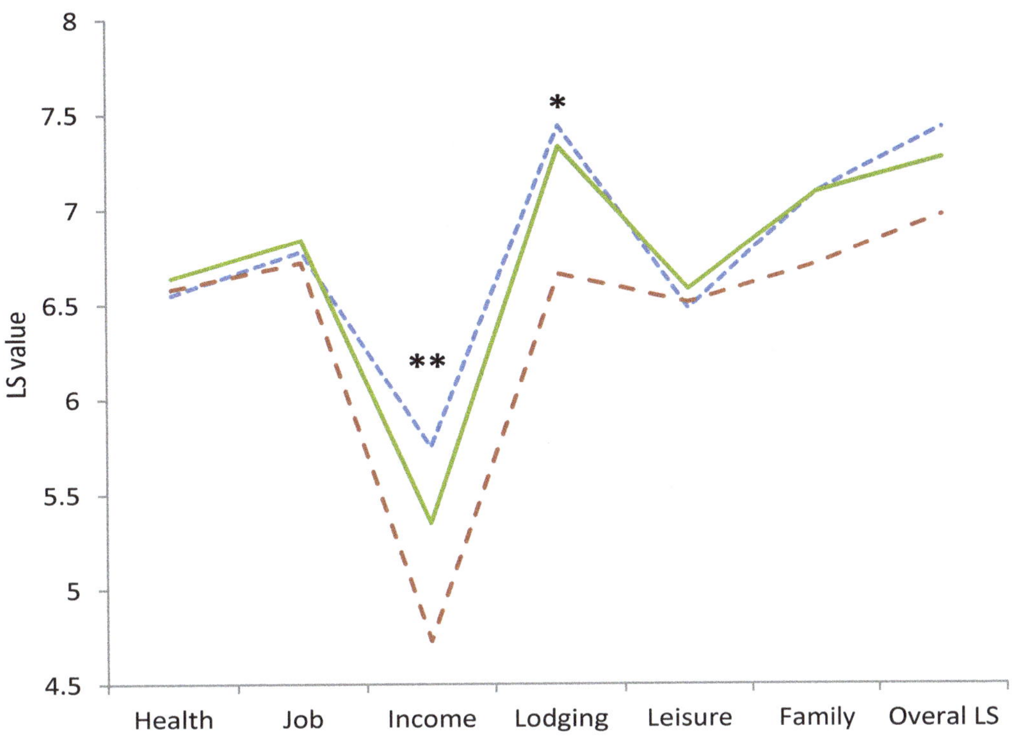

Figure 1. Life satisfaction values depending on commuting status: (BC) business-commuter (dotted blue line), (NC) non-commuters (solid green line), and (PC) private-commuters (dashed red line); * $p = 0.01$, ** ($p < 0.001$) significant differences between all three groups.

The sample sizes used in the analyses for all groups considering commuting status and gender are summarized in Table 3. Age was not associated with commuting status ($r = 0.003$, $p = 0.834$).

Table 3. Sample sizes depending on commuting status and gender.

Sample	B/P *-Commuting	Non-Commuting	Business-Commuting	Private-Commuting
Complete $N = 5039$	409	3774	676	180
Female $N = 3477$	270	2684	391	132
Male $N = 1562$	139	1090	285	48

* B/P: Business and Private.

3.3. *Perception of Stress and Overall Attitude Towards Commuting*

For the total sample, the CSM and ATC variable ("Commuting stresses me"; "Attitude towards commuting") was negatively correlated with all life satisfaction variables in the business-commuters group but not in the private-commuters group. The same result was found when differentiating for gender; however, for both females and males all correlations between CSM/ATC and life satisfaction variables were negative (or not present) in the business-commuting group and nonexistent for females in the private-commuting group. In the private-commuting group we observed one significant negative correlation for males between CSM and overall LS ($r = -0.39$, $p = 0.006$, after Bonferroni correction for multiple testing; corrected alpha: 0.05/8=0.00625). All correlations are summarized in Table 4.

Table 4. Correlations between CSM ("Commuting stresses me"), ATC ("Attitude towards commuting"; 4 item scale), and life satisfaction variables.

Commuting Status	Health	Job	Income	Lodging	Leisure	Family	Overall LS
BC	−0.11 **/−0.13 **	−0.25 **/−0.28 **	−0.22 **/−0.22 **	−0.16 **/−0.18 **	−0.21 **/−0.26 **	−0.10 **/-0.16 **	−0.14 **/−0.19 **
PC	−0.02/−0.01	−0.06/−0.10	0.01/0.03	−0.10/−0.11	−0.07/−0.09	0.01/0.02	−0.11/−0.11
BC (male)	−0.15 */−0.18 **	−0.28 **/−0.33 **	−0.22 **/−0.23 **	−0.12 */−0.15 *	−0.24 **/−0.34 **	−0.14 */−0.23 **	−0.17 **/−0.25 **
BC (female)	−0.07/−0.09	−0.24 **/−0.26 **	−0.21 **/−0.20 **	−0.19 **/−0.20 **	−0.19 **/−0.20 **	−0.07/−0.12 *	−0.14 **/−0.16 **
PC (male)	−0.14/−0.14	−0.41 */−0.39 *	0.03/0.10	−0.17/−0.03	−0.14/−0.01	−0.03/0.16	−0.39 **/−0.31 *
PC (female)	0.02/0.03	0.03/−0.04	0.04/0.05	−0.08/−0.15	−0.03/−0.11	0.00/−0.05	−0.03/−0.05

BC = business-commuting, PC = private commuting, CSM/ATC; * $p < 0.05$, ** $p < 0.001$.

An ANOVA revealed that CSM scores were significantly higher for females ($M_{female} = 3.00$, $SD_{female} = 1.17$) compared to males ($M_{male} = 2.68$, $SD_{male} = 1.20$); $F_{(1674)} = 12.13$, $p = 0.001$) within the business-commuting group and the private-commuting group ($M_{female} = 3.05$, $SD_{female} = 1.19$; $M_{male} = 2.33$, $SD_{male} = 1.19$; $F_{(1178)} = 12.59$, $p < 0.001$). We observed no significant gender differences for the CSM score between business-commuting group, private-commuting group and non-commuting-group. However, ATC scores were significantly higher for females ($M_{female} = 11.09$, $SD_{female} = 3.88$) compared to males ($M_{male} = 10.19$, $SD_{male} = 3.80$); $F_{(1674)} = 9.19$, $p = 0.003$) within the business-commuting group and the private-commuting group ($M_{female} = 11.14$, $SD_{female} = 3.81$; $M_{male} = 9.13$, $SD_{male} = 3.92$; $F_{(1178)} = 9.76$, $p = 0.002$). No differences were observed between the business-, private-, and non-commuting groups (CSM: $F_{(2,1001)} = 0.01$, $p = 0.994$; ATC: $F_{(2,1001)} = 1.58$, $p = 0.207$).

3.4. *Association of Internet Use, Attitude Towards Commuting, Stress, and Life Satisfaction*

The s-IAT was positively associated with the attitude towards commuting (ATC) and stress perception (CSM) but only in the business-commuting group. For females, the association between CSM and IAT was $r = 0.14$, $p = 0.005$, and between ATC and IAT $r = 0.12$, $p = 0.015$. Males showed an association of $r = 0.18$, $p = 0.003$ between CSM and IAT score, and $r = 0.18$, $p = 0.002$ between ATC and IAT values. A positive correlation between ATC/CSM scores and CMD ("because of commuting I use digital devices more often") was observed, again only in the business-commuter group. For females, the association between ATC and CMD was $r = 0.24$, $p < 0.001$ (males: $r = 0.22$, $p < 0.001$), while the association for CSM and CMD was $r = 0.21$, $p < 0.001$ (males: $r = 0.22$, $p < 0.001$). For females in the non-commuting group, the correlation between excessive Internet use and overall life satisfaction was $r = -0.17$, $p < 0.001$, while for males the correlation was $r = -0.11$, $p < 0.001$. For business and private commuters, we found significant associations between Internet addiction and life satisfaction only for females (business: $r = -0.13$, $p = 0.009$; private: $r = -0.23$, $p = 0.009$).

4. Discussion

The aim of this research was to extend already existing research on the association between personality, life satisfaction, and stress perception as a function of commuting status. No differences for personality were found between non-commuters, business-commuters, and private-commuters (see Supplementary Material as well as Baretta et al. [42] and Ruedl [43]). Significant associations were observed between income and lodging depending on commuting status. The business-commuting group showed the highest scores, while the private-commuting group the lowest scores for these areas of life satisfaction. As expected, stress perception was higher for females in the business-commuting group than males. In the private-commuting group the stress perception of females stayed high, whereas the stress perception of males decreased. However, a significant gender effect in relation to CSM/ATC was found only within the business and private-commuting group, i.e., not between the business- and private-commuting group or in the non-commuting group. A positive association was found between Internet addiction and both ATC and CSM, in the business-commuting group, regardless of gender. Moreover, a negative association between Internet addiction and overall life satisfaction (females and males) was found in the complete sample under investigation, as well as a negative association between Internet addiction and overall life satisfaction in the business and private-commuter groups, but for females only.

The association between life satisfaction and commuting [4,15,16,18] was also investigated. For two areas of life satisfaction, namely income and lodging, significant results were found. Interestingly, private-commuters showed lower and business-commuters higher life satisfaction scores than non-commuters for income and lodging. This finding is somewhat unexpected, as our rationale was that lower self-determination in the business-commuter group would lead to lower life satisfaction scores. However, one can infer that this emphasizes the distinct categorization between business-commuters and private-commuters. We discuss two possible explanations for this finding: First, self-determination might not be as a prominent predictor of life satisfaction as expected (at least in the context of commuting), and second, the presence or absence of a financial compensation in a commuting situation influences life satisfaction (life satisfaction scores for income shows the highest effects in our analyses). According to Erikson [44] and Newman et al. [17] self-determination represents an important factor that promotes higher life satisfaction scores. This, in fact, should lead to higher life satisfaction scores in the private-commuter group since within this group, the freedom of choice whether to commute or not should be higher as in the business-commuter group (as discussed above). The main reason why this is not the case and life satisfaction scores are higher for business-commuters could be due to the distinctiveness of the commuting situation: Business-commuters receive a financial compensation from the job, whereas private-commuters have only costs without any compensation. In this context, we propose that the monetary effect on life satisfaction, especially on income, could be much stronger than the influence of self-determination. Further analyses considering gender effects revealed that significant differences for lodging were present but only for females. Those who commuted for private reasons exhibited not only the lowest scores for income but also the lowest satisfaction scores in lodging. Considering that lodging is more important for females than males [45], it seems comprehensible that satisfaction scores for females in lodging are lowest for private commuters; the money they have spent on their private commute is no longer available to adequately furnish a home. Again, for business-commuting there is, at least, a financial compensation, which potentially enhances life satisfaction in this area.

Our findings regarding stress perception were mostly in accordance with previous findings asserting that females experience more stress in a commuting situation than males [8,46]. Interestingly, the level of perceived stress of females remained almost stationary regardless of whether they commuted for business or private reasons, whereas the stress level of males was much lower in the private-commuting group. Roberts et al. [13] proposed that the larger responsibility of females compared to males for daily household tasks could be the reason for higher stress levels of commuting females. In this case, it would be plausible that the reason for commuting (business or private) would have no influence on the female's perception of stress because the outcome (possible neglect of household tasks due to commuting) is independent from the reason of commuting. The fact that significantly higher stress levels for females compared to males were present within the commuting groups, but not in the non-commuting group, further exacerbates findings concerning the detrimental effects of commuting, especially for females.

Also noticeable is the association between the attitude towards commuting/stress and Internet addiction [47]. Our findings point to a possible compensation of a negative attitude towards commuting by increased excessive Internet use. Interestingly, this association was only present in the business-commuter group and was independent of gender. Moreover, for the business-commuter group, again independent of gender, we observed a positive association between stress perception (attitude towards commuting) and CMD ("because of commuting I use digital devices more often"), which further supports this observation. The findings concerning the association between overall life satisfaction and Internet addiction, where females show more robust and stronger negative associations between Internet addiction and life satisfaction, also support earlier findings [48]. In this study, different thresholds have been suggested for females and males with respect to negative effects on life satisfaction because of high Internet use. Considering the present Internet addiction and commuting findings, one can denote forthcoming benefits from future studies examining what kinds of activities are done while commuting, and at what frequency. For instance, commuting time can be spent on work or learning new skills (e.g., via massive open online courses [49]) and should not be seen as fostering addictive tendencies towards digital technologies, per se. As previously mentioned, the diagnosis of Internet addiction depends on many criteria, but in the current research, it is merely the stressed commuter that is taken into account with regards to having higher Internet addiction tendencies.

The present study has strengths and also limitations worth noting. Firstly, using a cross-sectional design refrain us from causal inferences. It would be desirable to support the results of this study by replicating the main findings in longitudinal and experimental studies. Secondly, despite collecting a rather large sample, some group sizes (particularly the private-commuting group) used in the analyses are relatively small (see results section). Nevertheless, based on our considerations and findings we state that the discrimination between business and private commuters' data can be used in a meaningful way to shed further light on the intriguing association between psychological (and even physiological) variables and commuting behavior. In addition to this, our data collection was accomplished by means of self-report questionnaires, which usually inherits a certain chance for biases. Future studies could minimize this potential shortcoming by using multiple approaches, such as peer reports or data logging to collect data. Furthermore, it should be noted that statements about the generalization of our findings should be done so with caution, since it is difficult to precisely pinpoint the locations of the respondents. On the other hand, the present study was promoted nationwide in Germany and relies on a fairly large sample, which adds to the validity of the findings. In addition, it is important to consider that the ratio of participants (non-commuters, business-commuters, private-commuters) simply reflects the response-rate of the participants from a nationwide promotional campaign. Naturally, this ratio may not be fully representative of the general population. Lastly, a concern of the present study was to learn more about the association between commuting, life satisfaction and Internet addiction. Therefore, we focused on the motivation to commute (private and business) rather than the association between duration/distance and life satisfaction, which has previously been investigated. Since there is evidence that some commuters possibly consider commuting as a fulfilling activity (independent of the duration/distance of the commute) this may be a consideration for further studies to shed light on.

5. Conclusions

In conclusion, the present study underlines the association between life satisfaction, stress perception, and commuting. Extending previous findings in literature, our results show that the reason to commute (business or private) has the potential to explain differences in life satisfaction variables, namely income and lodging. We also replicated previous findings concerning the gender specific role of stress in a commuting situation and its specific impact on females. Furthermore, we demonstrated that this association (in contrast to life satisfaction and commuting) did not vary, regardless of whether the commute was due to business or private reasons. Finally, the current study finds an association between the attitude towards commuting/stress and Internet addiction. Here, a more negative attitude towards commuting was associated with higher tendencies towards excessive use of the Internet. For future research, it would be beneficial to further investigate the association between the frequency and type of commuting behavior with Internet addiction. Moreover, strong insights can be provided by the use of applications to track activity on ubiquitous smartphones, while allowing access to specific questionnaires, and having GPS tracking activated. Essentially, this would mean combining self-reports with objective data directly collected from the smartphone. This research methodology will be complimentary to the emerging research discipline of Psychoinformatics [50]. Furthermore, this design would allow longitudinal studies to be conducted in an accessible and efficient way. Finally, future studies should aim to assess smartphone addiction, as inclinations of an overlap between Internet and smartphone addiction have been shown to exist [51,52], though they are not synonymous. Moreover, smartphones are clearly of high relevance in a commuter's life, and recently, associations between smartphone addiction and lower productivity have also been reported [53].

Acknowledgments: The present study was funded by the German Research Foundation (MO 2363/2-1). Moreover, the position of Christian Montag is funded by a Heisenberg grant awarded to him by the German Research Foundation (MO 2363/3-2).

Author Contributions: Bernd Lachmann and Christian Montag designed the study. Moreover they developed the attitude towards commuting (ATC) items. Christopher Kannen programmed the online platform and preprocessed the data. Bernd Lachmann performed statistical analyses. Bernd Lachmann wrote the manuscript. Christian Montag, Bernd Lachmann, Rayna Sariyska and Maria Stavrou critically worked on the manuscript. Moreover, Maria Stavrou checked the manuscript for language. All authors contributed substantially to the final version of the paper.

References

1. Becker, R.; Cáceres, R.; Hanson, K.; Isaacman, S.; Loh, J.M.; Martonosi, M.; Rowland, J.; Urbanek, S.; Varshavsky, A.; Volinsky, C. Human mobility characterization from cellular network data. *Commun. ACM* **2013**, *56*, 74–82. [CrossRef]
2. Mokhtarian, P.L.; Salomon, I. Travel for the fun of it. *ACCESS Mag.* **1999**, *15*, 26–31.
3. Stutzer, A.; Frey, B.S. Commuting and life satisfaction in Germany. *Small* **1992**, *44*, 179–189.
4. Pfaff, S. Pendelentfernung, Lebenszufriedenheit und Entlohnung/Commuting Distance, Life Satisfaction, and Wages. *Z. Soziol.* **2014**, *43*, 113–130. [CrossRef]
5. Stutzer, A.; Frey, B.S. Stress that doesn't pay: The commuting paradox. *Scand. J. Econ.* **2008**, *110*, 339–366. [CrossRef]
6. Hoehner, C.M.; Barlow, C.E.; Allen, P.; Schootman, M. Commuting distance, cardiorespiratory fitness, and metabolic risk. *Am. J. Prev. Med.* **2012**, *42*, 571–578. [CrossRef] [PubMed]
7. Urhonen, T.; Lie, A.; Aamodt, G. Associations between long commutes and subjective health complaints among railway workers in Norway. *Prev. Med. Rep.* **2016**, *4*, 490–495. [CrossRef] [PubMed]
8. Gottholmseder, G.; Nowotny, K.; Pruckner, G.J.; Theurl, E. Stress perception and commuting. *Health Econ.* **2009**, *18*, 559–576. [CrossRef] [PubMed]
9. Friedman, H.S.; Kern, M.L. Personality, Well-Being, and Health. *Annu. Rev. Psychol.* **2014**, *65*, 719–742. [CrossRef] [PubMed]
10. Gana, K.; Bailly, N.; Saada, Y.; Joulain, M.; Trouillet, R.; Hervé, C.; Alaphilippe, D. Relationship between life satisfaction and physical health in older adults: A longitudinal test of cross-lagged and simultaneous effects. *Health Psychol.* **2013**, *32*, 896–904. [CrossRef] [PubMed]
11. Künn-Nelen, A. Does commuting affect health? *Health Econ.* **2016**, *25*, 984–1004. [CrossRef] [PubMed]
12. Feng, Z.; Boyle, P. Do long journeys to work have adverse effects on mental health? *Environ. Behav.* **2014**, *46*, 609–625. [CrossRef]
13. Roberts, J.; Hodgson, R.; Dolan, P. "It's driving her mad": Gender differences in the effects of commuting on psychological health. *J. Health Econ.* **2011**, *30*, 1064–1076. [CrossRef] [PubMed]
14. Lyons, G.; Chatterjee, K. A human perspective on the daily commute: Costs, benefits and trade-offs. *Transp. Rev.* **2008**, *28*, 181–198. [CrossRef]
15. Fichter, C. Mobilität: Macht Pendeln unglücklich? Wirtschaftspsychol. Aktuell. 2015, pp. 23–26. Available online: http://www.wirtschaftspsychologie-aktuell.de/files/wirtschaftspsychologie-aktuell-2-2015-fichter.pdf (accessed on 13 September 2017).
16. Morris, E.A. Should we all just stay home? Travel, out-of-home activities, and life satisfaction. *Transp. Res. Part A Policy Pract.* **2015**, *78*, 519–536. [CrossRef]
17. Newman, D.B.; Tay, L.; Diener, E. Leisure and subjective well-being: A model of psychological mechanisms as mediating factors. *J. Happiness Stud.* **2014**, *15*, 555–578. [CrossRef]

18. Olsson, L.E.; Gärling, T.; Ettema, D.; Friman, M.; Fujii, S. Happiness and satisfaction with work commute. *Soc. Indic. Res.* **2013**, *111*, 255–263. [CrossRef] [PubMed]
19. Ostovar, S.; Allahyar, N.; Aminpoor, H.; Moafian, F.; Nor, M.B.M.; Griffiths, M.D. Internet addiction and its psychosocial risks (depression, anxiety, stress and loneliness) among Iranian adolescents and young adults: A structural equation model in a cross-sectional study. *Int. J. Ment. Health Addict.* **2016**, *14*, 257–267. [CrossRef]
20. Lepp, A.; Li, J.; Barkley, J.E.; Salehi-Esfahani, S. Exploring the relationships between college students' cell phone use, personality and leisure. *Comput. Hum. Behav.* **2015**, *43*, 210–219. [CrossRef]
21. Riedl, R.; Kindermann, H.; Auinger, A.; Javor, A. Technostress from a neurobiological perspective. *Bus. Inf. Syst. Eng.* **2012**, *4*, 61–69. [CrossRef]
22. Montag, C.; Reuter, M. *Internet Addiction: Neuroscientific Approaches and Therapeutical Implications Including Smartphone Addiction*; Springer: Berlin, Germany, 2017.
23. Brand, M.; Young, K.S.; Laier, C.; Wölfling, K.; Potenza, M.N. Integrating psychological and neurobiological considerations regarding the development and maintenance of specific Internet-use disorders: An Interaction of Person-Affect-Cognition-Execution (I-PACE) model. *Neurosci. Biobehav. Rev.* **2016**, *71*, 252–266. [CrossRef] [PubMed]
24. Petry, N.M.; O'brien, C.P. Internet gaming disorder and the DSM-5. *Addiction* **2013**, *108*, 1186–1187. [CrossRef] [PubMed]
25. Young, K.S. Internet addiction: The emergence of a new clinical disorder. *Cyberpsychol. Behav.* **1998**, *1*, 237–244. [CrossRef]
26. Young, K.S. Psychology of computer use: XL. Addictive use of the Internet: A case that breaks the stereotype. *Psychol. Rep.* **1996**, *79*, 899–902. [CrossRef] [PubMed]
27. Tao, R.; Huang, X.; Wang, J.; Zhang, H.; Zhang, Y.; Li, M. Proposed diagnostic criteria for internet addiction. *Addiction* **2010**, *105*, 556–564. [CrossRef] [PubMed]
28. Rumpf, H.; Meyer, C.; Kreuzer, A.; John, U.; Merkeerk, G. Prävalenz der Internetabhängigkeit (PINTA). Available online: https://www.bundesgesundheitsministerium.de/fileadmin/Dateien/5_Publikationen/Drogen_und_Sucht/Berichte/PINTA-Kurzbericht-Endfassung_140711_korr.pdf (accessed on 13 September 2017).
29. Montag, C.; Bey, K.; Sha, P.; Li, M.; Chen, Y.; Liu, W.; Zhu, Y.; Li, C.; Markett, S.; Keiper, J. Is it meaningful to distinguish between generalized and specific Internet addiction? Evidence from a cross-cultural study from Germany, Sweden, Taiwan and China. *Asia Pac. Psychiatry* **2015**, *7*, 20–26. [CrossRef] [PubMed]
30. Pontes, H.; Griffiths, M. Internet addiction disorder and internet gaming disorder are not the same. *J. Addict. Res. Ther.* **2014**, *5*, e124. [CrossRef]
31. Davis, R.A. A cognitive-behavioral model of pathological Internet use. *Comput. Hum. Behav.* **2001**, *17*, 187–195. [CrossRef]
32. Hosseinkhanzadeh, A.A.; Taher, M. The relationship between personality traits with life satisfaction. *Sociol. Mind* **2013**, *3*, 99–105. [CrossRef]
33. Specht, J.; Egloff, B.; Schmukle, S.C. Examining mechanisms of personality maturation the impact of life satisfaction on the development of the big five personality traits. *Soc. Psychol. Personal. Sci.* **2013**, *4*, 181–189. [CrossRef]
34. Steel, P.; Schmidt, J.; Shultz, J. Refining the relationship between personality and subjective well-being. *Psychol. Bull.* **2008**, *134*, 138–161. [CrossRef] [PubMed]
35. Gutiérrez, J.L.G.; Jiménez, B.M.; Hernández, E.G.; Pcn, C. Personality and subjective well-being: Big five correlates and demographic variables. *Personal. Individ. Differ.* **2005**, *38*, 1561–1569. [CrossRef]
36. Rammstedt, B.; John, O.P. Measuring personality in one minute or less: A 10-item short version of the Big Five Inventory in English and German. *J. Res. Personal.* **2007**, *41*, 203–212. [CrossRef]
37. John, O.P.; Donahue, E.M.; Kentle, R.L. *The Big Five Inventory: Versions 4a and 54, Institute of Personality and Social Research*; University of California: Berkeley, CA, USA, 1991.
38. Diener, E.; Emmons, R.A.; Larsen, R.J.; Griffin, S. The satisfaction with life scale. *J. Personal. Assess.* **1985**, *49*, 71–75. [CrossRef] [PubMed]
39. Siedler, T.; Schupp, J.; Spiess, C.K.; Wagner, G.G. The German socio-economic panel as reference data set. *Schmollers Jahrb.* **2009**, *129*, 367–374. [CrossRef]

40. Pawlikowski, M.; Altstötter-Gleich, C.; Brand, M. Validation and psychometric properties of a short version of Young's Internet Addiction Test. *Comput. Hum. Behav.* **2013**, *29*, 1212–1223. [CrossRef]
41. Field, A.; Miles, J. *Discovering Statistics Using SAS*; SAGE Publications Ltd.: Thousand Oaks, CA, USA, 2011.
42. Baretta, D.; Greco, A.; Steca, P. Understanding performance in risky sport: The role of self-efficacy beliefs and sensation seeking in competitive freediving. *Personal. Individ. Differ.* **2017**, *117*, 161–165. [CrossRef]
43. Ruedl, G.; Abart, M.; Ledochowski, L.; Burtscher, M.; Kopp, M. Self reported risk taking and risk compensation in skiers and snowboarders are associated with sensation seeking. *Accid. Anal. Prev.* **2012**, *48*, 292–296. [CrossRef] [PubMed]
44. Erikson, R. Descriptions of Inequality: The Swedish Approach to Welfare Research. In *The Quality of Life*; Clarendon Press: Oxford, UK, 1993; pp. 67–87.
45. Tomaszewski, W.; Perales, F. Who settles for less? Subjective dispositions, objective circumstances, and housing satisfaction. *Soc. Indic. Res.* **2014**, *118*, 181–203. [CrossRef]
46. Koslowsky, M.; Aizer, A.; Krausz, M. Stressor and personal variables in the commuting experience. *Int. J. Manpow.* **1996**, *17*, 4–14. [CrossRef]
47. Riedl, R. Mensch-Computer-Interaktion und Stress. *HMD Prax. Wirtsch.* **2013**, *50*, 97–106. [CrossRef]
48. Lachmann, B.; Sariyska, R.; Kannen, C.; Cooper, A.; Montag, C. Life satisfaction and problematic Internet use: Evidence for gender specific effects. *Psychiatry Res.* **2016**, *238*, 363–367. [CrossRef] [PubMed]
49. Sun, G.; Cui, T.; Yong, J.; Shen, J.; Chen, S. MLaaS: A cloud-based system for delivering adapative micro learning in mobile MOOC learning. *IEEE Trans. Serv. Comput.* **2015**. [CrossRef]
50. Montag, C.; Duke, É.; Markowetz, A. Toward Psychoinformatics: Computer science meets psychology. *Comput. Math. Methods Med.* **2016**, *2016*. [CrossRef] [PubMed]
51. Duke, É.; Montag, C. Smartphone Addiction. In *Internet Addiction*; Springer: Cham, Switzerland, 2017; pp. 359–372.
52. Montag, C.; Sindermann, C.; Becker, B.; Panksepp, J. An affective neuroscience framework for the molecular study of Internet addiction. *Front. Psychol.* **2016**, *7*, 1906. [CrossRef] [PubMed]
53. Duke, É.; Montag, C. Smartphone addiction, daily interruptions and self-reported productivity. *Addict. Behav. Rep.* **2017**, *6*, 90–95. [CrossRef]

16

Social Exclusion, Surveillance Use and Facebook Addiction: The Moderating Role of Narcissistic Grandiosity

Myungsuh Lim

Department of Business Administration, Sangji University, Wonju 26339, Korea; mslim@sangji.ac.kr

Abstract: One hundred and eighty-eight participants completed the online questionnaire with items on demographics (age and gender), social exclusion, surveillance use, Facebook addiction, and narcissistic grandiosity. The findings showed that social exclusion was positively associated with Facebook addiction (B = 0.237, $p < 0.001$) and surveillance use was significantly positively associated with Facebook addiction (B = 0.211, $p < 0.01$). The surveillance use of Facebook was found to be a significant mediator between the risk of social exclusion on Facebook and Facebook addiction (B = 0.054, CI [0.20, 0.113]). Narcissistic grandiosity significantly moderated the associations between social exclusion and Facebook addiction (B = 0.079, $p = 0.012$). These findings suggest that the risk of social exclusion could serve as facilitator of Facebook addiction depending on narcissistic grandiosity.

Keywords: social exclusion; surveillance; Facebook addiction

---

1. Introduction

Although the use of Facebook has helped increase social capital and build relationships [1], "unfriending" on Facebook leads to negative emotions [2], promotes social media ostracism, and inhibits well-being [3]. A root cause of these negative effects is that Facebook is not always used to maintain or develop relationships. For example, voyeurism, a positive driver of Facebook use, is a form of social surveillance that fulfills the need to belong but attempts to avoid negative feelings and experiences; those who engage in it do not aim to maintain relationships with those they observe [1]. Moreover, Facebook is a platform that makes it easy to self-promote, allowing others to easily surveil the extensive content produced.

On the other hand, cyber-ostracism, which causes social exclusion on the Internet, has been found to be a threat to fundamental human needs, such as the needs of belonging and high self-esteem [4]. The negative effects of feeling excluded are not significantly different whether they arise in the context of a remote communication method or through in-person situations [5]. To cope with their online social exclusion, Facebook users may search for social information to restore their affiliation with other users [6], which facilitates their addiction to Facebook. On the other hand, people with narcissistic tendencies may be more likely to cope with social exclusion in order to maintain their ego-centric aspect [7], although the affiliation need is low [8].

Previous studies have shown that Facebook overuse to fill the need to belong can lead to Facebook addiction [9]. However, there is a lack of research identifying the mediation variables in the process of social exclusion and Facebook addiction and investigating social network attachment in social exclusion situations that do not meet the need to belong [10]. In addition, the self-presentation need [11] and the need for admiration [9] have been cited as the main reasons for using Facebook. Narcissism, in particular, has drawn attention as a major personality characteristic associated with problematic Facebook use [12]. The present research, therefore, investigated the following hypothetical relationships: (1) whether social exclusion on Facebook is positively related to addiction to Facebook;

(2) whether those with a narcissistic personality trait have a greater tendency to become addicted to Facebook as a way to avoid social exclusion; and (3) whether the use of Facebook for surveillance in response to social exclusion leads to Facebook addiction.

2. Hypotheses Development

2.1. Social Exclusion and Facebook Addiction

One of the main reasons that people use the Internet is to reveal themselves and to gain a sense of belonging [13]. A human being is innately motivated to belonging as a fundamental impetus to form and maintain relationships with others [14]. Social exclusion, which undermines the social affiliation that occurs on Facebook, happens when people are restricted from producing content or are unable to receive responses from others [15]. Addiction to social network services (SNS) is classified as Internet-related relationship addiction [16]. While whether SNS addiction should actually be classified as addiction is still debated, it does display relevant symptoms similar to other substance and behavioral addictions, such as mood-repair experience and salience (e.g., full attention to usage) [17]. Facebook is the leading SNS and has been shown to have strong correlations with symptoms classified as Internet addiction [18]. Addiction to Facebook interferes with vital activities in life, and virtual relationships dominate actual relationships [19].

Social exclusion may lead to Facebook addiction for the following reasons. First, social exclusion causes social anxiety. Socially anxious people are prone to becoming immersed in the Internet. According to the social skill model, high levels of social anxiety lead to the increased use of the Internet in order to elevate the sense of self-worth [13]. The fear of social exclusion increases the user's social risk, which leads to the pathological use of the Internet [13].

Second, users who feel socially excluded are motivated to restore their social affiliation, which may lead to Facebook addiction. They want to feel that they belong to a group, which includes affiliation and companionship [20]. Considering that the aim to identify one's social identity within the group to which one belongs and fulfill the need to belong is a significant predictor of the increase in SNS usage [12], social exclusion may make users more obsessed with SNSs. Hence, the lack of relatedness is connected to Facebook addiction [21].

Third, a primary driver of social media use is the fear of being excluded and forgotten, which increases the frequency of Facebook use [10,22]. For example, those snubbed by others on the phone attach to social networks to regain the feeling of social inclusion [10]. Both positive and negative feedback from other users affect Facebook users' well-being, and so does failure to receive feedback because FOMO (Fear of Missing Out) increases the Facebook-related stress stemming from not being popular or involved with peers on Facebook [23].

Hypothesis 1 (H1). *The higher the degree of social exclusion on Facebook is, the greater the Facebook addiction is.*

2.2. Social Exclusion and Surveillance Use

Interpersonal electronic surveillance refers to the use of communication technologies to observe another people's behavior both online and offline. The subjects of surveillance can be close friends, romantic partners, business associates, and family members [24]. Surveillance also allows users to maintain a healthy interpersonal relationship by constantly engaging with others [25]. However, it also compromises privacy settings [24]. Because SNSs, including Facebook, are repositories of messages, pictures, and videos, they provide an environment that facilitates surveillance. In the present study, surveillance concerns the use of surveillance in horizontal relationships between ordinary people [24].

Social exclusion may promote surveillance for the following reasons. Social exclusion promotes the heightened attention to social information and the processing of social information [26]. Social exclusion motivates both the need for belonging and the use of surveillance to cope with the sense of isolation [27] for successful social survival. Social exclusion induces the feeling of not belonging to a group, which generates negative effects, such as anxiety, loneliness, and antisocial behaviors [14]. Users who fear social exclusion continuously monitor their social status to maintain their feeling of social inclusion [28]. This behavior reduces the sense of loneliness caused by social exclusion [29], thus resolving social anxiety. This social monitoring system extends to the social environment and social opportunities [27]. This goal-directed behavior is motivated by the need for social affiliation. The sense of belonging is the innate, evolutionarily adaptive human motive [14]. People seek social information to classify the relationship with another party, to distinguish information that should be strategically stored for the relationship, and to verify the extent to which the social relationship is related to the event, when forming attribution [6]. In addition, the level of information processing at this time can be influenced by the degree of concern about the relationship [6]. Similarly, the social exclusion that users identify on Facebook forces them to face their uncertain social status [30] and to pursue goal-relevant behavior to restore their sense of social affiliation. Users who feel socially excluded are sensitive to social information and actively process it [6]. Based on the above discussion, the following hypothesis is stated:

Hypothesis 2 (H2). *The higher the degree of social exclusion is on Facebook is, the higher the use of Facebook for surveillance is.*

2.3. Surveillance Use and Facebook Addiction

Surveillance use may lead to Facebook addiction for the following reasons. First, remote technologies such as the Internet increase the effect of disinhibition effect on users [31]. Therefore, the effects of social exclusion online to users can be just as powerful as those of social exclusion offline [32]. Because social exclusion online motivates the need to belong [33], Facebook is frequently used for surveillance [34]. People who feel lonely because of social exclusion exhibit higher levels of social monitoring and scanning the environment for social cues [27].

Second, the function of mutual surveillance on Facebook enhances addiction. Facebook's surveillance function keeps people informed about their connections and personal information [35]. Therefore, when social exclusion occurs, people can access social information on Facebook, which increases the number of alternative actions that can compensate for the lack of social relationships. Users pursue surveillance gratification by viewing photographs or newsfeeds on Facebook, which may be associated with the fear of "missing out" [36]. Individuals who have experienced social exclusion may become addicted to Facebook by using Facebook's informative functions to overcome the sense of isolation. Based on the above discussion, the following hypothesis is stated.

Hypothesis 3 (H3). *The higher the use of Facebook for surveillance is, the greater Facebook addiction is.*

2.4. The Mediating Role of Surveillance Use

This study supports recent findings that anxiety about social exclusion (e.g., FOMO) causes surveillance use [37]. As discussed, the FOMO and the need to belong motivate people to overcome uncertainty about their social positions by seeking social information, which encourages surveillance use of Facebook. A lack of a sense of social belonging thus can result from being addicted to Facebook through passive, continuous monitoring of relationships rather than being stimulated to actively form relationships. The Facebook environment also promotes disinhibition in individuals, and the mutual surveillance function of Facebook leads to addiction among those using it for surveillance. Based on this theoretical review, the following hypothesis is proposed:

Hypothesis 4 (H4). *Surveillance use mediates the relationship between social exclusion and Facebook addiction.*

2.5. Moderating Effects of Grandiosity on Social Exclusion and Facebook Addiction

There may be individual differences in the responses to social exclusion [38]. Narcissistic grandiosity is characterized by arrogant, conceited, and domineering attitudes and behaviors based on maladaptive self-enhancement. Unlike others, narcissists have heightened needs for recognition and admiration [39]. In addition, individuals who exhibit the characteristics of narcissistic grandiosity are highly concerned about impression management [40], which frequently occurs on Facebook [41]. If social exclusion occurs on Facebook, the grandiose narcissist will try to find ways to maintain self-enhancement.

Therefore, narcissistic grandiosity may become a variable that has a moderating effect on personal differences in the relation between social exclusion and Facebook addiction. The reasons are as follows. First, the primary reason that narcissists use Facebook is self-exhibition. Therefore, they continuously pursue their intention to use Facebook even in the context of social exclusion. Narcissists have low affiliation needs [8]. Their reason for social networking is not to build social relationships but to present themselves as superior to others [1]. Despite their social exclusion, they can still be addicted to social networking without the surveillance intention and the need to acquire social information about others. Furthermore, they tend to have a high propensity for addiction to SNSs per se [12]. Exhibitionism is a powerful motivator for narcissists to use SNSs [42]. They seek a wide audience rather than social interaction [43]. Their behavior to attract attention becomes stronger when they are socially excluded, which leads to SNS addiction.

Second, a high degree of narcissistic grandiosity promotes unstable self-esteem [44]. Those with unstable self-esteem respond more sensitively to social exclusion than others do [45]. They think that they can stabilize their self-esteem by immersing themselves in online activity [46]. Persons with a high narcissistic tendency and high inconsistency between explicit and implicit self-esteem continually monitor their position because they are insecure and prone to self-doubt [47]. In this case, perceived social anxiety is a major factor in the problematic use of the Internet [13]. In addition, social anxiety is related to low self-esteem [17].

Third, narcissists tend to respond more strongly to social exclusion than others do [48]. They want to avoid the negative result of social exclusion. Narcissists perceive exclusion, such as social rejection, as a serious threat to their ego [48]. Furthermore, users with narcissistic grandiosity are impulsive, which exacerbates their addiction to SNS [49]. Based on the foregoing theoretical review, the following hypothesis is stated.

Hypothesis 5 (H5). *The direct effect of social exclusion on Facebook addiction is contingent on narcissistic grandiosity such that the effect is stronger in those who are high in narcissistic grandiosity.*

2.6. The Research Model

The current study aims to examine the association between social exclusion and Facebook addiction. The research model derived from the findings of the literature review is based on the following assumptions: (1) a positive association exists between social exclusion as predictor variable (X) and Facebook addiction as the dependent variable (Y); (2) this association is mediated by positive surveillance use as mediator variable (M); and (3) grandiosity as moderator variable (W) moderates the direct associations hypothesized, and associations are stronger in individuals with higher grandiosity.

3. Materials and Methods

3.1. Participants and Procedure

Upon their agreement to participate in the study, the participants were informed that they would be asked to discuss their personal experiences regarding Facebook. No conflicts of interest were reported in the current study. The participants recruited from CrowdFlower (Figure eight, San Francisco, USA), a crowdsourcing data collection platform, completed the survey (Mean age = 32.64,

Standard Deviation (SD) = 23.16; females = 60.6%; n = 188). The area of data collection was limited to inside the United States. The average survey completion time was 3.51 min (SD = 3.07). The online introduction explained the policy on privacy protection to all participants before the survey began. The survey introduction described the monetary reward, and after completing the survey, the participants were paid through virtual accounts. All procedures followed were in accordance with the ethical standards of the responsible institutional committee on human experimentation.

3.2. Measures

A 26-item, English-language survey was designed using Qualtrics.com (https://www.qualtrics.com). Before they answered the questions, the survey asked the participants to recall a real interaction with a Facebook friend, such as a romantic partner, co-worker, colleague, virtual friend, etc., whom we named 'X'. While the participants were recalling the relationship with 'X', they indicated the extent of their social exclusion from X, the extent of their use of Facebook for surveillance and the extent of their Facebook addiction. They then checked whether they had the propensity for narcissistic grandiosity (see the Appendix A). Finally, the participants marked gender and age according to their demographic.

Unless otherwise indicated, the measures are based on a 7-point Likert-type scale (1 = strongly disagree, 7 = strongly agree). Social exclusion was measured using four of the six items on the Perceived Risk of Exclusion Scale [50]. Because the two excluded items were assumed to concern social exclusions offline, they were not suitable for the study of social exclusion on Facebook. An example is "I wonder if X might try to avoid me". The participants responded on scales regarding the extent to which the Facebook user perceived the possible risk of exclusion and avoidance by the Facebook friend. The items were summed (Cronbach's $\alpha = 0.921$). Facebook surveillance was measured using four items [51]. These items were selected to assess the extent to which the participants agreed with the behaviors of paying attention to and monitoring the Facebook friend. An example of an item is "I view this person's profile to monitor his/her interactions and watch out for his/her best interests". The participant's responses were averaged (Cronbach's $\alpha = 0.725$). Facebook addiction was measured with six items [19]. These items assess addiction in SNS use. An example is "Since I have been on Facebook my grades/success on work have deteriorated/my performance at work is worse". The participants' responses were averaged (Cronbach's $\alpha = 0.867$). Narcissistic grandiosity was assessed by ten items. These items were used to measure the degree of the propensity for grandiose exhibition according to the Narcissistic Personality Inventory [52], the standard measure of subclinical narcissistic traits. An example is "I really like to be center of attention". The participants responded on a scale ranging from 1 = "Not at all like me" to 7 = "Very much like me". Higher scores indicated higher narcissistic grandiosity. The summed items showed good reliability ($\alpha = 0.921$). Additionally, factor analysis was performed by applying varimax rotation to confirm the validity of the measure. In the results, the set of four factors accounted for 65.348% of the variance. The factor loading of the items ranged from 0.505 to 0.811, and all the items used had acceptable validity.

3.3. Statistical Analyses

The hypotheses were tested using model 5 in PROCESS macro [53], which allows statistical direct, indirect, and conditional direct effects to be assessed simultaneously. In testing the indirect effect of X on Y through M, the conditional direct effect of W was accounted for; furthermore, the conditional direct effect of W on the relationship between X and Y was tested while controlling for M. To test the indirect effects, 5000 bootstrapped resamples were used which generated a bias correction of 95% and adjusted confidence intervals (CI). The CIs that excluded zero demonstrated a statistically significant indirect effect. The two indirect effects were tested simultaneously using the same model that was used to test the conditional direct effect. To test the conditional direct effects, the predictor and moderator variables were mean-centered, and the significant conditional direct effects were decomposed by plotting the slopes at ±1 standard deviation [54].

4. Results

4.1. Preliminary Analyses

First, all the main study variables were tested for non-normality. All measures of skewness (−0.242 to 1.213) and kurtosis (−1.827 to 0.942) were below the cutoff of satisfaction. Second, Mahalanobis distance was used to check for multivariate outliers in the main study variables. Because no participant was found to be a multivariate outlier, the final study sample was 188 participants. Lastly, to decide what, if any, demographic control variables to include in the model testing, the bivariate correlations between the study variables and the demographic characteristics (for age and gender) were examined. The correlations were based on the demographic variable and the study variables. Therefore, age and gender were included as a control variable in all subsequent analyses. The means, standard deviations, and bivariate correlations of the study variables used in the analysis are shown in Table 1. All study variables were intercorrelated in the predicted directions.

Table 1. Means, standard deviations, correlations, and alpha reliabilities [a] for variables.

Variables	M	SD	1	2	3	4
Social Exclusion	3.545	1.612	(0.921)			
Surveillance Use	4.026	1.273	0.328 **	(0.752)		
Facebook Addiction	2.756	1.434	0.515 **	0.455 **	(0.867)	
Grandiosity	3.131	1.333	0.405 **	0.421 **	0.610 **	(0.921)

Note: [a] on diagonal in parentheses, ** $p < 0.01$.

4.2. Testing the Research Model

The results showing the unstandardized regression coefficients are presented in Figure 1. This study first hypothesized that social exclusion is positively associated with Facebook addiction (H1). Figure 1 shows that social exclusion and Facebook addiction were indeed significantly and positively related, indicating that as social exclusion increased, so did Facebook addiction (B = 0.237, t = 4.508, $p < 0.001$, CI [0.133, 0.341]. Thus, H1 was supported. Next, social exclusion was positively associated with surveillance use (B = 0.259, t = 4.524, $p < 0.01$, 95% CI = [0.146, 0.371]). Thus, H2 was supported. In addition, surveillance use was positively associated with Facebook addiction (B = 0.211, t = 3.160, $p < 0.01$, 95% CI = [0.079, 0.342]). Thus, H3 was supported. This study predicted that the mediation model of social exclusion would be related to Facebook addictive tendencies through Facebook surveillance use (H4). The results showed that the indirect effect of social exclusion on Facebook addiction through Facebook surveillance use was significant (B = 0.054, CI [0.020, 0.113]). That is, when Facebook users reported higher levels of social exclusion, they also reported higher levels of Facebook surveillance use. Similarly, as Facebook surveillance use increased, Facebook addiction also increased. Thus, H4 was supported.

Lastly, this study hypothesized the conditional direct effect of narcissistic grandiosity on the relationship between social exclusion and Facebook addiction (H5). The results revealed that narcissistic grandiosity significantly moderated the relationship between social exclusion and Facebook addiction (B = 0.079, t = 2.526, $p = 0.012$, CI [0.017, 0.140]). Figure 2 illustrates this interaction, showing that there were differences between Facebook addiction at high levels of narcissistic grandiosity, at medium levels of narcissistic grandiosity, and at low levels of narcissistic grandiosity, Facebook users reported the highest levels of Facebook addiction when they also reported high levels of social exclusion. Thus, H5 was supported (see Table 2).

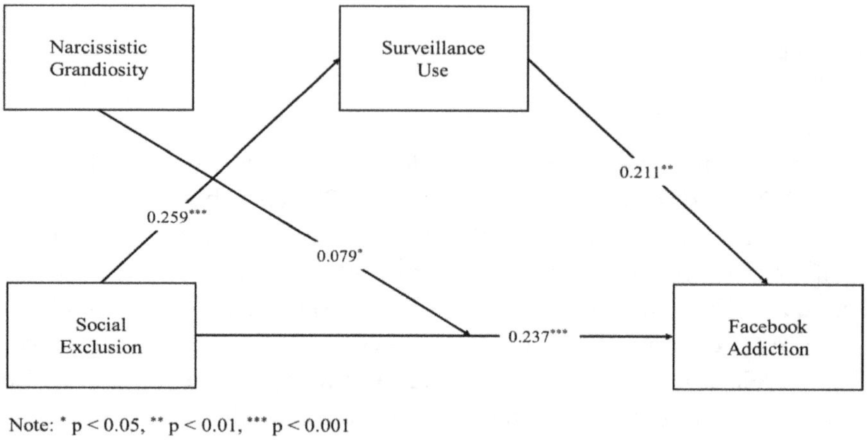

Figure 1. The indirect effect of surveillance use modeling and the conditional direct effect of narcissistic grandiosity on the relationship between social exclusion and Facebook addiction.

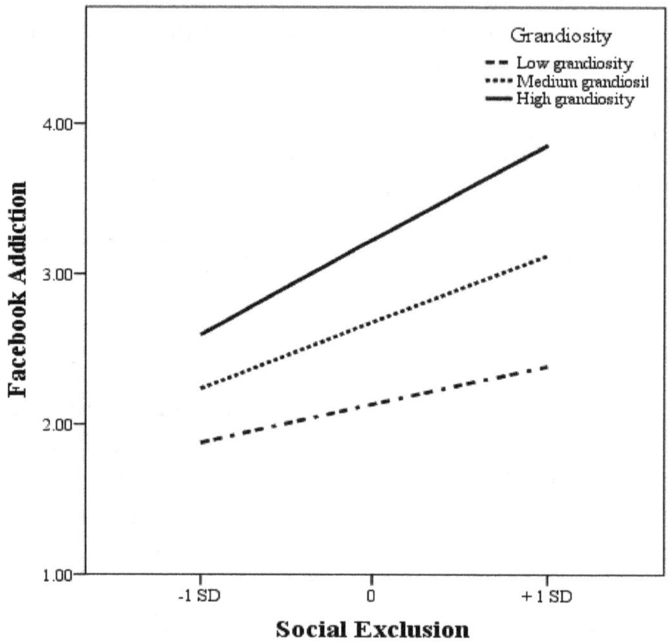

Figure 2. The conditional direct effect of narcissistic grandiosity on social exclusion and Facebook addiction.

Table 2. Conditional direct association of social exclusion on Facebook addiction (N = 188).

Narcissistic Grandiosity	Effect (Slope for Social Exclusion)	SE	*t*	*p*	LLCI	ULCI
Low (1.8)	0.131	0.064	2.073	0.040	0.006	0.257
Medium (3.13)	0.237	0.053	4.508	<0.001	0.133	0.341
High (4.46)	0.342	0.070	4.865	<0.001	0.203	0.481

Note: SE (Standard Error), LLCI & ULCI (Low and Upper Levels for Confidence Interval).

5. Discussion

The theoretical contributions of this research are as follows. This study elaborated an earlier study of Filipkowski and Smyth [5] that confirmed that the effects of online social exclusion on anxiety and emotions were as harmful as social exclusion in personal communication. This result of the present study indicated that the recent phenomenon of social exclusion on SNSs, which is highly common, can lead to surveillance behaviors and result in addiction.

The mediational role of surveillance use can be explained by the social connection theory and the environmental characteristics provided by Facebook. According to the social connection theory [55], social exclusion means that the need of social connection is not met. The loss of an SNS relationship increases the stress regarding social exclusion and further immerses the user in SNS use [56]. From an evolutionary perspective, humans have a basic need to attend to resources that provide social connections and satisfy the affiliation motivation [14,57]. On Facebook, user-generated content is stored through various forms, such as location data, status and mood messages, comments to profiles, videos, and pictures [58]. These resources facilitate surveillance and may also be linked to Facebook addiction behaviors.

The present research refers to a negative aspect of SNS use, but other studies assert that the use of social resources through SNSs can improve user well-being [59,60]. Authentic behavior showing true self-presentation on an SNS can act as a predictor of well-being to enhance the longitudinal health of the user. However, it may not offer appropriate social capital, such as social support, to a person in a low state of well-being due to positivity bias in SNS communication [61]. The narcissistic tendencies this study examines as individual differences are characteristics found in SNS personalities [62], and also narcissistic tendencies are those of a disagreeable extrovert [63]. Therefore, narcissists who do not communicate through their true selves may attempt to pursue relational interests because they do not receive sufficient social support in SNSs where positive bias occurs. In this situation, the previous research on cyber-ostracism related to narcissism focused on aggression as a maladaptive behavior caused by social exclusion [4]. These results of the present study demonstrated that the higher the level of narcissistic grandiosity is, the more severe the Facebook addiction is as another form of maladaptive behavior.

The present study has several limitations that may serve as directions for future research. First, this research did not distinguish among the types of social exclusion and relationships (e.g., romantic partners, co-workers, colleagues, and virtual friends) on Facebook. The typical Facebook friends recalled in the survey comprised heterogeneous groups that differed in the strength of their ties, intimacy, and emotional bonding [64]. Distinguishing these friend groups can produce different results. For example, information processing differs according to whether the social exclusion is caused by collective rejection or dyadic rejection [6]. This distinction could also influence Facebook addiction, so it would be meaningful to distinguish the types of rejection that cause social exclusion. In addition, the intensity of the relationships between romantic partners, coworkers and virtual friends differed. For example, according to the relationship type, social exclusion may result in different anti-social behaviors. Offensive behavior due to social exclusion is more frequent in easily replaced relationships than close relationships [65]. For example, in the case of strong ties (e.g., romantic partners) facing increased relational uncertainty, surveillance can be pursued as negative maintenance of romantic partnerships [66]. Meanwhile, the weak ties among some acquaintances (e.g., work colleagues) may benefit more from direct interactions. Thus, under weak ties, Facebook surveillance in social exclusion can be intensified [64]. Therefore, in the present study, the intensity of the relationship could have affected the causal relationship between the research variables. However, this study did not consider social exclusion and the correlations arising from different type of relationships because it evaluated various relationship types simultaneously in the survey condition. Therefore, in future research, the differences in the indirect effects of surveillance use should be distinguished in the relation with social exclusion and Facebook addiction depending on the type of relationship.

Second, demographic variables including individual differences were not used to confirm the correlations in the model, but future research should introduce them as crucial variables. Individuals have different reactions to social exclusion. For example, individuals with feelings of loneliness or a high need for social belonging are likely to monitor social information [27]. Those in closed romantic relationships might seek information about ex-partners through Facebook surveillance to reduce relational uncertainty, which causes emotional distress [67]. Thus, to deeply understand the specific personal relationship situations (e.g., romantic break-ups) that affect Facebook surveillance use and addiction, the current research model should reflect the characteristics of the users' networks. For example, do other users in Facebook users' networks actively use SNS in terms of the generation? Are there gender differences in responses to relational problems? The results suggested that females respond more negatively than males to interpersonal stressors such as social exclusion [68]. How important are the formation and dissolution of relationships in the life cycle as marital status varies by individual choice? After all, users' personal characteristics can affect their Facebook networks. To increase the validity of this research model, therefore, it is necessary to follow changes in the relationships between the variables by including individual difference variables.

Third, attention should be paid to the interpretation of the narcissistic personal trait, which serves as a moderating variable in this study. This study used narcissistic grandiosity to measure the subclinical narcissistic trait rather than the index to evaluate narcissistic personality disorder. These items used by Gentile et al. [69] reflect the tendency of college students to show more narcissistic personal traits than morbidity than did those of previous decade and also limit the ability of the results to track Facebook usage patterns. Even considering narcissistic tendencies as a minor trait, the amount of time a user takes editing on Facebook before intentionally showing themselves [69] could affect the use of Facebook. In the DSM-5 [70], histrionic personality and narcissistic personality overlap in their pursuit of attention and focus on impression management. In this study, the narcissistic tendencies are framed by emphasis on self-enhancement based on grandiose gestures. On the other hand, research on histrionic disorder tendencies on SNSs explores behavior such as exaggeration of the attractiveness of the selfie [71]. However, there is also a study that defines a focus on selfies as narcissistic behavior [72]. Therefore, it is necessary for future SNS-user research to more clearly discuss differences between the behaviors exhibited by the users with these disorders.

Fourth, to generalize the research results, it is necessary to attempt to reduce future sampling errors. First of all, the number of samples should be increased. Fewer samples were used compared with the items used. Attention, therefore, should be paid to the interpretation of the results. As the sample size decreases, the standard deviation may increase, resulting in less accurate results and a non-response bias as some subjects might not be able to complete the survey. Additionally, if, in a small sample, only those interested in a topic participate in a survey, voluntary response bias occurs, increasing the chances of skewness in the responses [73]. Future studies, therefore, should have more survey participants to be able to generalize the measurement model. Also, this study validated the model limited to Facebook. To generalize the research results, it is necessary to confirm them by collecting variables from various SNS platforms.

Fifth, the constructs of the study were dependent on self-reported data, which are prone to bias [74]. Hence, future researchers are encouraged to employ objective measures to collect data from various sources to strengthen the reliability of the findings.

6. Conclusions

The purpose of this study was to identify the mediation role of surveillance use and the moderating effect of narcissistic grandiosity in the relationship between social exclusion and Facebook addiction. The study yielded several important findings, which have the following implications. First, social exclusion in Facebook is positively associated with Facebook addiction. Second, when social exclusion occurs on Facebook, the higher the degree of narcissistic grandiosity is, the stronger the Facebook addiction is. Third, when social exclusion is a factor that promotes Facebook addiction, surveillance use plays a mediating role to monitor social information between social exclusion and addiction.

Author Contributions: All parts were contributed by M.L.

Informed Consent: All procedures followed were in accordance with the ethical standards of the responsible committee on human experimentation (institutional and national) and with the Helsinki Declaration of 1975, as revised in 2000 (5). Informed consent was obtained from all patients for being included in the study.

Human and Animal Rights: All procedures performed in studies involving human participants were in accordance with the ethical standards of the institutional and/or national research committee and with the 1964 Helsinki declaration and its later amendments or comparable ethical standards.

Appendix A

Social exclusion

I sometimes feel as though X might ignore me.
I wonder if X might try to avoid me.
I suspect I might be shut out of conversation by X.
I think it is possible that X might treat me as if I am not there.

Surveillance use of Facebook

I view X's Facebook profile to monitor his/her interactions and watch out for his/her best interests.
I feel like monitoring X's Facebook page is sufficient to maintain this relationship.
I pay attention to X's Facebook updates as a way to know what he/she is doing w/o actually paying attention to him/her.
I pay attention to X's Facebook updates when I am scrolling through the newsfeed so I feel up-to-date on his/her life.

Facebook addiction

Since I have been on Facebook my grades/success on work have deteriorated/my performance at work is worse.
It happens to me that I sleep much less than usually because I stay longer with Facebook.
Sometimes I have an impression that I live two lives: one private and another virtual.
I would rather spend an afternoon and/or evening on Facebook than devote that time to any other activities.
I have better time with people that I have met over Facebook than with those that I know in person.
I fear that I might meet some of my virtual Facebook friends in real life.

Narcissistic grandiosity

I know that I am good because everybody keeps telling me so.
I like to be the center of attention.
I like to display my body.
I like to look at my body.
I am apt to show off if I get the chance.
I like to be complimented.
I like to start new fads and fashions.
I like to look at myself in the mirror.
I really like to be the center of attention.
I get upset when people don't notice how I look when I go out in public.

References

1. Mäntymäki, M.; Islam, A.N. The Janus face of Facebook: Positive and negative sides of social networking site use. *Comput. Hum. Behav.* **2016**, *61*, 14–26. [CrossRef]
2. Bevan, J.L.; Pfyl, J.; Barclay, B. Negative emotional and cognitive responses to being unfriended on Facebook: An exploratory study. *Comput. Hum. Behav.* **2012**, *28*, 1458–1464. [CrossRef]

3. Schneider, F.M.; Zwillich, B.; Bindl, M.J.; Hopp, F.R.; Reich, S.; Vorderer, P. Social media ostracism: The effects of being excluded online. *Comput. Hum. Behav.* **2017**, *73*, 385–393. [CrossRef]
4. Poon, K.-T.; Chen, Z. Assuring a sense of growth: A cognitive strategy to weaken the effect of cyber-ostracism on aggression. *Comput. Hum. Behav.* **2016**, *57*, 31–37. [CrossRef]
5. Filipkowski, K.B.; Smyth, J.M. Plugged in but not connected: Individuals' views of and responses to online and in-person ostracism. *Comput. Hum. Behav.* **2012**, *28*, 1241–1253. [CrossRef]
6. Gardner, W.L.; Pickett, C.L.; Brewer, M.B. Social exclusion and selective memory: How the need to belong influences memory for social events. *Pers. Soc. Psychol. Bull* **2000**, *26*, 486–496. [CrossRef]
7. Gabriel, M.T.; Critelli, J.W.; Ee, J.S. Narcissistic illusions in self-evaluations of intelligence and attractiveness. *J. Pers.* **1994**, *62*, 143–155. [CrossRef]
8. Elliot, A.J.; Thrash, T.M. Narcissism and motivation. *Psychol. Inq.* **2001**, *12*, 216–219.
9. Casale, S.; Fioravanti, G. Why narcissists are at risk for developing Facebook addiction: The need to be admired and the need to belong. *Addict. Behav.* **2018**, *76*, 312–318. [CrossRef]
10. David, M.E.; Roberts, J.A. Phubbed and alone: Phone snubbing, social exclusion, and attachment to social media. *J. Assoc. Consum. Res.* **2017**, *2*, 155–163. [CrossRef]
11. Nadkarni, A.; Hofmann, S.G. Why do people use Facebook? *Pers. Indiv. Differ.* **2012**, *52*, 243–249. [CrossRef] [PubMed]
12. Kuss, D.J.; Griffiths, M.D. Online social networking and addiction—A review of the psychological literature. *Int. J. Environ. Res. Public Health* **2011**, *8*, 3528–3552. [CrossRef] [PubMed]
13. Lee-Won, R.J.; Herzog, L.; Park, S.G. Hooked on Facebook: The role of social anxiety and need for social assurance in problematic use of Facebook. *Cyberpsych. Beh. Soc. N.* **2015**, *18*, 567–574. [CrossRef] [PubMed]
14. Baumeister, R.F.; Leary, M.R. The need to belong: Desire for interpersonal attachments as a fundamental human motivation. *Pol. Psychol. Bull* **1995**, *117*, 497–529. [CrossRef]
15. Tobin, S.J.; Vanman, E.J.; Verreynne, M.; Saeri, A.K. Threats to belonging on Facebook: Lurking and ostracism. *Soc. Influ.* **2015**, *10*, 31–42. [CrossRef]
16. Young, K.S. Internet addiction: Evaluation and treatment. *BMJ* **1999**, *7*, 351–352. [CrossRef]
17. Hong, F.Y.; Huang, D.H.; Lin, H.Y.; Chiu, S.L. Analysis of the psychological traits, Facebook usage, and Facebook addiction model of Taiwanese university students. *Telemat. Inform.* **2014**, *31*, 597–606. [CrossRef]
18. Lopez-Fernandez, O. Generalised Versus Specific Internet Use-Related Addiction Problems: A Mixed Methods Study on Internet, Gaming, and Social Networking Behaviours. *Int. J. Environ. Res. Public Health* **2018**, *15*, 2913. [CrossRef]
19. Milošević-Đorđević, J.S.; Žeželj, I.L. Psychological predictors of addictive social networking sites use: The case of Serbia. *Comput. Hum. Behav.* **2014**, *32*, 229–234. [CrossRef]
20. Pillow, D.R.; Malone, G.P.; Hale, W.J. The need to belong and its association with fully satisfying relationships: A tale of two measures. *Pers. Indiv. Differ.* **2015**, *74*, 259–264. [CrossRef]
21. Masur, P.K.; Reinecke, L.; Ziegele, M.; Quiring, O. The interplay of intrinsic need satisfaction and Facebook specific motives in explaining addictive behavior on Facebook. *Comput. Hum. Behav.* **2014**, *39*, 376–386. [CrossRef]
22. Przybylski, A.K.; Murayama, K.; DeHaan, C.R.; Gladwell, V. Motivational, emotional, and behavioral correlates of fear of missing out. *Comput. Hum. Behav.* **2013**, *29*, 1841–1848. [CrossRef]
23. Beyens, I.; Frison, E.; Eggermont, S. "I don't want to miss a thing": Adolescents' fear of missing out and its relationship to adolescents' social needs, Facebook use, and Facebook related stress. *Comput. Hum. Behav.* **2016**, *64*, 1–8. [CrossRef]
24. Tokunaga, R.S. Social networking site or social surveillance site? Understanding the use of interpersonal electronic surveillance in romantic relationships. *Comput. Hum. Behav.* **2011**, *27*, 705–713. [CrossRef]
25. Lampe, C.; Ellison, N.; Steinfield, C. A Face (book) in the crowd: Social searching vs. social browsing. In *Paper Presented at the Proceedings of the 2006 20th Anniversary Conference On Computer Supported Cooperative Work*; ACM Publications: New York, NY, USA, 2006; pp. 167–170.
26. Warburton, W.A.; Williams, K.D.; Cairns, D.R. When ostracism leads to aggression: The moderating effects of control deprivation. *J. Exp. Soc. Psychol.* **2006**, *42*, 213–220. [CrossRef]
27. Pickett, C.L.; Gardner, W.L.; Knowles, M. Getting a cue: The need to belong and enhanced sensitivity to social cues. *Pers. Soc. Psychol. Bull* **2004**, *30*, 1095–1107. [CrossRef]
28. Leary, M.R. Making sense of self-esteem. *Curr. Dir. Psychol. Sci.* **1999**, *8*, 32–35. [CrossRef]

29. Peplau, L.A. *Loneliness: A Sourcebook of Current Theory, Research, and Therapy*; John Wiley & Sons Inc.: New York, NY, USA, 1982; Volume 36.
30. Emmers, T.M.; Canary, D.J. The effect of uncertainty reducing strategies on young couples' relational repair and intimacy. *Commun. Q.* **1996**, *44*, 166–182. [CrossRef]
31. Suler, J. The online disinhibition effect. *Cyberpsychol. Behav.* **2004**, *7*, 321–326. [CrossRef]
32. Karlen, C.E.; Daniels, J.R. Cyberostracism and social monitoring: Social anxiety's effects on reactions to exclusion and inclusion online. In *Honors Projects 147*; Digital Commons@IWU: Bloomington, IN, USA, 2011.
33. Mäntymäki, M.; Islam, A.N. Voyeurism and exhibitionism as gratifications from prosuming social networking sites. In *Paper Presented at the 22nd European Conference on Information Systems (ECIS2014)*; Association for Information Systems: Atlanta, GA, USA, 2014.
34. Zhang, Y.; Tang, L.S.-T.; Leung, L. Gratifications, collective self-esteem, online emotional openness, and traitlike communication apprehension as predictors of Facebook uses. *Cyberpsychology Behav. Soc. Netw.* **2011**, *14*, 733–739. [CrossRef]
35. Trottier, D. Interpersonal surveillance on social media. *Can. J. Commun.* **2012**, *37*, 319–332. [CrossRef]
36. Ryan, T.; Chester, A.; Reece, J.; Xenos, S. The uses and abuses of Facebook: A review of Facebook addiction. *J. Behav. Addict.* **2014**, *3*, 133–148. [CrossRef] [PubMed]
37. Blackwell, D.; Leaman, C.; Tramposch, R.; Osborne, C.; Liss, M. Extraversion, neuroticism, attachment style and fear of missing out as predictors of social media use and addiction. *Pers. Individ. Differ.* **2017**, *116*, 69–72. [CrossRef]
38. Williams, K.D. Ostracism. *Annu. Rev. Psychol.* **2007**, *58*, 425–452. [CrossRef] [PubMed]
39. Pincus, A.L.; Cain, N.M.; Wright, A.G. Narcissistic grandiosity and narcissistic vulnerability in psychotherapy. *Pers. Disord. Theory Res. Treat.* **2014**, *5*, 439–443. [CrossRef] [PubMed]
40. Hart, W.; Adams, J.; Burton, K.A.; Tortoriello, G.K. Narcissism and self-presentation: Profiling grandiose and vulnerable Narcissists' self-presentation tactic use. *Pers. Individ. Differ.* **2017**, *104*, 48–57. [CrossRef]
41. Hall, J.A.; Pennington, N.; Lueders, A. Impression management and formation on Facebook: A lens model approach. *New Media Soc.* **2014**, *16*, 958–982. [CrossRef]
42. Panek, E.T.; Nardis, Y.; Konrath, S. Mirror or Megaphone: How relationships between narcissism and social networking site use differ on Facebook and Twitter. *Comput. Hum. Behav.* **2013**, *29*, 2004–2012. [CrossRef]
43. Carpenter, C.J. Narcissism on Facebook: Self-promotional and anti-social behavior. *Pers. Individ. Differ.* **2012**, *52*, 482–486. [CrossRef]
44. Cain, N.M.; Pincus, A.L.; Ansell, E.B. Narcissism at the crossroads: Phenotypic description of pathological narcissism across clinical theory, social/personality psychology, and psychiatric diagnosis. *Clin. Psychol. Rev.* **2008**, *28*, 638–656. [CrossRef] [PubMed]
45. Onoda, K.; Okamoto, Y.; Nakashima, K.I.; Nittono, H.; Yoshimura, S.; Yamawaki, S.; Ura, M. Does low self-esteem enhance social pain? The relationship between trait self-esteem and anterior cingulate cortex activation induced by ostracism. *Soc. Cogn. Affect. Neur.* **2010**, *5*, 385–391. [CrossRef] [PubMed]
46. Krämer, N.C.; Winter, S. Impression management 2.0: The relationship of self-esteem, extraversion, self-efficacy, and self-presentation within social networking sites. *J. Media Psychol.* **2008**, *20*, 106–116. [CrossRef]
47. Zeigler-Hill, V. Discrepancies between implicit and explicit self-esteem: Implications for narcissism and self-esteem instability. *J. Pers.* **2006**, *74*, 119–144. [CrossRef] [PubMed]
48. Twenge, J.M.; Campbell, W.K. "Isn't it fun to get the respect that we're going to deserve?" Narcissism, social rejection, and aggression. *Pers. Soc. Psychol. Bull* **2003**, *29*, 261–272. [CrossRef] [PubMed]
49. Wu, A.M.S.; Cheung, V.I.; Ku, L.; Hung, E.P.W. Psychological risk factors of addiction to social networking sites among Chinese smartphone users. *J. Behav. Addict.* **2013**, *2*, 160–166. [CrossRef] [PubMed]
50. Thau, S.; Derfler-Rozin, R.; Pitesa, M.; Mitchell, M.S.; Pillutla, M.M. Unethical for the sake of the group: Risk of social exclusion and pro-group unethical behavior. *J. Appl. Psychol.* **2015**, *100*, 98–113. [CrossRef] [PubMed]
51. McEwan, B. Sharing, caring, and surveilling: An actor–partner interdependence model examination of Facebook relational maintenance strategies. *Cyberpsychology Behav. Soc. Netw.* **2013**, *16*, 863–869. [CrossRef]
52. Ackerman, R.A.; Witt, E.A.; Donnellan, M.B.; Trzesniewski, K.H.; Robins, R.W.; Kashy, D.A. What does the Narcissistic Personality Inventory really measure? *Assessment* **2010**, *18*, 67–87. [CrossRef]

53. Hayes, A.F. *Introduction to Mediation, Moderation, and Conditional Process Analysis: A Regression-Based Approach*; Guilford Press: New York, NY, USA, 2013.
54. Aiken, L.S.; West, S.G.; Reno, R.R. *Multiple Regression: Testing and Interpreting Interactions*; Sage: New York, NY, USA, 1991.
55. Maner, J.K.; DeWall, C.N.; Baumeister, R.F.; Schaller, M. Does social exclusion motivate interpersonal reconnection? Resolving the "porcupine problem". *J. Pers. Soc. Psychol.* **2007**, *92*, 42–55. [CrossRef]
56. Chiou, W.-B.; Lee, C.-C.; Liao, D.-C. Facebook effects on social distress: Priming with online social networking thoughts can alter the perceived distress due to social exclusion. *Comput. Hum. Behav.* **2015**, *49*, 230–236. [CrossRef]
57. Buss, D.M. Evolutionary personality psychology. *Annu. Rev. Psychol.* **1991**, *42*, 459–491. [CrossRef] [PubMed]
58. Fuchs, C. New media, web 2.0 and surveillance. *Sociol. Compass* **2011**, *5*, 134–147. [CrossRef]
59. Kim, J.; Lee, J.E.R. The Facebook paths to happiness: Effects of the number of Facebook friends and self-presentation on subjective well-being. *Cyberpsychology Behav. Soc. Netw.* **2011**, *14*, 359–364. [CrossRef] [PubMed]
60. Steinfield, C.; Ellison, N.B.; Lampe, C. Social capital, self-esteem, and use of online social network sites: A longitudinal analysis. *J. Appl. Dev. Psychol.* **2008**, *29*, 434–445. [CrossRef]
61. Reinecke, L.; Trepte, S. Authenticity and well-being on social network sites: A two-wave longitudinal study on the effects of online authenticity and the positivity bias in SNS communication. *Comput. Hum. Behav.* **2014**, *30*, 95–102. [CrossRef]
62. Buffardi, L.E.; Campbell, W.K. Narcissism and social networking web sites. *Pers. Soc. Psychol. Bull* **2008**, *34*, 1303–1314. [CrossRef]
63. Paulhus, D.L. Normal narcissism: Two minimalist accounts. *Psychol. Inq.* **2001**, *12*, 228–230.
64. Koban, K.; Krüger, S. Out of sight, (Not yet) out of mind: The impact of tie strength on direct interaction and social surveillance among geographically close and long-distance Facebook friends. *Commun. Res. Report* **2018**, *35*, 74–84. [CrossRef]
65. Elshout, M.; Nelissen, R.; van Beest, I.; Elshout, S.; van Dijk, W. Situational precursors of revenge: Social exclusion, relationship type, and opportunity. *Pers. Relatsh.* **2017**, *24*, 291–305. [CrossRef]
66. Dainton, M.; Goodboy, A.K.; Borzea, D.; Goldman, Z.W. The dyadic effects of relationship uncertainty on negative relational maintenance. *Commun. Rep.* **2017**, *30*, 170–181. [CrossRef]
67. Tong, S.T. Facebook use during relationship termination: Uncertainty reduction and surveillance. *Cyberpsychology Behav. Soc. Netw.* **2013**, *16*, 788–793. [CrossRef] [PubMed]
68. Leary, M.R.; Tambor, E.S.; Terdal, S.K.; Downs, D.L. Self-esteem as an interpersonal monitor: The sociometer hypothesis. *J. Pers. Soc. Psychol.* **1995**, *68*, 518–530. [CrossRef]
69. Gentile, B.; Twenge, J.M.; Freeman, E.C.; Campbell, W.K. The effect of social networking websites on positive self-views: An experimental investigation. *Comput. Hum. Behav.* **2012**, *28*, 1929–1933. [CrossRef]
70. American Psychiatric Association. *Diagnostic and Statistical Manual of Mental Disorders (DSM-5®)*; American Psychiatric Pub.: Washington, DC, USA, 2013.
71. Sorokowski, P.; Sorokowska, A.; Frackowiak, T.; Karwowski, M.; Rusicka, I.; Oleszkiewicz, A. Sex differences in online selfie posting behaviors predict histrionic personality scores among men but not women. *Comput. Hum. Behav.* **2016**, *59*, 368–373. [CrossRef]
72. Arpaci, I.; Yalçın, S.B.; Baloğlu, M.; Kesici, Ş. The moderating effect of gender in the relationship between narcissism and selfie-posting behavior. *Per. Indiv. Differ.* **2018**, *134*, 71–74. [CrossRef]
73. The Disadvantages of a Small Sample Size. Available online: https://sciencing.com/disadvantages-small-sample-size-8448532.html (accessed on 17 September 2019).
74. Straub, D.; Limayem, M.; Karahanna-Evaristo, E. Measuring system usage: Implications for IS theory testing. *Manag. Sci.* **1995**, *41*, 1328–1342. [CrossRef]

17

A Phenotype Classification of Internet Use Disorder in a Large-Scale High-School Study

Katajun Lindenberg [1,*], Katharina Halasy [1], Carolin Szász-Janocha [1] and Lutz Wartberg [2]

1 Institute for Psychology, University of Education Heidelberg, 69120 Heidelberg, Germany; halasy@ph-heidelberg.de (K.H.); szaszc@ph-heidelberg.de (C.S.-J.)
2 German Center for Addiction Research in Childhood and Adolescence, University Medical Center Hamburg-Eppendorf, 20246 Hamburg, Germany; lwartberg@uke.de
* Correspondence: lindenberg@ph-heidelberg.de

Abstract: Internet Use Disorder (IUD) affects numerous adolescents worldwide, and (Internet) Gaming Disorder, a specific subtype of IUD, has recently been included in DSM-5 and ICD-11. Epidemiological studies have identified prevalence rates up to 5.7% among adolescents in Germany. However, little is known about the risk development during adolescence and its association to education. The aim of this study was to: (a) identify a clinically relevant latent profile in a large-scale high-school sample; (b) estimate prevalence rates of IUD for distinct age groups and (c) investigate associations to gender and education. *N* = 5387 adolescents out of 41 schools in Germany aged 11–21 were assessed using the Compulsive Internet Use Scale (CIUS). Latent profile analyses showed five profile groups with differences in CIUS response pattern, age and school type. IUD was found in 6.1% and high-risk Internet use in 13.9% of the total sample. Two peaks were found in prevalence rates indicating the highest risk of IUD in age groups 15–16 and 19–21. Prevalence did not differ significantly between boys and girls. High-level education schools showed the lowest (4.9%) and vocational secondary schools the highest prevalence rate (7.8%). The differences between school types could not be explained by academic level.

Keywords: Internet Use Disorder; prevalence; epidemiology; adolescence; latent profile analysis

---

1. Introduction

Internet Use Disorder (IUD) describes mental disorders due the problematic use of the Internet. Internet Gaming Disorder (IGD), a specific subtype of IUD characterized by the persistent and recurrent use of the Internet to engage in games, has been included in the DSM-5 section "conditions for further studies" [1] because of its significant health importance. The World Health Organization stated recently that Gaming disorder (GD) will be listed as independent diagnosis in the upcoming ICD-11 and defined GD as "a pattern of recurrent video-gaming" (online or offline), manifested by impaired control over gaming, increasing priority of gaming over other life interests and daily activities and continuation of gaming despite the occurrence of negative consequences, which results in significant impairment in personal, family, social, educational, occupational or other important areas of functioning and should be evident over a period of at least 12 months [2].

Non-gaming subtypes, such as problematic social media use, were not included in DSM-5 due to lack of empirical research. In ICD-11, however, other (non-gaming) Internet-related disorders can be classified as other specific disorders due to addictive behaviors. It is discussed that gaming and non-gaming IUD should be defined using the same criteria. Facing the multiple severe comorbidities and impairments which are associated with IUD, the early diagnosis is of particular interest [3–5]. Moreover, it is essential not only to identify but also to differentiate between adolescents with IUD and high-risk Internet use in order to tailor preventive interventions and treatments for those individuals most in need.

The DSM-5 group has noted that the majority of studies lack of a standard definition from which to derive prevalence data and called for further research [1]. The use of various conceptualizations, assessment tools and cut-off scores for estimating the prevalence of IUD led to widely heterogeneous findings of prevalence rates. International prevalence estimates for IUD in adolescents vary between 0.8% in Italy [6] and 26.7% in China [7]. A multinational meta-analysis of 31 nations revealed a global prevalence of 6.0% [8]. The estimate was based on the Young Diagnostic Questionnaire (YDQ) [9] and the Internet Addiction Test (IAT) [10]. The highest prevalence rates were reported in the Middle East and the lowest prevalence rates in Northern and Western Europe. Recent studies investigating IGD in Germany reported prevalence rates of 1.2% in adolescents aged 11–18 years [11] to 5.7% in adolescents and young adults aged 12–25 years [12].

In Europe, several studies have used the Compulsive Internet Use Scale (CIUS) to estimate the prevalence of IUD [13–15], which resulted in more homogeneous findings. The CIUS is a widely used questionnaire for assessing IUD [16,17] and for the German version of the instrument good psychometric properties were reported [18]. However, a sound cut-off score of the CIUS has not yet been identified to classify IUD and high-risk Internet users (HR-IU). The authors have suggested a cut-off score of 28 to identify IUD [17]. A study comparing the CIUS with the IAT proposed a cut-off value of 18 for case finding and 21 for prevalence estimates [19]. Furthermore, empirical data of a representative German sample suggested a cut-off score of 30 for prevalence estimates and a cut-off score of 24 for the detection of HR-IU [13]. As a methodological superior alternative to cut-off scores, previous research [14,15,20,21] has suggested to empirically identify distinct groups based on latent profiles to estimate the prevalence of clinically relevant IUD. Latent profile analysis (LPA) is a powerful method to classify phenotypes based on latent mixture modeling. It allows identification of underlying (or latent) groups of individuals on the basis of their response pattern across a set of indicators for IUD and thus, identifying the prevalence of the group characterized by clinically relevant IUD symptoms.

Applying LPA to CIUS data, Rumpf et al. [14] found a prevalence rate of 4.0% in German adolescents aged 14–16 years in a general population sample. In the total sample (14 to 64 years) the prevalence rate was 1.0%. In line with these results, a similar rate of 4.7% was classified as IUD based on latent profiles indicated by the CIUS [22]. In this large school survey, the latent profile classifying individuals with IUD showed a mean sum score of 30. Another empirically driven LPA using the CIUS revealed a prevalence of 3.2% in adolescents aged 14 to 17 years and a CIUS mean score of 31.93 in the profile group of adolescents with IUD [15]. These prevalence rates were confirmed by another representative study investigating prevalence based on external ratings by parents [20].

Findings about sociodemographic variables associated with IUD are inconsistent. Some studies assessing the relationship between gender and IUD reported higher prevalence rates in males [6,23–27]. Despite these, other studies found no difference between males and females e.g., [28] or higher prevalence rates in females e.g., [22]. Moreover, empirical research shows a higher association between males and gaming related IUD and females and non-gaming IUD including the use of social networking and other applications of the Internet [13,22,29]. Rehbein and Mößle [22] investigated gaming related IUD and non-gaming IUD separately and emphasized the need for differentiation in a number of ways. They reported a female preponderance of non-gaming IUD and a male preponderance of gaming related IUD. Furthermore, in students of grades 7 to 10, higher risk of non-gaming IUD was found in older students and higher risk of gaming related IUD in younger students. Although prevalence rates indicate that compared to adults adolescents seem to be particularly affected by IUD e.g., [14], currently it remains unclear how the risk for IUD develops (e.g., decreases or increases) over the course of adolescence. According to Cerniglia et al. [30] concerning this matter the specific neuro-developmental plasticity in adolescence is an important aspect.

Bakken et al. [31] conducted a prevalence study in a large representative Norwegian sample aged 16 to 74 years. They found highest prevalence rates among males aged 16–29 years. Furthermore, achieved high education level (university level vs. senior high school and junior high school) was positively associated with Internet addiction. In line with these results, other studies [27,32,33] showed a positive relationship between the current academic level (lower vs. higher degree of current education) and IUD. However, parental education level has shown to be negatively correlated with IUD [34].

Studies assessing the effects of age on IUD show inconsistent findings. A recent longitudinal study [26] revealed a decrease of IUD symptoms between 16 and 18 years. Another study [24] conducted in Croatia, Finland and Poland surveyed an adolescent sample of n = 1078 aged 11 to 18 years and reported the lowest risk of IUD among the 11–12 year old participants and the highest risk among the 15–16 year old participants. It was discussed that this peak was driven by a greater level of independence and less parental control over free time and social activities.

In sum, research assessing IUD, i.e., non-gaming IUD and (I)GD, show inconsistent findings with regard to epidemiology and sociodemographic risk factors. Therefore, it is a public health challenge to understand risk factors and upholding conditions which are associated with IUD in order to develop effective prevention programs and bring them to broader dissemination. Although research supported first evidence for an increase of risk in middle adolescence with a peak at the ages of 15 and 16, little is known about the development in late adolescence until the age of 21.

The purpose of this study was to: (a) empirically derive a clinically relevant latent profile characterized by an IUD phenotype in a large epidemiological sample of children and adolescents using LPA; (b) to estimate prevalence of IUD and HR-IU in adolescence; (c) to estimate the differential risk of IUD for distinct age groups from 11 to 21 years separately; (d) to identify effects of gender on risk of IUD and (e) to assess the associations between academic career and risk of IUD. To the best of our knowledge, this is the first large-scale epidemiological study investigating the prevalence rate for distinct age groups from early to late adolescence. We explored the following research questions: (1) How many different profile groups of adolescent Internet users can be identified in our sample by a LPA? (2) Is the number of profile groups comparable with the findings in previous studies? (3) What is the prevalence estimate of Internet Use Disorder (IUD) and high-risk Internet use (HR-IU) in our sample? (4) Are there gender differences in the prevalence of IUD and HR-IU? (5) Are there differences in the prevalence rates of IUD or HR-IU between different age groups? (6) Are there differences in the prevalence rates of IUD or HR-IU between different school types?

2. Materials and Methods

2.1. Data Collection

Data were collected within the PROTECT study (ClinicalTrials.gov: NCT02907658). Ethical approval was obtained from the University of Education Heidelberg Research Ethics Committee on 3 September 2015 (Az.: 7741.35-13). Approval from the Regierungspräsidium Karlsruhe was obtained on 19 October 2015 (Az.: 71c2-6499.25) for school-wide screenings and thus, individual written consent was not necessary. The study was supported by the Dietmar Hopp foundation, thus, in line with the funding priority we focused on schools in the Rhine-Neckar region and adjoining areas. Data collection was conducted in schools during regular school hours between September 2015 and February 2017. Target groups were students aged 11–21 from 41 secondary schools (convenience sample of schools). All types of schools within the German school system were included, i.e., low education level (Werkrealschule), middle education level (Realschule), high education level (Gymnasium), comprehensive schools (Gemeinschaftsschule), vocational school (Berufsschule) and vocational upper secondary school (Berufliches Gymnasium). Data collection was conducted by a team of trained psychologists. Teachers were present in the classroom during completion of the survey, but were not involved in the data collection. Total time for introduction and data collection in each class took approximately 20 min.

2.2. Measures

We used the German version of the Compulsive Internet Use Scale [18] for investigating the severity of IUD. The questionnaire consists of 14 items with a 5-level Likert-scale ranging from 0 = never to 4 = very often. Hence 0 to 56 points can be obtained in the total score. Internal consistency lies between Cronbach's $\alpha = 0.89–0.90$ [17]. The questionnaire has been translated to various languages and examined empirically. The German version was psychometrically validated in a representative sample of adolescents [18]. The majority of research supports a one dimensional structure of the scale [18,35,36]. We applied the same model as Meerkerk et al. [17], correlating the error variances of items 1 and 2, items 6 and 7, items 8 and 9, items 10 and 11 as well as items 12 and 13, and could confirm the one-dimensional structure of the instrument in our sample (RMSEA = 0.047, CFI = 0.962, TLI = 0.952) with standardized factor loadings between 0.33 (Item 8) and 0.64 (Item 14). Cronbach's α was 0.87 in our sample.

According to the authors, the CIUS assesses the symptoms loss of control, withdrawal symptoms, coping with unpleasant mood, mental and behavioral preoccupation as well as inter- and intrapersonal conflicts CIUS (see Table 1; [17,35,36]).

Table 1. Symptoms assessed by CIUS items.

	Symptoms Assessed by CIUS Items
1	Loss of control (LOC)
	1. How often do you find it difficult to stop using the Internet when you are online? 2. How often do you continue to use the Internet despite your intention to stop? 5. How often are you short of sleep because of the Internet? 9. How often have you unsuccessfully tried to spend less time on the Internet?
2	Withdrawal symptoms (WS)
	14. How often do you feel restless, frustrated, or irritated when you cannot use the Internet?
3	Coping with unpleasant mood (C)
	12. How often do you go on the Internet when you are feeling down? 13. How often do you use the Internet to escape from your sorrows or get relief from negative feelings?
4	Mental and behavioral preoccupation (MBP)
	4. How often do you prefer to use the Internet instead of spending time with others (e.g., partner, children, parents, friends *)? 6. How often do you think about the Internet, even when not online? 7. How often do you look forward to your next Internet session?
5	Inter- and intrapersonal conflicts (IIC)
	3. How often do others (e.g., partner, children, parents, friends *) say you should use the Internet less? 8. How often do you think you should use the Internet less often? 10. How often do you rush through your (home) work in order to go on the Internet? 11. How often do you neglect your daily obligations (work, school, or family life) because you prefer to go on the Internet?

Note: * "friends" was not mentioned in the original version by Meerkerk et al. [17] but was included in the German translation by Gürtler et al. [35] and Peukert et al. [36].

The five symptom scales were calculated by the means of respective variables (range 0–4). In addition to the CIUS, we recorded sociodemographic data consisting of age, gender, grade and school type.

2.3. Sample

Overall, 5549 students from 41 schools participated in the study (range 11–52 years). The high range in age was due to the inclusion of vocational schools. We excluded all students older than 21 years ($n = 162$), because our focus was to study IUD in adolescence. Remaining sample size was 5387 with a mean age of 14.72 ($SD = 1.96$). Gender ratio was 51.4% male, 47.3% female and 1.3% without information on their gender ($n = 68$). The age distribution was 613 11- to 12-year olds (11.4% of the sample), 2185 13- to 14-year olds (40.6%), 1526 15- to 16-year olds (28.3%), 865 17- to 18-year olds (16.1%), 198 19- to 21-year olds (3.7%). Overall, 11.6% of the pupils attended the "Werkrealschule" (low educational level), 11.4% "Realschule" (middle educational level), 40.4% "Gymnasium" (high educational level), 5.8% "Gesamtschule" (comprehensive school), 17.6% "Berufsschule" (vocational school) and 13.1% attended "berufliches Gymnasium" (vocational upper secondary school).

2.4. Statistical Analyses

All statistical analyses were conducted with SPSS Statistics for Windows version 24.0 (IBM, Armonk, NY, USA) and MPlus version 8 (Muthén & Muthén, Los Angeles, CA, USA). Because our aim was to empirically classify phenotypes based on the underlying latent profile, we chose LPA as statistical method. LPA is a person-centered approach which allows "... to classify individuals into distinct groups or categories based on individual response patterns so that individuals within a group are more similar than individuals between groups" [37] (p. 309). We tested six models including 1–6 latent profiles and used the Akaike information criterion (AIC), Bayesian information criterion, BIC, the entropy value as well as the Lo-Mendell-Rubin likelihood ratio test [38] as fit indices to compare the models. The BIC was given priority among the criteria as it has been found to be superior [39]. In line with prior studies [15], we allowed within-class correlations in the LPA between the CIUS items because of the given one-dimensionality [17], which we confirmed in our data. However, within-class correlations were restricted to be equal across classes. This procedure was equal to the study conducted by Wartberg et al. [15]. For comparison of the different profile groups, we used the Kruskal Wallis test due to disparity of variances and chi-square test for comparison of frequencies.

3. Results

3.1. Phenotype Classification Using LPA

LPA models varying the number of latent profiles from 1–6 were evaluated. BIC was lowest for a 5-profile solution, thus, the 5-profile solution was found to be the best-fitting model (see Table 2). The Lo-Mendell-Rubin likelihood ratio test for 4 (H0) versus 5 indicated that five profiles resulted in a significantly better model fit that four profiles ($p < 0.001$), whereas the Lo-Mendell-Rubin likelihood ratio test for five (H0) versus six profiles was no longer significant ($p = 0.51$), i.e., the inclusion of a sixth profile did not result in a better model fit. Of the total sample, $n = 134$ (2.5%) were members of latent profile group (LPG) 1, $n = 2483$ (46.1%) were members of LPG2, $n = 1695$ (31.5%) were members of LPG3, $n = 748$ (13.9%) were members of LPG4 and $n = 327$ (6.1%) were members of LPG5.

Table 2. Fit indices of the LPA.

Profile No.	AIC	BIC	Entropy	p (LMR-LRT)	Persons Per Profile Group, n	Relative Frequency
1	203,864.875	204,649.292			5387	
2	202,484.369	203,367.662	0.869	0.0000	4112 1275	0.76 0.24
3	201,610.314	202,592.484	0.948	0.0000	2510 2373 504	0.47 0.44 0.09
4	192,946.834	194,027.880	1.000	0.0000	2617 748 1695 327	0.49 0.14 0.31 0.06
5	192,753.95	193,933.868	0.975	0.0000	134 2483 1695 748 327	0.02 0.46 0.31 0.14 0.06
6	192,716.38	193,995.181	0.951	0.5069	2401 132 748 83 1696 327	0.45 0.02 0.14 0.02 0.31 0.06

Note: AIC = Akaike information criterion; BIC = Bayesian information criterion; LMR-LRT = Lo-Mendell-Rubin likelihood ratio test.

3.2. Comparison of Latent Profile Groups

A comparison of the CIUS total scores showed significant differences ($H = 1968.65$, $df = 4$, $p = 0.000$) between the 5 LPGs. Post hoc tests, with Bonferroni correction for multiple tests, showed significant differences between each of the five groups. The largest profile (LPG2) was characterized by a CIUS total score of $M = 12.07$ ($SD = 6.72$), loss of control $M = 0.96$ ($SD = 0.61$), withdrawal symptoms $M = 0.57$ ($SD = 8.84$), coping with unpleasant mood $M = 1.18$ ($SD = 1.02$), mental and behavioral preoccupation $M = 0.81$ ($SD = 0.68$), inter- and intrapersonal conflicts $M = 0.73$ ($SD = 0.53$). The differences in symptom severity across profile groups can be found in Table 3.

LPG5 was characterized by the highest CIUS total scores ($M = 32.16$, $SD = 9.01$). The values of all symptom scales were significantly higher in LPG5 as compared to all other profiles (loss of control $M = 2.28$, $SD = 0.78$; withdrawal symptoms $M = 2.06$, $SD = 1.33$; coping with unpleasant mood $M = 2.57$, $SD = 1.26$; mental and behavioral preoccupation $M = 2.11$, $SD = 0.97$; inter- and intrapersonal conflicts $M = 2.40$, $SD = 0.67$).

The LGP with the second highest burden was LPG4 (CIUS total score $M = 24.64$, $SD = 7.55$; loss of control $M = 1.84$, $SD = 0.70$; withdrawal symptoms $M = 1.39$, $SD = 1.14$; coping with unpleasant mood $M = 2.08$, $SD = 1.16$; mental and behavioral preoccupation $M = 1.55$, $SD = 0.80$; inter- and intrapersonal conflicts $M = 1.79$, $SD = 0.58$).

3.3. Prevalence Estimates of IUD and HR-IU

Based on the profile characteristics, LPG5 was found to be the group that comprises individuals with IUD. It consisted of 327 adolescents. Thus, the prevalence of IUD was found to be 6.1% in the total sample. LPG4 was defined as HR-IU group. It included 748 adolescents and accounted for 13.9% of the total sample. Clinically relevant IUD symptoms were absent in LPG1, LPG2 and LPG3, thus, these groups are defined as unproblematic Internet users.

Table 3. Symptom severity across profile groups: mean CIUS symptom scales and total score.

Parameter	TS	PG1	PG2	PG3	PG4 HR-IU	PG5 IUD	*H*	*df*	*p*
N	5387	134	2483	1695	748	327			
Mean age	14.72 (1.96)	14.31 (1.95)	14.48 (1.95)	14.89 (1.93)	15.06 (1.98)	15.14 (1.91)	108.80	4	0.000
CIUS total score	17.24 (9.27)	20.60 (6.87)	12.07 (6.72)	18.40 (7.35)	24.64 (7.55)	32.16 (9.01)	1968.65	4	0.000
Loss of control (LOC)	1.34 (0.78)	1.99 (0.72)	0.96 (0.61)	1.43 (0.69)	1.84 (0.70)	2.28 (0.78)	1410.05	4	0.000
Withdrawal symptoms (WS)	0.90 (1.07)	0.93 (1.09)	0.57 (0.84)	0.96 (1.03)	1.39 (1.14)	2.06 (1.33)	698.56	4	0.000
Coping with unpleasant mood (C)	1.53 (1.15)	1.74 (1.09)	1.18 (1.02)	1.60 (1.08)	2.08 (1.16)	2.57 (1.26)	615.27	4	0.000
Mental and behavioral preoccupation (MBP)	1.11 (0.81)	1.08 (0.71)	0.81 (0.68)	1.17 (0.72)	1.55 (0.80)	2.11 (0.97)	937.37	4	0.000
Inter- and intrapersonal conflicts (IIC)	1.16 (0.74)	1.28 (0.59)	0.73 (0.53)	1.27 (0.56)	1.79 (0.58)	2.40 (0.67)	2127.43	4	0.000

Notes: Profiles were compared using Kruskal-Wallis *H*-test. Values are presented as means (with *SD* in parentheses). TS = total sample, LPG = latent profile group, HR-IU = high risk Internet use, IUD = Internet Use Disorder, *H* = Kruskal Wallis test statistic.

3.4. Differential Risk for Distinct Age Groups

We found significant difference in the distribution of age across the five profile groups ($H = 108.80$, $df = 4$, $p = 0.000$). Post hoc tests showed significant differences between profile group 1 compared to profile groups 3, 4, 5 ($p = 0.002$, $p = 0.000$, $p = 0.000$), profile group 2 and profile groups 3, 4, 5 ($p = 0.000$ respectively). Relative frequencies of LPG 5 (IUD) increased with rising age, with prevalence peaks at the age groups of 15- to 16-year-olds and 19- to 21-year-olds (see Figure 1). The prevalence of IUD was 2.8% for the 11- to 12-year-olds (17 of 613), 5.5% for the 13- to 14-year-olds (121 of 2185), 7.6% for the 15- to 16-year-olds (116 of 1526), 6.4% for the 17- to 18-year-olds (55 of 865) and 9.1% for the 19- to 21-year-olds (18 of 198) adolescents. The same pattern was found in LGP4 (HR-IU). Relative frequencies increased with rising age, with prevalence peaks at the age groups of 15- to 16-year-olds and 19- to 21-year-olds. The prevalence of HR-IU was 10.0% for the 11- to 12-year-olds (61 of 613),

12.4% for the 13- to 14-year-olds (272 of 2185), 16.1% for the 15- to 16-year-olds (246 of 1526), 14.6% for the 17- to 18-year-olds (126 of 865) and 21.7% for the 19- to 21-year-olds (43 of 198) adolescents.

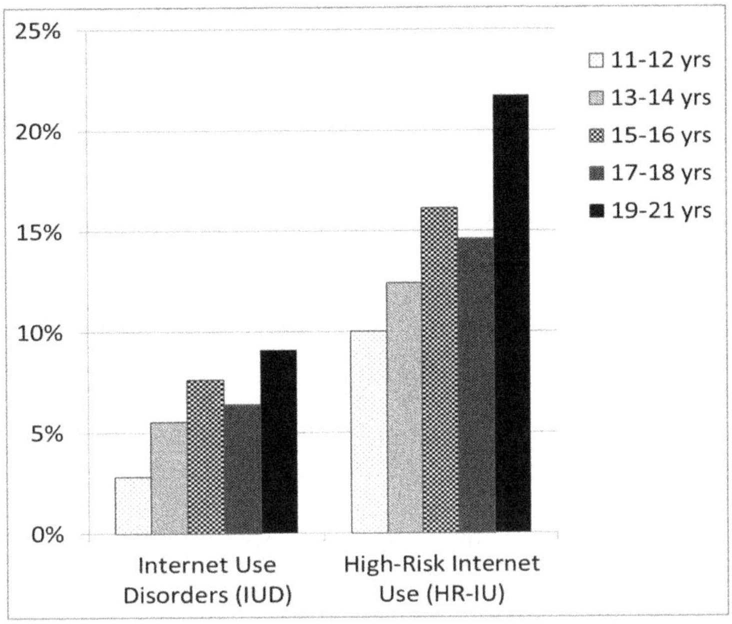

Figure 1. Changes in prevalence rates from early to late adolescence in IUD: two peaks at 15–16 and 19–21 years.

3.5. Gender Effects

We did not find significant gender effects in profile group membership (LPG1 2.2% males vs. 2.8% females; LPG2 45.8% males vs. 46.5% females; LPG3 32.8% males vs. 30.2% females; LPG4 13.4% males vs. 14.4% females; LPG5 5.9% males vs. 6.2% females; χ^2 (4) = 6.27, p = 0.18).

3.6. Associations between Education and IUD

Because age groups were not equally distributed across school types in the German school system, we analyzed associations between education and IUD or HR-IU for different age groups. As presented in Table 4, prevalence rates of IUD and HR-IU differed between school types. Within the same school type, risk increased with age.

Table 4. Associations of school type (separated by age group) and prevalence of IUD/HR-IU.

		11–12 Years	13–14 Years	15–16 Years	17–18 Years	19–21 Years
Low Educational Level	**IUD**	1.2%	7.9%	7.9%	-	-
	HR-IU	19.5%	14.2%	15.8%	-	-
Middle Educational Level	**IUD**	5.7%	6.7%	11.4%	-	-
	HR-IU	13.8%	13.1%	18.6%	-	-
High Educational Level	**IUD**	2.4%	4.8%	6.5%	-	-
	HR-IU	7.1%	12.6%	18.5%	-	-
Comprehensive School	**IUD**	-	4.8%	-	-	-
	HR-IU	-	9.6%	-	-	-
Vocational School	**IUD**	-	6.2%	6.3%	5.8%	7.4%
	HR-IU	-	4.6%	11.9%	9.8%	18.9%
Vocational Upper Secondary School	**IUD**	-	-	9.4%	7.0%	14.3%
	HR-IU	-	-	15.1%	18.0%	30.6%

Notes: Cell counts below n = 40 within age group per school type are not reported.

4. Discussion

The primary objective of this study was to use a phenotype classification approach to estimate prevalence rates of clinically relevant IUD in a large-scale high-school sample including both gaming and non-gaming subtypes. Moreover, we aimed at identifying the differences in phenotypes between problematic and unproblematic Internet users. The LPA was based on the response pattern of the CIUS, indicating the severity of the symptoms (1) loss of control; (2) withdrawal symptoms; (3) coping with unpleasant mood; (4) mental and behavioral preoccupation; and (5) inter- and intrapersonal conflicts. These symptoms cover most of the diagnostics criteria as proposed by DSM-5 and ICD-11 for (I)GD.

Specifically, we identified distinct profile groups characterized by IUD and HR-IU as compared to unproblematic users. The prevalence estimate was 6.1% for IUD in adolescents aged 11–21. The impairment of individuals classified to the IUD group (CIUS total $M = 32.16$) was comparable to the clinically relevant groups identified by Rumpf et al. ($M > 28.00$) [21], Rumpf et al. ($M = 34.24$) [14] and Wartberg et al. ($M = 31.93$) [15]. Thus, the definition of illness underlying the prevalence estimates is comparable across the previous and our studies. As a second clinically relevant group, we identified 13.9% of all adolescents characterized by high-risk behavior (LPG4: HR-IU). The impairment of this sub-threshold pathology group (CIUS total $M = 24.64$) was also comparable to the sub-clinical group identified by Rumpf et al. ($M = 23.09$) [14]. We observed no significant gender effect on profile group membership for IUD and HR-IU. This finding is in line with several studies reporting no differences in the estimated IUD prevalence between German female and male adolescents in representative samples [14,15,20].

Comparing the phenotypes of profile members, the largest differences between IUD and functional Internet use can be observed for the symptom inter- and intrapersonal conflicts (see Table 4), followed by loss of control, mental and behavioral preoccupation coping with unpleasant mood and withdrawal symptoms. In other words, having inter- and intrapersonal conflicts due to recurrent Internet use seems to be the best factor to differentiate between functional and dysfunctional Internet use. This is an important finding in the discussion about the specificity of symptoms defining the disorder.

Another important result was that risk of IUD and HR-IU was significantly associated with age. Distribution of age showed an increase for the IUD and HR-IU groups from 11 to 21. We identified two peaks, showing the largest prevalence rates at the ages of 15–16 (IUD = 7.6%, HR-IU = 16.1%) and 19–21 years (IUD = 9.1%, HR-IU = 21.7%). Few studies have found similar results showing an increased risk at the ages of 15–16 [24,26]. However, the age group of 19–21, which was found to be the group of highest risk in our study, was not investigated separately. Most studies that investigated prevalence rates in adolescents either summarized the findings over age groups because of fewer sample sizes [21,22,31] or investigated fewer age groups that were analyzed separately [24,26].

One finding that requires further attention is the significant difference of risk across school types. The findings must be interpreted carefully, because school types and age groups are intercorrelated. Specific school types exclude higher age groups (e.g., low level education and middle level education schools), whereas other school types exclude lower age groups (e.g., vocational school and vocational upper secondary school). Therefore, we analyzed the effects of school type separately for each age group. It was notable that even within each school type, prevalence increased with age. However, the base rates were highly different across schools and the differences could not be explained by the level of education per se. More research is needed to investigate, if specific school characteristics (i.e., humanistic vs. vocational track) might be associated with IUD. e.g., in the age group 15–16, risk of IUD seems to be highest in middle education level (11.4%) followed by vocational upper secondary school (9.4%), low educational level (7.9%), high educational level (6.5%) and vocational school (6.3%). A quite similar pattern was found for HR-IU, with the highest risk in middle educational level (18.6%) followed by high educational level (18.5%), low educational level (15.8%), vocational upper secondary school (15.1%) and vocational school (11.9%).

Strengths of the present study are the large number of cases and the broad age range of the sample, but of course, the survey has also several limitations. Although we used the same instrument (CIUS) and methods as Rumpf et al. [14] and Wartberg et al. [15], our prevalence rate (6.1%) was higher than previously reported (i.e., 4.0% [14] and 3.2% [15]) in representative samples of adolescents. This might be due to several reasons: First, it is assumable that prevalence rates have increased over time. Second, prevalence estimates have been found to be very sensitive to effects of age, school type and probably some more factors which have not yet been identified. Although our sample size was larger than most of the studies that have been conducted in this age group, it was based on an ad-hoc sample of schools that agreed to participate within a specific region and the distribution of school types (e.g., regarding Gymnasium and Gesamtschule) was not representative for the Rhine-Neckar region or for Germany. Further limitations of our study were the focus on self-report measures, the absence of external ratings of parents, teachers or peers and the absence of diagnostic interviews ("gold standard"). Nonetheless, to our knowledge this is the first study that estimates prevalence rates of IUD and HR-IU in a large adolescent sample for distinct age groups ranging from early to late adolescence.

5. Conclusions

IUD was found to affect 6.1% of German adolescents aged 11–21. The risk of IUD increased with age, ranging from 2.8% to 9.1%. The course of prevalence rates over adolescence showed two peaks at age groups 15–16 and 19–21. Gender was equally distributed across all phenotype profiles. Inter- and intrapersonal conflicts were identified to be the symptom to differentiate most specifically between functional and dysfunctional Internet use.

One finding which needs further attention was the fact prevalence rates differed significantly between school types, which could not be explained by the level of education. Future research on school characteristics and education is needed to identify factors that explain these considerable differences in risk of illness and academic career. Longitudinal designs are needed to investigate causality.

Our results indicate that IUD is a major health challenge that increases over the course of adolescence and it should be a public health policy priority to identify individuals most in need that might benefit from effective preventive approaches and treatments.

Acknowledgments: The data were collected within the PROTECT study (ClinicalTrials.gov: NCT02907658), which is supported by the Dietmar Hopp Foundation. No conditions were imposed by the financing. We thank all students who participated in the study and the headmaster, teacher and social worker which supported us at the schools.

Author Contributions: K.L. was principle investigator, conceived and designed the study, analyzed the data and wrote the paper. K.H. was involved in data collection, data analysis and writing. C.S.-J. was involved was involved in data collection, data analysis and writing. L.W. was involved in data analysis and writing.

References

1. American Psychiatric Association. *Diagnostic and Statistical Manual of Mental Disorders: DSM-5*, 5th ed.; American Psychiatric Association: Washington, DC, USA, 2013.
2. ICD-11 Beta Draft. Available online: https://icd.who.int/dev11/l-m/en (accessed on 27 February 2018).
3. Ho, R.C.; Zhang, M.W.B.; Tsang, T.Y.; Toh, A.H.; Pan, F.; Lu, Y.; Cheng, C.; Yip, P.S.; Lam, L.T.; Lai, C.-M.; et al. The association between internet addiction and psychiatric co-morbidity: A meta-analysis. *BMC Psychiatry* **2014**, *14*, 183. [CrossRef] [PubMed]
4. Ko, C.H.; Yen, J.Y.; Yen, C.F.; Chen, C.S.; Chen, C.C. The association between Internet addiction and psychiatric disorder: A review of the literature. *Eur. Psychiatry* **2012**, *27*, 1–8. [CrossRef] [PubMed]
5. Carli, V.; Durkee, T.; Wasserman, D.; Hadlaczky, G.; Despalins, R.; Kramarz, E.; Wasserman, C.; Sarchiapone, M.; Hoven, C.W.; Brunner, R.; et al. The association between pathological internet use and comorbid psychopathology: A systematic review. *Psychopathology* **2013**, *46*, 1–13. [CrossRef] [PubMed]
6. Poli, R.; Agrimi, E. Internet addiction disorder: Prevalence in an Italian student population. *Nordic J. Psychiatry* **2012**, *66*, 55–59. [CrossRef] [PubMed]
7. Shek, D.T.L.; Yu, L. Internet addiction phenomenon in early adolescents in Hong Kong. *Sci. World J.* **2012**, *2012*, 104304. [CrossRef] [PubMed]

8. Cheng, C.; Li, A.Y.L. Internet addiction prevalence and quality of (real) life: A meta-analysis of 31 nations across seven world regions. *Cyberpsychol. Behav. Soc. Netw.* **2014**, *17*, 755–760. [CrossRef] [PubMed]
9. Young, K.S. Internet Addiction: The Emergence of a New Clinical Disorder. *Cyber Psychol. Behav.* **1998**, *1*, 237–244. [CrossRef]
10. Young, K.S. *Caught in the Net: How to Recognize the Signs of Internet Addiction—And a Winning Strategy for Recovery*; John Wiley & Sons: New York, NY, USA, 1998.
11. Rehbein, F.; Kliem, S.; Baier, D.; Mößle, T.; Petry, N.M. Prevalence of Internet gaming disorder in German adolescents: Diagnostic contribution of the nine DSM-5 criteria in a state-wide representative sample. *Addict. Abingd. Engl.* **2015**, *110*, 842–851. [CrossRef] [PubMed]
12. Wartberg, L.; Kriston, L.; Thomasius, R. The Prevalence and Psychosocial Correlates of Internet Gaming Disorder. *Dtsch. Arzteblatt Int.* **2017**, *114*, 419–424. [CrossRef]
13. Bischof, G.; Bischof, A.; Meyer, C.; John, U.; Rumpf, H.J. *Prävalenz der Internetabhängigkeit—Diagnostik und Risikoprofile (PINTA-DIARI)*; Report to the German Federal Ministry of Health: Lübeck, Germany, 2013.
14. Rumpf, H.J.; Vermulst, A.A.; Bischof, A.; Kastirke, N.; Gürtler, D.; Bischof, G.; Meerkerk, G.J.; John, U.; Meyer, C. Occurence of internet addiction in a general population sample: a latent class analysis. *Eur. Addict. Res.* **2014**, *20*, 159–166. [CrossRef] [PubMed]
15. Wartberg, L.; Kriston, L.; Kammerl, R.; Petersen, K.U.; Thomasius, R. Prevalence of pathological Internet use in a representative German sample of adolescents: Results of a latent profile analysis. *Psychopathology* **2015**, *48*, 25–30. [CrossRef] [PubMed]
16. Laconi, S.; Rodgers, R.F.; Chabrol, H. The measurement of Internet addiction: A critical review of existing scales and their psychometric properties. *Comput. Hum. Behav.* **2014**, *41*, 190–202. [CrossRef]
17. Meerkerk, G.-J.; Van Den Eijnden, R.J.J.M.; Vermulst, A.A.; Garretsen, H.F.L. The Compulsive Internet Use Scale (CIUS): Some psychometric properties. *Cyber Psychol. Behav.* **2009**, *12*, 1–6. [CrossRef] [PubMed]
18. Wartberg, L.; Petersen, K.-U.; Kammerl, R.; Rosenkranz, M.; Thomasius, R. Psychometric Validation of a German Version of the Compulsive Internet Use Scale. *Cyberpsychol. Behav. Soc. Netw.* **2014**, *17*, 99–103. [CrossRef] [PubMed]
19. Guertler, D.; Rumpf, H.J.; Bischof, A.; Kastirke, N.; Petersen, K.U.; John, U.; Meyer, C. Assessment of problematic internet use by the Compulsive Internet Use Scale and the Internet Addiction Test: A sample of problematic and pathological gamblers. *Eur. Addict. Res.* **2014**, *20*, 75–81. [CrossRef] [PubMed]
20. Wartberg, L.; Kriston, L.; Bröning, S.; Kegel, K.; Thomasius, R. Adolescent problematic Internet use: Is a parental rating suitable to estimate prevalence and identify familial correlates? *Comput. Hum. Behav.* **2017**, *67*, 233–239. [CrossRef]
21. Rumpf, H.J.; Meyer, C.; Kreuzer, A.; John, U. *Prävalenz der Internetabhängigkeit (PINTA)*; Report to the German Federal Ministry of Health: Lübeck, Germany, 2011.
22. Rehbein, F.; Mößle, T. Video Game and Internet Addiction: Is there a Need for Differentiation? *SUCHT* **2013**, *59*, 129–142. [CrossRef]
23. Anderson, E.L.; Steen, E.; Stavropoulos, V. Internet use and Problematic Internet Use: A systematic review of longitudinal research trends in adolescence and emergent adulthood. *Int. J. Adolesc. Youth* **2016**, *22*, 430–454. [CrossRef]
24. Karacic, S.; Oreskovic, S. Internet Addiction through the Phase of Adolescence: A Questionnaire Study. *JMIR Mental Health* **2017**, *4*, e11. [CrossRef] [PubMed]
25. Ostovar, S.; Allahyar, N.; Aminpoor, H.; Moafian, F.; Nor, M.B.M.; Griffiths, M.D. Internet Addiction and its Psychosocial Risks (Depression, Anxiety, Stress and Loneliness) among Iranian Adolescents and Young Adults: A Structural Equation Model in a Cross-Sectional Study. *Int. J. Ment. Health Addict.* **2016**, *14*, 257–267. [CrossRef]
26. Stavropoulos, V.; Griffiths, M.D.; Burleigh, T.L.; Kuss, D.J.; Doh, Y.Y.; Gomez, R. Flow on the Internet: A longitudinal study of Internet addiction symptoms during adolescence. *Behav. Inf. Technol.* **2018**, 1–14. [CrossRef]
27. Xu, J.; Shen, L.X.; Yan, C.H.; Hu, H.; Yang, F.; Wang, L.; Kotha, S.R.; Zhang, L.N.; Liao, X.P.; Zhang, J.; et al. Personal characteristics related to the risk of adolescent internet addiction: A survey in Shanghai, China. *BMC Public Health* **2012**, *12*, 1106. [CrossRef] [PubMed]

28. Jackson, L.A.; von Eye, A.; Biocca, F.A.; Barbatsis, G.; Fitzgerald, H.E.; Zhao, Y. Personality, cognitive style, demographic characteristics and Internet use—Findings from the HomeNetToo project. *Swiss J. Psychol.* **2003**, *62*, 79–90. [CrossRef]
29. Riedl, D.; Stöckl, A.; Nussbaumer, C.; Rumpold, G.; Sevecke, K.; Fuchs, M. Nutzungsmuster von Internet und Computerspielen. *Neuropsychiatrie* **2016**, *30*, 181–190. [CrossRef] [PubMed]
30. Cerniglia, L.; Zoratto, F.; Cimino, S.; Laviola, G.; Ammaniti, M.; Adriani, W. Internet Addiction in adolescence: Neurobiological, psychosocial and clinical issues. *Neurosci. Biobehav. Rev.* **2017**, *76*, 174–184. [CrossRef] [PubMed]
31. Bakken, I.J.; Wenzel, H.G.; Götestam, K.G.; Johansson, A.; Oren, A. Internet addiction among Norwegian adults: A stratified probability sample study. *Scand. J. Psychol.* **2009**, *50*, 121–127. [CrossRef] [PubMed]
32. Kuss, D.J.; van Rooij, A.J.; Shorter, G.W.; Griffiths, M.D.; van de Mheen, D. Internet addiction in adolescents: Prevalence and risk factors. *Comput. Hum. Behav.* **2013**, *29*, 1987–1996. [CrossRef]
33. Stavropoulos, V.; Alexandraki, K.; Motti-Stefanidi, F. Recognizing internet addiction: Prevalence and relationship to academic achievement in adolescents enrolled in urban and rural Greek high schools. *J. Adolesc.* **2013**, *36*, 565–576. [CrossRef] [PubMed]
34. Tsitsika, A.; Janikian, M.; Schoenmakers, T.M.; Tzavela, E.C.; Olafsson, K.; Wójcik, S.; Macarie, G.F.; Tzavara, C.; Richardson, C. Internet addictive behavior in adolescence: A cross-sectional study in seven European countries. *Cyberpsychol. Behav. Soc. Netw.* **2014**, *17*, 528–535. [CrossRef] [PubMed]
35. Gürtler, D.; Rumpf, H.-J.; Bischof, A.; Kastirke, N.; Meerkerk, G.J.; John, U.; Meyer, C. Psychometrische Eigenschaften und Normierung der deutschen Version der Compulsive Internet Use Scale (CIUS). *Diagnostica* **2014**, *61*, 210–221. [CrossRef]
36. Peukert, P.; Steffen, S.; ElKasmi, J.; Barth, G.M.; Meerkerk, G.J.; Batra, A. Faktorielle Struktur der deutschen Version der Compulsive Internet Use Scale (CIUS) nach konfirmatorischer Faktorenanalyse. *Z. Klin. Psychol. Psychother.* **2012**, *41*, 101–108. [CrossRef]
37. Jung, T.; Wickrama, K.A.S. An Introduction to Latent Class Growth Analysis and Growth Mixture Modeling. *Soc. Personal. Psychol. Compass* **2008**, *2*, 302–317. [CrossRef]
38. Lo, Y. Testing the number of components in a normal mixture. *Biometrika* **2001**, *88*, 767–778. [CrossRef]
39. Nylund, K.L.; Asparouhov, T.; Muthen, B.O. Deciding on the number of classes in latent class analysis and growth mixture modeling: A Monte Carlo simulation study. *Struct. Equ. Model.* **2007**, *14*, 535–569. [CrossRef]

Permissions

All chapters in this book were first published by MDPI; hereby published with permission under the Creative Commons Attribution License or equivalent. Every chapter published in this book has been scrutinized by our experts. Their significance has been extensively debated. The topics covered herein carry significant findings which will fuel the growth of the discipline. They may even be implemented as practical applications or may be referred to as a beginning point for another development.

The contributors of this book come from diverse backgrounds, making this book a truly international effort. This book will bring forth new frontiers with its revolutionizing research information and detailed analysis of the nascent developments around the world.

We would like to thank all the contributing authors for lending their expertise to make the book truly unique. They have played a crucial role in the development of this book. Without their invaluable contributions this book wouldn't have been possible. They have made vital efforts to compile up to date information on the varied aspects of this subject to make this book a valuable addition to the collection of many professionals and students.

This book was conceptualized with the vision of imparting up-to-date information and advanced data in this field. To ensure the same, a matchless editorial board was set up. Every individual on the board went through rigorous rounds of assessment to prove their worth. After which they invested a large part of their time researching and compiling the most relevant data for our readers.

The editorial board has been involved in producing this book since its inception. They have spent rigorous hours researching and exploring the diverse topics which have resulted in the successful publishing of this book. They have passed on their knowledge of decades through this book. To expedite this challenging task, the publisher supported the team at every step. A small team of assistant editors was also appointed to further simplify the editing procedure and attain best results for the readers.

Apart from the editorial board, the designing team has also invested a significant amount of their time in understanding the subject and creating the most relevant covers. They scrutinized every image to scout for the most suitable representation of the subject and create an appropriate cover for the book.

The publishing team has been an ardent support to the editorial, designing and production team. Their endless efforts to recruit the best for this project, has resulted in the accomplishment of this book. They are a veteran in the field of academics and their pool of knowledge is as vast as their experience in printing. Their expertise and guidance has proved useful at every step. Their uncompromising quality standards have made this book an exceptional effort. Their encouragement from time to time has been an inspiration for everyone.

The publisher and the editorial board hope that this book will prove to be a valuable piece of knowledge for researchers, students, practitioners and scholars across the globe.

List of Contributors

Kai Dou, Lin-Xin Wang, Guo-Dong Wang, Yan-Yu Li and Yi-Ting Huang
Department of Psychology and Research Center of Adolescent Psychology and Behavior, School of Education, Guangzhou University, Guangzhou 510006, China

Jian-Bin Li
Department of Early Childhood Education, The Education University of Hong Kong, Hong Kong, China

Li Chen, Ruiyi Liu, Huan Zeng, Xianglong Xu, Rui Zhu and Yong Zhao
School of Public Health and Management, Chongqing Medical University, Chongqing 400016, China
Research Center for Medicine and Social Development, Chongqing Medical University, Chongqing 400016, China
The Innovation Center for Social Risk Governance in Health, Chongqing Medical University, Chongqing 400016, China

Manoj Sharma
Department of Behavioural and Environmental Health, Jackson State University, Jackson, MS 39213, USA
Health for All, Omaha, NE 68144, USA
College of Health Sciences, Walden University, Minneapolis, MN 55401, USA

Sarah E. Domoff
Department of Psychology, Central Michigan University, Mount Pleasant, MI 48859, USA

Emma Q. Sutherland
School of Public Health, University of Michigan, Ann Arbor, MI 48109, USA

Sonja Yokum
Oregon Research Institute, Eugene, OR 97403, USA

Ashley N. Gearhardt
Department of Psychology, University of Michigan, Ann Arbor, MI 48109, USA

Arnold Alejandro Tafur-Mendoza
Research Center (CIUP), Universidad del Pacífico, Lima 15072, Peru

Julio César Acosta-Prado
School of Accounting, Economic and Business Sciences, Universidad de Manizales, Manizales 170001, Colombia
School of Business Science, Universidad del Pacífico, Lima 15072, Peru

Duván Emilio Ramírez-Ospina
School of Accounting, Economic and Business Sciences, Universidad de Manizales, Manizales 170001, Colombia

Rodrigo Arturo Zárate-Torres
Colegio de Estudios Superiores de Administración, Bogota 111071, Colombia

Ningyuan Guo, Tzu Tsun Luk, Jung Jae Lee, Sophia Siu-Chee Chan and Man Ping Wang
School of Nursing, University of Hong Kong, Hong Kong, China

Sai Yin Ho and Tai Hing Lam
School of Public Health, University of Hong Kong, Hong Kong, China

Chen Shen
Department of Epidemiology and Biostatistics, Imperial College London, London W2 1PG, UK

John Oliffe
School of Nursing, University of British Columbia, Vancouver, BC V6T 2B5, Canada

Seung-Yup Lee, Min-Hyeon Park and Kyu-In Jung
Department of Psychiatry, Eunpyeong St. Mary's Hospital, College of Medicine, The Catholic University of Korea, Seoul 03312, Korea

Yong-Sil Kweon and Hae Kook Lee
Department of Psychiatry, Uijeongbu St. Mary's Hospital, College of Medicine, The Catholic University of Korea, Seoul 06591, Korea

Jung-Seok Choi
Department of Psychiatry, SMG-SNU Boramae Medical Center, Seoul 07061, Korea

Soo-young Bang
Department of Psychiatry, College of Medicine, Eulji University, Seoul 01830, Korea

Ju-Yu Yen
Department of Psychiatry, Faculty of Medicine, College of Medicine, Kaohsiung Medical University, Kaohsiung City 807, Taiwan
Department of Psychiatry, Kaohsiung Municipal Ta-Tung Hospital, Kaohsiung Medical University, Kaohsiung City 812, Taiwan

Wei-Po Chou and Tai-Ling Liu
Department of Psychiatry, Kaohsiung Medical University Hospital, Kaohsiung Medical University, Kaohsiung City 807, Taiwan

Huang-Chi Lin
Department of Psychiatry, Faculty of Medicine, College of Medicine, Kaohsiung Medical University, Kaohsiung City 807, Taiwan
Department of Psychiatry, Kaohsiung Medical University Hospital, Kaohsiung Medical University, Kaohsiung City 807, Taiwan

Chih-Hung Ko
Department of Psychiatry, Kaohsiung Medical University Hospital, Kaohsiung Medical University, Kaohsiung City 807, Taiwan
Department of Psychiatry, Kaohsiung Municipal Siaogang Hospital, Kaohsiung Medical University, Kaohsiung 801, Taiwan
Substance and Behavior addiction Research Center, Kaohsiung Medical University, Kaohsiung City 807, Taiwan

Sheila Yu
Department of Preventive Medicine, University of Southern California, 2001 N Soto St., Los Angeles, CA 90032, USA

Steve Sussman
Department of Preventive Medicine, University of Southern California, 2001 N Soto St., Los Angeles, CA 90032, USA
Department of Psychology, University of Southern California, 3620 South McClintock Ave, Los Angeles, CA 90089, USA

Maria Stavrou
Department of Psychology, Goldsmiths, University of London, London SE14 6NW, UK

Ela Ari
Istanbul Medipol University, Faculty of Humanities and Social Sciences, Psychology Department, 34810 Istanbul, Turkey

Siti Rubiaehtul Hassim, Wan Nor Arifin and Yee Cheng Kueh
Biostatistics and Research Methodology Unit, School of Medical Sciences, Universiti Sains Malaysia, Kubang Kerian 16150, Malaysia

Nor Azwany Yaacob
Department of Community Medicine, School of Medical Sciences, Universiti Sains Malaysia, Kubang Kerian 16150, Malaysia

Yi-Ping Hsieh
Department of Social Work, College of Nursing and Professional Disciplines, University of North Dakota, Grand Forks, ND 58202, USA

Cheng-Fang Yen
Department of Psychiatry, School of Medicine, and Graduate Institute of Medicine, College of Medicine, Kaohsiung Medical University, Kaohsiung 807, Taiwan

Wen-Jiun Chou
Department of Child and Adolescent Psychiatry, Chang Gung Memorial Hospital, Kaohsiung Medical Center and College of Medicine, Chang Gung University, Kaohsiung 833, Taiwan

Xavier Carbonell, Ursula Oberst, Beatriz Rodrigo and Mariona Prades
FPCEE Blanquerna, Universitat Ramon Llull, 08022 Barcelona, Spain

Andrés Chamarro
Departamento de Psicología, Universitat Autónoma de Barcelona, Cerdanyola del Vallès, 08193 Barcelona, Spain
Serra Hunter Program, Generalitat de Catalunya, 08029 Barcelona, Spain

Jean-Jacques Rémond and Lucia Romo
Psychology Department, Laboratory EA CLIPSYD 4430, Paris Nanterre University, 92000 Nanterre, France

Anna Faltýnková, Lukas Blinka and Anna Ševčíková
Faculty of Social Studies, Masaryk University, Brno 601 77, Czech Republic

Daniela Husarova
Department of Health Psychology and Methodology Research, Faculty of Medicine, P.J. Safarik University in Kosice, Košice 040 01, Slovakia

Bernd Lachmann and Rayna Sariyska
Molecular Psychology, Institute of Psychology and Education, Ulm University, Helmholtzstrasse 8/1, 89081 Ulm, Germany

Adnan Veysel Ertemel
Istanbul Commerce University, Faculty of Business Administration, International Trade Department, 34445 Istanbul, Turkey

Christopher Kannen
Department of Informatics, University of Bonn, 53012 Bonn, Germany

Christian Montag
Molecular Psychology, Institute of Psychology and Education, Ulm University, Helmholtzstrasse 8/1, 89081 Ulm, Germany
Key Laboratory for NeuroInformation/Center for Information in Medicine, School of Life Science and Technology, University of Electronic Science and Technology of China, Chengdu 611731, China

Myungsuh Lim
Department of Business Administration, Sangji University, Wonju 26339, Korea

Katajun Lindenberg, Katharina Halasy and Carolin Szász-Janocha
Institute for Psychology, University of Education Heidelberg, 69120 Heidelberg, Germany

Lutz Wartberg
German Center for Addiction Research in Childhood and Adolescence, University Medical Center Hamburg-Eppendorf, 20246 Hamburg, Germany

Index

www.ingramcontent.com/pod-product-compliance
Lightning Source LLC
LaVergne TN
LVHW081413160926
848178LV00067B/94